ORTHOPAEDIC BIOMECHANICS

ORTHOPAEDIC

BIOMECHANICS

by

H. M. FROST, M.D.

Department of Orthopaedic Surgery
Henry Ford Hospital
Detroit, Michigan

Orthopaedic Lectures
Volume V

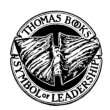

CHARLES C THOMAS   PUBLISHER
Springfield, Illinois, U.S.A.

Published and Distributed Throughout the World by

CHARLES C THOMAS • PUBLISHER

Bannerstone House

301–327 East Lawrence Avenue, Springfield, Illinois, U.S.A.

© *1973, by* **CHARLES C THOMAS • PUBLISHER**

ISBN 0-398-02824-9

Library of Congress Catalog Card Number: 72-11612

With THOMAS BOOKS *careful attention is given to all details of manufacturing and design. It is the Publisher's desire to present books that are satisfactory as to their physical qualities and artistic possibilities and appropriate for their particular use.* THOMAS BOOKS *will be true to those laws of quality that assure a good name and good will.*

Printed in the United States of America

CC-11

Preface

Primarily for orthopaedists, but also for engineers, metallurgists, prosthetists, veterinarians, dentists, oral surgeons, physiologists and other physicians, this fifth volume in the Orthopaedic Lecture Series introduces biomechanics, a relatively new field in medicine and of still poorly defined scope.

In a general way biomechanics attempts to fuse the science and technology of engineering with biology and physiology. Surgeons who implant artificial devices in the human body, or who operate to correct and/or prevent musculoskeletal defects of congenital and acquired origin, need to familiarize themselves with many aspects of the man-evolved engineering sciences. Besides that fairly conventional body of knowledge, they must learn the *twists* or new emphases and solutions that we find living biological organisms have evolved for familiar engineering challenges. Here we stand on uncertain ground because we have just begun to recognize those twists and can hardly claim to an even elementary understanding of any one of them as yet.

On the other hand, engineers who design and/or make devices (and materials) for use in or on the body must learn some of the special needs of and limitations imposed by the biological organism, as well as how to resolve conflicts arising between contemporary engineering practice and biological necessity.

This work does not deal with all biomechanics and so does not purport to be a text book; it focusses on selected aspects of the design and function of the musculoskeletal system, and brings in only some engineering knowledge, and only where it seems useful. It makes only elementary use of mathematics for its purpose consists of *communicating*, effectively and clearly to the orthopaedist reader, some essential ideas and facts of use in clinical practice.

The book has three parts.

PART I deals with nonbiological matters such as stress, strain, matter and materials properties. Engineers will find these chapters pretty elementary and may wish to skip them; they will understand that that part of the text attempts to introduce nonmathematical and usually very busy orthopaedists to mechanics, and their background requires using a format familiar to them to succeed.

PART II of the book deals primarily with some of the biological aspects of orthopaedic biomechanics, and it includes a fair amount of new material, unavailable in any other text in any language at this writing. In both of the first two parts a series of test questions appear at the end of each chapter, which should allow the reader to test his own biomechanical-educational progress.

This part of the text draws heavily upon material in the preceding four volumes of this series which, in fact, were conceived originally to lay its groundwork. Rather than increase this book's length by repeating or reproducing all of that material here, we will merely identify its source and then abstract it here.

PART III: Here the reader will find a series of nine *Appendices* which review some of the elementary mathematics, physics and mechanics required to solve simple biomechanical problems; 19 *Special Tables* also required to solve biomechanical problems (clinical as well as theoretical); Glossary, of many of the mechanical and biological terms employed in order that we may communicate more accurately across some of the interdisciplinary boundaries; *Answers* to the test questions given at the end of each chapter; a *Bibliography*; and an *Index*. And, last of all, a postscript addressed to all of my former residents and colleagues.

Contents

vii

PART III
APPENDICES

ORTHOPAEDIC BIOMECHANICS

PART I

MECHANICS

Some of the Mechanics in Biomechanics

ORTHOPAEDIC RESIDENTS AND colleagues should find much interesting material herein, for by its nature it intrigues the gadgeteer and orthopaedists are great ones. This part of the book deals with the mechanical and physical properties of matter, mostly as one finds it in the liquid and solid states. The resident may at times find it bewildering simply because technical and scientific usage of some words differs from the lay usage to which all of us obtained first exposure. Clinicians will find that a knowledge of mechanics provides an essential backbone to any realistic grasp of musculoskeletal system functions, diseases and how we treat them.

Convention: All tables, figures and equations in the text carry two numbers. The first designates the chapter in which it appears, the second its numerical order in that chapter. Thus Table *3.01* signifies the first table in Chapter 3; figure *10.07* the seventh figure in Chapter 10; equation *5.02* the second equation in Chapter 5. Figures and tables in Part III however receive numbers in simple numerical order.

Chapter 1

Forces, Loads, Energy and Work

W̲ₑ ᴡɪʟʟ ᴅᴇғɪɴᴇ the meaning of *force* before that of *loads*.

I: FORCE

1) Tʜᴇ Fᴏʀᴄᴇ-Aᴄᴄᴇʟᴇʀᴀᴛɪᴏɴ Rᴇʟᴀᴛɪᴏɴ: When one drops a glass above a concrete floor it falls with progressively increasing speed and upon impacting on the floor probably shatters. It falls because a force called gravity exists which pulls the earth towards the glass and vice versa. But because the mass and thus the inertia of the earth enormously exceeds that of the glass the glass alone seems to do the moving or dropping when one releases it. If we applied another pull of the same identical strength as gravity but acting sideways on the glass it would then begin to move sideways also, and again with equal (and progressively increasing) speed. Given that both forces acted simultaneously, then after any time interval the sideways speed of the glass would equal exactly its downward speed.

Note that the longer the force acts on it the faster the glass moves, ignoring the effects of air resistance. In other words, the force accelerates the glass or changes its speed of motion in space. A glass held securely in the hand does not fall simply because that hand exerts an upward force on it exactly equal to the downward-pulling force of gravity but opposite to it in direction; that situation causes these two forces to cancel out as far as the glass is concerned. Since the *net* force acting on it then becomes zero, the glass does not accelerate.

Dᴇғɪɴɪᴛɪᴏɴ: *acceleration: A change in an object's speed and/or direction of motion.*

Newton observed that in the absence of all applied forces a given object or mass maintains an absolutely uniform speed and direction of motion.

7

When we say the glass weighs 100 gm, this means that the earth pulled downwards on this chunk of matter (i.e., this amount of mass) with 100 gm of force. If applied by some other suitable means (such as springs, rubber bands, compressed air) to other chunks of matter able to move freely in response, this identical force will cause them to accelerate too. Just so do the hip muscles in S. Stanisavljevic's babies move their lower limbs (254). And as long as a force acts in the absence of a counterforce, it will continue to accelerate a mass.

Obviously, before a 100 gm force a 1000 gm weight would not undergo as much acceleration as a one gm weight. This leads to two ways of defining a force which, while equivalent, represent different points of view:

DEFINITION: *Force:* (a) *that which can accelerate matter.**
Or, (b) *the resistance of matter to acceleration.*†

As a matter of interest, in the field of physics the second definition establishes a rigorous and universally applicable definition of *mass* which differs slightly in meaning from that of *weight*; the latter term signifies the earth's particular attraction for a given mass, and that identical and unchanging (or invariant) mass would weigh less on our moon or Mars, and more on Jupiter or Saturn, than it does here on the earth (and it will not weigh *exactly* the same in London as in New York) simply because those bodies exert different gravitational pulls on the same identical mass (70).

DEFINITION: *Mass: a resistance of matter to acceleration by a force of unit magnitude.*

DEFINITION: *Weight: the pull on some body of matter or on some object of the earth's gravitational field.* Or, in ordinary language if you prefer: *the earth's attraction for that object or matter.*

If a force known to act on an object causes no visible acceleration of it, this can mean only one thing: that an equal

---

* The conventional definition.
† Conventionally known as inertia.

but opposite force (s) exists and also acts on the object in such a way as to cancel or nullify the effects of the first one. For example, in his latter years my father had a boat which floated rather than sank (good thing too—Maine seas are *cold!*) because the sea exerted upwards on its hull a total force equal to but opposite in direction to that of the earth, meaning its weight. Thus the forces of the sea and its weight cancelled. Furthermore if, while it sat in the boat house on its ways during the winter, one pushed sideways on it with the hand, it would fail to move (note that it would have moved were it floating on the water). This failure to accelerate means that an equal but opposite force to the hand's must have existed, which in this instance constituted something known as "starting friction" which we will deal with later on. Table 1.01 lists some types of forces, of which we recognize quite a variety. And we generalize the concept to sociological, emotional and still other spheres which do not properly concern this text.

TABLE 1.01
SOME TYPES OF FORCES

Loads (compression, tension, shear, torque, flexure)	Centrifugal force
Stresses (compression, tension, shear)	Magnetic field
	Electric field
Fluid friction	Hydrostatic pressure
Starting friction	Barometric pressure
Gravity	Van der Waal's
Covalent bond	Ionic bond
Centripetal force	Radiation pressure
	Wind pressure

2) THE FORCE-MASS RELATION: The above remarks should by now have suggested that force, mass and acceleration relate to each other in some particular way. And they do; in the field of physics, acceleration a, force F, and mass m, relate to each other as follows:

Force equals mass multiplied by acceleration.

Or to express it in more compact algebraic symbols and format which, nevertheless, mean and say exactly the same thing:

$$F = ma$$ *Equation 1.01*

Thus if one knows the values of the mass and acceleration in a given situation he can "plug" them into this formula or equation to obtain the value of the force. To actually solve any such relation for one of its terms, given numerical values of the remaining ones, one must take care to use the same system of units (i.e., *consistent units*) in all of them. In other words, always use the same units of length (such as mm, meter, inch or yard), time (such as second, hour or year) and mass (such as gram, pound or ton). For use later on, let us here explain how to solve such a relation for any one of its terms. "Solving for a term" simply means getting that term alone on one side of the equals sign in such a way that what remains on the other side truly represents the solution. Assume we know both F and *m* in a given situation; we wish to find out the value of *a* that corresponds to them. We need to get rid of the *m* on the right side of equation 1.01 somehow to leave the *a* standing alone. Simple: divide both sides through by *m*. Since both sides equal each other (the mathematician says: "they are identically equal"), dividing two equals by the same quantity leaves the result still equal. Thus we have:

$$\frac{F}{m} = \frac{m}{m} a$$

Now on the right side, *m* divided by *m* equals unity, i.e., the number one. So that expression simply means:

$$\frac{F}{m} = 1 \times a$$

Since any quantity multiplied by the number one remains unchanged, we need not bother to write the number one; it becomes a redundant term. So our expression now becomes:

$$\frac{F}{m} = a \qquad\qquad\qquad \textit{Equation 1.02}$$

Or, reversing right and left now:

$$a = \frac{F}{m}$$

Appendix 1 goes into this procedure in greater detail for the physician who needs to brush up on this.

3) THE EQUATIONS OF MOTION: Let us review briefly here some of the relationships between speed, acceleration and distance, for use later on. The velocity v, attained by an object under a given acceleration a, acting for a duration of time t, constitutes acceleration times time, or:

$$v = a\,t \qquad\qquad Equation\ 1.03$$

In that same period of time and given that uniform acceleration persisted throughout it, then the distance s, that object traversed while attaining that velocity v, becomes:

$$s = \frac{v}{2}\,t \qquad\qquad Equation\ 1.04$$

It also forms:

$$s = \tfrac{1}{2}\,at^2 \qquad\qquad Equation\ 1.05$$

If you have trouble understanding how we got that result, note that equation 1.03 stated that v equalled at; thus one may substitute the latter for v in the present equation to get $s = \tfrac{1}{2}\,at \times t = \tfrac{1}{2}\,at^2$.

And we have elsewhere recorded that the force applied to a mass causes it to accelerate according to this relation:

$$F = ma \qquad\qquad Equation\ 1.01$$

4) MAGNITUDE AND DIRECTION: Forces have two fundamentally different properties which one must keep always in mind in discussing them and their effects. One property, the amount or size of some force, represents its *magnitude*. Mathematicians call a parameter possessing the property of magnitude alone a *scalar quantity*. One would express the magnitude of a force in terms such as dynes (the rigorous form) or grams (the layman's equally acceptable and useful form), poundals or slugs (see Part III, Table 19) (rigorous) or pounds (ordinary), and so on. Table 1.02 defines some of these and other units used in biomechanical work and in reporting research results.

TABLE 1.02

DEFINITIONS OF SOME PHYSICAL UNITS

Unit System	Parameter
c.g.s	*dyne:* that force which will accelerate a 1 gm mass to a speed of 1cm/sec by acting upon it for 1 sec. *gm. force:* the attraction of the earth for a mass of one gram: = 980 dynes.
m.k.s.	*Newton:* that force which in one second's time will accelerate a mass of one kilogram to a speed of one meter per second, written: 1 M/sec equals 9.8 × 10⁷ dynes. *kg. force:* the attraction of the earth for a one kilogram mass = 9.8 newtons.
ft. lb. sec.	*poundal:* that force which in one second will accelerate a one lb. mass to a speed of one foot per second, written: 1 ft/sec. *pound:* the attraction of the earth for a one pound mass, = 32.16 poundals.
c.g.s.	*g:* the gravitational constant: 980 cm/sec/sec; also written 980 cm/sec².
m.k.s.	*g:* the gravitational constant: 9.8 m/sec²
ft. lb. sec.	*g:* the gravitational constant: 32.16 ft/sec²
c.g.s.	*erg:* the amount of work done in accelerating a one gram mass to a speed of 1 cm/sec. *gm-cm:* the work done in lifting one gram a height of one cm against earth's gravitational pull, equals 980 ergs. *Joule:* 10⁷ (i.e., 10 million) ergs; equals 1/9.8 Newton.
ft. lb. sec.	*ft-lb:* the work done in lifting a one lb. mass one foot against earth's gravity.

This table defines some of the more commonly used units of force, mass and work. You will need to understand them in order to understand contemporary and future biomechanical research reports, literature and textbooks. Special Tables 3–14 in Part III allow you to convert easily from any one system of units to any other. Memorize these abbreviations now: c.g.s.: centimeter-gram-second system of units. m.k.s.: meter kilogram-second system of units. ft.lb.sec.: foot-pound-second (English) system of units.

[Taken from references (4, 39, 111, 123, 173, 280)].

Forces can also have a second property, that of *directionality,* meaning they can act in some particular direction or sense in three dimensional space. And engineers term parameters possessing that property in addition to magnitude, as *vectorial quantities.** For some purposes in this text we need only to know the scalar aspect of forces (i.e., their magni-

---

* We need not learn here the mathematician's rigorous difinition of a vectorial quantity; this high school physics one suffices for all of our needs, well enough in fact that most biomechanicians and many engineers do not even know that this represents a special case definition rather than a general and rigorous one.

tudes) , while for others we will also need to know their vectorial nature too (i.e., their direction or "line of action," as well as their magnitudes) . The wordings should make clear which case obtains.

In mechanics generally and in biomechanics too, we recognize at least two different and, for our needs, important subcategories of forces: *(a)* those forces that *come from outside* of a structure and which act upon it in some way, which we will call *loads*; *(b)* those forces generated or *developed within the substance* of a structure's matter in response to those loads, which we will call *stresses*. Note then that force represents a very general and all-inclusive term, while the terms loads and stresses signify particular subcategories of forces. Note too that the distinction between the terms loads and stresses simply implies different points of view, employed because they have proven quite useful in explaining and understanding mechanical things. Thus in one problem one may define some forces as loads and others as stresses, and in the very next hour in another problem the former loads may become the stresses of current concern, and the former stresses now become the loads. So at this juncture let us discuss briefly some attributes of loads.

II: LOADS

DEFINITION: *Load: any force or combination of forces, applied to the outside of a structure, and therefore sustained or carried by the matter in the structure.*

We can define a few kinds or arrangements of loads for frequent use throughout the remainder of the book, and they appear in a diagram form in Figure 1.01. For example, the pull of a muscle on a bone represents a load applied to and carried by the bone.† The injection of blood through the nutrient artery into the marrow cavity of a bone increases the pressure inside the cavity, tending to burst or bulge the bony wall or casing, and it represents another load applied to and

---

† With equal validity, we can consider the bone's resistance to the muscle pull as a load on the muscle. The choice of what point of view one adopts will depend on what he studies.

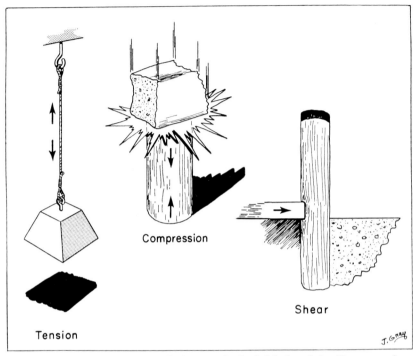

Figure 1.01. The meaning of three principal kinds of loading: tension, compression and shear. This figure also conveys the meanings of the three principal stresses (as forces arising within the materials which resist the deforming actions of those loads), and the three principal strains (as the kinds of deformations these loads tend to induce in matter). (Reprinted by permission of author and publisher, ref. no. 94.)

carried by the bone. The twist on the crankshaft of an auto engine, generated by a piston pushed by burning gasoline expanding in the combustion chamber, forms a load on that shaft. So also does the weight of the body on the bones of the foot, the pressure of the sun's radiation on a satellite, and the motion of magnetic lines of force through the coils of wire in an electric motor or generator.

While a load comes within our general definition of a force (because it can accelerate matter), its special property of interest to us derives from the effects it exerts on the structures we work with. And when applied loads do not cause resulting accelerations, forces of equal magnitudes but acting in the opposite direction to those loads must exist to account for this, and we say the object exists in a state of *static equilibrium*.

1) Specification of Forces and Loads: In order to measure and compare forces and loads, and to derive them or related quantities in experimental situations or in designing new gadgets, we need some consistent and universal way or ways of expressing them. Conventionally, engineers express forces and loads in basically two different ways (see Fig. 1.02).

(a) *Unit Force and Unit Load*: Assume an area of one square centimeter carries a 10 kilogram (kg) load distributed evenly over that area; then the load on that unit of area equals 10 kg per square cm, written thus: 10 kg/cm². Now assume another situation in which five cm² carry a total of 50 kg: the unit load still equals 10 kg/cm². Here we have the "unit load" context or format, in which we express forces and loads per unit of cross sectional area of the structural member carrying it. This unit can constitute the inch, foot, centimeter, millimeter, micron or kilometer, as examples. One usually gives the loads in consistent systems of units. Thus one uses pounds with inches in English measure, and grams with centimeters (or for some purposes kilograms with millimeters or meters) in metric measure.

Figure 1.02 illustrates this and the next-coming idea.

As for expressing the above algebraically, assume the A signifies the total cross section area of the structure carrying a given outside load, and P signifies the load. Then if σ (Greek lower case letter sigma; see Part III, Table 16) signifies the unit load, this expression applies:

$$\sigma = \frac{P}{A} \qquad\qquad \textit{Equation 1.06}$$

Then you can see that when P equals 10 kg, and A one cm², unit loading equals 10/1 equals 10 kg/cm²; or for a 50 kg load on a 5 cm² area, unit loading equals 50/5 equals-again-10 kg/cm².

All of the above state scalar properties.

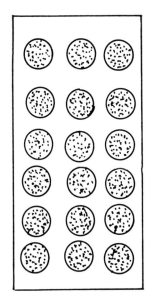
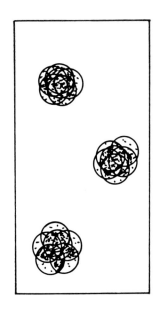

A   B

Figure 1.02. At A on the left the rectangular surface contains 18 one kilogram weights, each of 10 cm² cross section, sitting on it and each identical to all the others. Thus the total load on the rectangle equals 18 kg, but the unit loading equals 1 kg/10 cm² = 0.1 kg/cm² under each weight, and zero in the regions between them.

At B on the right we stack the weights on top of each other in groups of 6. The total load still equals 18 kg, the unit loading between them still equals zero but the unit loading under each stack now equals 6 kg/10 cm² = 0.6 kg/cm². The circles were purposely drawn not accurately concentric to convey the stacking concept.

(b) *Total Force and Total Load*: In the above examples, the total load or force in each example equalled respectively, 10 and 50 kg. Now take a situation in which a 1000 gm total load distributes over a cross section area of 10 square centimeters. While the total load equals 1000 gm, the unit load equals 100 gm/cm². Now put the same load on five square centimeters. The total load remains 1000 gm but now the unit load becomes 200 gm/cm².

All of the above state scalar properties.

In upcoming discussions, we will need a clear idea of the engineering meanings of several terms that relate to loads and other categories of forces in motion, so at this juncture let us define them; their lay usages often differ and/or suffer greatly from fuzzy meaning. For example, think how interesting a debate on the benefits of "capitalism" would become if done between an orthodox Marxist and an orthodox American. The same word conveys totally different meaning to each, which leads to heated misunderstandings.

2) MECHANICAL WORK: Lift a one pound weight against the earth's gravitational pull. You have exerted a known force over a measured distance to perform one foot-pound (written ft-lb) of "work." Or move an aeroplane one kilometer (i.e., 1000 meters) against an air resistance of 10,000 kg force; you have performed 10,000,000 kg-M of work. And equally, in moving electrons against some form of electrical resistance; in arising from a chair; in assembling various elementary organic molecules into the specialized biological building stuff known as collagen, and in whittling a point onto a tent stake for the benefit of your young son, you have done (or witnessed the performance of) work. In algebraic terms, using F to signify a force, L a distance and W the work, this equation expresses how these factors relate to each other:

$$W = F\ L \qquad\qquad Equation\ 1.07$$

In the above airplane example, 10,000 kg of force times 1000 meters equals 10 million kg-M of mechanical work, most of it expended in pushing air away from the advancing airframe.

3) MECHANICAL ADVANTAGE: A basic axiom in physics (one still unsuccessfully challanged by would-be inventors of perpetual motion machines) states that in a perfect machine one can obtain at the most only that amount of work or energy one puts into it, never any more. And in man-made and thus imperfect machines, one never achieves that; some loss of mechanical work always occurs to make the machine *inefficient* to varying degrees, ranging from 95%-plus efficiency for large electrical transformers to less than 5 percent efficiency for some motor bikes.

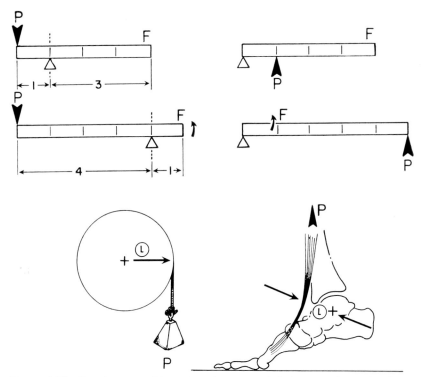

Figure 1.03. See the text. Note that the upper left lever reduces the force exerted at point F by the load P to one-third, while multiplying the distance traversed by F by three times over that at P. The ratios are one-fourth and four times at the upper right, four times and one-fourth at the middle left, and five times and one-fifth at the middle right.

At bottom left the same principle applies, as the load of a rope or driving belt acting on lever arm L, turns around a pulley or drum, and at the right in the human ankle, as the anterior tibial muscle contracts P to dorsiflex it, acting over the lever arm L.

But while one cannot obtain more work from a passive device than he put into it, he certainly can obtain a multiplication or reduction of either one (but *only* one) of the two other things that contribute to mechanical work: the magnitude of the force, or the speed and distance of its motion. Let us consider the force aspect first. Consult Figure 1.03.

(a) *Force division and multiplication*: In the top drawing a weight P, lies at the end of a lever so balanced over its fulcrum that it has a *lever arm* one meter long. The other end of the lever lies three meters from the fulcrum. What upwards force can it exert against a superimposed resistance? Simple, given only that that resistance prevents that end from rising, meaning that this system lies in static equilibrium. High school physics tell us that the moments must balance out (if that lost you, Appendix 9 and Chapter XI explain moments in somewhat more detail). Thus:

$$(P \times 1) - (F \times 3) = 0$$

We need to solve for F, the unknown. The solution proceeds thus (you may need to refer to *Part III: Appendices: Algebra Review,* if you do not understand these manipulations):

$$P \times 1 = F \times 3;$$

$$\frac{P \times 1}{3} = \frac{F \times 3}{3} \; ; \; \frac{P \times 1}{3} = F \times 1$$

$$\frac{P \times 1}{3} = F \; ; \; F = \tfrac{1}{3} \, P.$$

Hence at its output F, this system *reduces* to one third the force applied to its input at P, a situation that arises commonly in the human body where the source of the force F, represents a muscle pull, as shown in the top right and lower right drawings. Now in the lower drawing, simply by moving the fulcrum we now obtain a *force multiplying* system in which F = 4P, i.e., the reaction at the F end of the lever must exert four times the force exerted by P on its left, to maintain static equilibrium. Or by pushing down by hand 50 lb worth on the left, you could lift a 200 lb weight on the right. A numerically equal system lies in the middle right drawing but with the locations of fulcrum, load and reaction altered to represent a different class of lever (three classes are recognized, and each is shown in this figure but not named).

(b) *Distance division and multiplication*: Now for the same drawings consider a different aspect of the mechanical behavior: the vertical distance travelled by the point on the lever at which P acts, compared to the corresponding distance through which the point at F moves. Clearly the top two drawings diagram *distance multiplying* systems (and thus speed multiplying ones too). Note that at a sacrifice in force exerted at the output of these lever systems, we obtained an increased *speed* and *distance* of motion. This situation occurs frequently in our bodies.

In the middle two drawings the reverse obtains: the levers' outputs provide less distance and speed than goes into their inputs. One may look at this either as the necessary penalty paid for force multiplication, or (as occurs in micro-manipulators) a device for improving one's ability to control very fine motions by a distance dividing mechanism which markedly reduces the errors and tremors of the hand.

(c) *The Lever Arm*: In the above examples the distance between the point of application of the load P and the fulcrum constitutes the lever arm, signified here as L. The product of P × L represents the *moment,* which one would express (as in these illustrations) as kg-meters but could equally express as inch-pounds or gram-cm. The lowest two drawings illustrate on the left the lever arm of a pulley rope carrying a load P, and on the right an analogous situation found in different pulleys in the musculoskeletal system, here the ankle. The anterior tibial tendon shown here exerts a dorsiflexion force tending to rotate the ankle around its axis (here a virtual axis, where the pulley on the left has a real one) with a force equal—again—to P × L inch-pounds. To improve the mechanical advantage of this muscle it will do no good to move the attachment of its lower end further down on the foot. Instead one must increase the distance L, by making the tendon's point of closest approach to the ankle's virtual axis of rotation lie farther away. One could achieve this simply by sectioning the crural ligament which normally prevents that, and in fact this represents one perfectly good—if uncommon—means of increasing the mechanical advantage of ankle dorsiflexor muscles weakened by some prior injury or disease.

4) ENERGY: When forces act over distances, some new physical quantities develop. Here we will review briefly three such matters: *work, energy* and *power.*

(a) *Energy*: Energy represents some meaaureable quantity or amount of mechanical work, *or any equivalent amount of any other kind of energy expenditure* which, given perfectly efficient transducing mechanisms, can convert to that same quantity of mechanical work. Thus energy and work prove synonymous in the sense that the former term usually serves a more general sense, and the latter the specific subcase of mechanical forces acting over linear distances. Thus lifting a weight of one kg upwards one meter against the earth's gravitational attraction performs work equal to one kg-meter or 100 kg-cm of energy; it also constitutes any equivalent amount of any other form of energy, which one could express as kilogram-calories, or electric charge moved against an electric potential, or whatever. Similarly, lifting a gram one centimeter against the earth's gravitational field equals one gm-cm of work. If on the other hand, we exert one dyne of force against a mass of one gram for a period of one second, we have then performed a much smaller amount of work, a quantity known as one erg (which equals about 1/980 of one gm-cm). Note however that *time does not appear* in the work equation. Thus as already stated we may define work W as a force F, acting over a distance L, or :

$$W = F \, L \qquad\qquad Equation\ 1.07$$

When we deal with energy in motion, for example with the energy of a bullet headed for a target, or a hand throwing a ball, we call it *kinetic energy*. When we deal with stored energy, for example that in an elderly lady standing up but which, if she should fall down, may dissipate in her hip bone and fracture it, we deal with *potential energy*.

(b) *Power*: Time does enter into this parameter, for *it defines how quickly one performs work,* or how quickly one expends a given quantity of energy. Thus consider the 100 foot-lb of work done in lifting a one pound grapefruit 100 feet above a concrete walk in a period of one minute. The grapefruit of course sustained no damage during the process, which expended mechanical work on it at a rate or power of $\dfrac{100 \ \text{ft-lb}}{60 \ \text{sec}}$ = 1.66 ft-lb/sec. But upon impacting on the concrete walk after dropping it, it squashes and literally explodes. This occurs because the same identical total amount of mechanical work or energy (100 ft-lb, no more and no less) done in lifting it over some 60 seconds (a low power value), now returns to it in something like six milliseconds, i.e., in six one-thousands of one second. And the ratio of 60 seconds/.006 seconds or 10,000 to one means that during that impact, the sidewalk in arresting its fall (i.e., in decelerating it, exactly the same thing as a negative acceleration) did mechanical work upon it at a 10,000 times greater rate than you did by lifting it up. Or, the mechanical power tending to deform it during impact exceeded 10,000-fold the power acting on it during its original elevation. That high power generated such briefly acting but very large mechanical forces within its substance that its structure could not possibly withstand them; the chemical bonds holding its matter together proved weaker than those forces so it literally exploded. Similarly the rather small total amount of energy in an ordinary beam of red light shining on a piece of tool steel for 10 seconds has no visible effect upon it. But if one discharges exactly the same total amount of energy (i.e., of light) in an exceedingly small period of time such as one picosecond (one millionth of one millionth of a second) it can literally vaporize the steel and thereby burn a hole through it. The total energies absorbed by the steel in either case remain equal, but the *rate* of its absorption in the latter case exceeded by a factor of ten trillion that in the former, and that sufficed to break the intermolecular bonds holding the metal atoms together. Thus one aspect of the emerging usefulness of laser technology.

We will say more about this mechanically important phenomenon in Chapter II, under the heading of *impact*. Let us next discuss briefly several problems attendant to systems in which two or more forces act, and require some kind of analytical approach to derive or find their effects on the systems.

5) FORCE SYSTEMS:

(a) *Resultants*: Mechanical force has the property

of directionality in three dimensional space, so one can symbolize a given force as an arrow on a sheet of paper, its *orientation* signifying the *line of action* of the force, and its *length* the *magnitude*. Assume that two different forces act upon a body, as shown in Figure 1.04. Each has a magnitude (the scalar property) and each a line of action (the vectorial property). Furthermore their lines of action do not parallel each other, i.e., they diverge. Clearly, the body cannot go in two directions at once; rather it will respond to their sum as though it represented *a single force with its own line of action*.

Question: How might one obtain a meaningful statement of that single force and its line of action (which engineers term the *resultant,* a word you will encounter often hereafter)? One can do it without resorting to trigonometric calculations, as shown below, noting however that exactly that scheme serves as the basis for the trigonometric solution to such problems. The latter offsets the disadvantage of learning a new branch of math with the advantages of better accuracy, flexibility and rapidity of solution.

Solution: Draw a model parallelogram of the forces shown in Figure 1.04; each adjacent arm or arrow represents one of those forces, its angle signifying the direction and its length the magnitude. By simply duplicating them in mirror image fashion as shown (i.e., closing in the figure), a regular parallelogram results. *Then the connecting diagonal represents the resultant,* and with an accuracy limited only by the accuracy with which you constructed the figure and then measured the direction and length (which signifies the magnitude) of that resultant. Thus, if you adjusted the length of the arms to some useable scale such as one mm equals one kg, and correctly reproduced the angles of the line of action of each force, the resultant's line reveals with equal, and for all of our needs better than merely useful accuracy, both its magnitude and direction. For three or more coplanar forces one simply determines the resultant of any two, and then treats that resultant as a single new force with which to con-

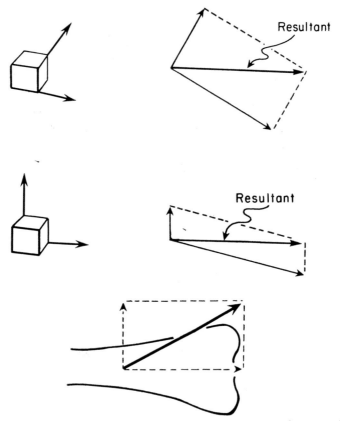

Figure 1.04. *Top Left:* A small cube of matter has two forces acting at an acute angle on it represented by the two arrows or vectors. The lines of action of these forces lie in the same plane as that of this sheet of paper, so we say they are *coplanar*. The entire discussion of multiple forces in this portion of the text deals with coplanar forces. Their lengths might signify the magnitude of each force according to any scale you choose (for example, one inch per lb, or one cm per kg), and their directions would signify their lines of actions.

To determine what resultant force acts on any such cube, construct a parallelogram of forces by drawing to scale the two forces, then adding the two right hand sides to close the figure, each accurately parallel to one on the left, and each originating from the very tip of one of the vectors. Then draw in the diagonal as shown; it represents the resultant force, meaning the cube behaves as though only a single force of the resultant's magnitude and direction acted upon it.

Middle: The same procedure for any two different forces diverging at an oblique angle still provides an accurately described resultant. Neat, eh?

Bottom: The converse also applies: given a force such as a muscle pull, find its two *orthogonal components* (this means simply lying at right angles) acting on the bone it attaches to. So construct the parallelogram shown. Then each arm of the resulting rectangle (which also forms a regular parallelogram but that special case of the class which has right angle corners) accurately portrays the components of the load transferred to bone the tendon. Even neater!

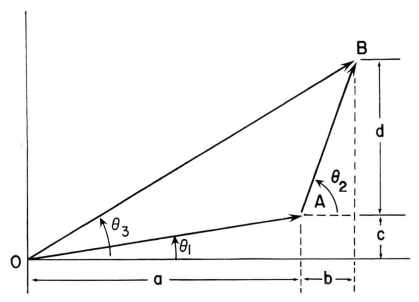

Figure 1.05. We have here two forces, represented by vectors OA and AB. Rather than use the parallelogram method shown in the previous figure, let us find their resultant mathematically. To do so, erect the orthogonal coordinates shown, their intersection to lie at the origin of OA. Don't worry; you could rotate the coordinates any amount, and place their intersection anywhere, and the method will still work; doing it as we have simply shortens and simplifies the arithmetic involved.

Then the text explains how to obtain the resultant. We needed orthogonal coordinates so we could use the Pythagorean theorem to obtain the answer, and you will find that theorem described in Appendix 5.

You can check this by filling in the parallelogram as in the previous figure, whereupon you will see that the resultant also equals the parallelogram's diagonal.

struct a new parallelogram with the / third force, determine therefrom their resultant, and likewise for a fourth, fifth and so on.

As for the third dimension of space, if one needs to work such matters out one simply repeats this process but now changing the plane of the graph paper to correspond to another aspect of the problem lying at 90° to the original one. Should you wish to compute such a resultant algebraically using trigonometry, Figure 1.05 illustrates the essence of the method, based upon the Pythagorean theorem. The magnitude of the resultant R, equals:*

$$R^2 = (a + b)^2 + (c + d)^2. \qquad \textit{Equation 1.08}$$

The angle or line of action of the resultant with respect to the Cartesian coordinate axes shown equals:

$$\text{Tan}^{-1}\ \theta_3 = \frac{c + d}{a + b} \qquad \textit{Equation 1.09}$$

You will find some trigonometric refresher material in Appendix 4 in Part III of this book.

(b) *Resolution of Forces*: We sometimes, in fact very commonly, need to do the opposite of the previous function: given the line of action and magnitude of some particular force (such as a muscle pull or a joint reaction), break it or the stresses it introduces in some structure down into its component elements. For example, the bottom of Figure 1.04 diagrammed the line of action of the semitendinosus tendon on the tibia as seen from the front. One can resolve the load it applies to that bone, and in the plane of that drawing, into two components, one parallel to the longitudinal axis of the bone, the other perpendicular to it, as shown in that drawing. The drawing in Fig. 1.06 also illustrates how to do it both graphically and for anyone capable of handling the trigonometry, how to do it mathematically. The drawing shows a force of unit magnitude, O A, acting along a line aligned θ degrees from the horizontal graph coordinate. The value of that horizontal component equals the cosine of the angle θ times the value of O A (see the table of trigonometric functions, in Part III). Since that cosine actually equates to side O B divided by side O A, or $\dfrac{O\ B}{O\ A}$, one solves the expression for OB to obtain: OB $=$ O A cos θ.

---

* If you want to obtain square roots—you need the square root of R^2 here— look up the logarithm of R^2 (after you have found its numerical value) in the table of ordinary logarithms in Special Table 1, Part III, divide by 2 (or by 3 to get a cube root), and then find the number corresponding to that logarithm. Cheer up—Appendix 3 also explains logarithms!

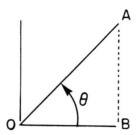

Figure 1.06. *Given:* the force represented by vector OA. *Problem:* find its horizontal component both graphically and trigonometrically.

Graphic solution: drop a perpendicular from the tip of OA to the horizontal axis at point B. Then the length of OB represents the magnitude of the horizontal component. So simple! By drawing in the remaining side from the vertical axis of the graph to A, and parallel to the horizontal axis, you can see that again we have a simple rectangular parallelogram.

Trigonometric solution: (Consult Appendix 5 if you need to refresh your trig.) The cosine of the angle θ equals $\frac{OB}{OA}$, or $\cos \theta = \frac{OB}{OA}$; solve for OB to obtain:

$$OB = \cos \theta \ OA.$$

Now do the necessary arithmetic, using actual values for the angle, and for the magnitude of OA.

(c) *The Parallelogram Laws:* We can list here and memorize two of them for future use.

1) *The sum of two vectors acting in a common plane equals the diagonal of a parallelogram whose adjacent sides represent the two vectors.* We will call this *vectorial addition*; it differs from ordinary addition as we illustrate shortly.

2) *The sum of three vectors equals the resultant of any two summed vectorially with the third. And likewise with any number of further vectors.*

Note that in adding 3 to 4, whether in the abstract sense or as batches of acorns or orthopaedic residents, the sum always equals 7. These represent *scalar* identities which have only one property (here, magnitude). But a force has at least two properties simultaneously: its magnitude, and its direction. Identities which represent two or more properties simultaneously do not add by ordinary scalar addition laws;

rather they add by the parallelogram laws, according to which
3 + 4 can equal any whole number from −1 to +7, and any
direction of the compass, as Figure 1.07 illustrates.

We express *speed*, a scalar quantity, in terms such as ft/
sec, cm/sec, and so on. One may add and subtract speed

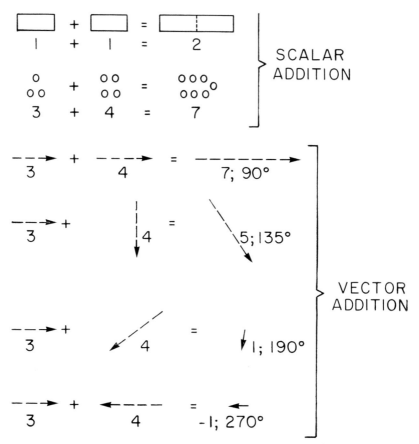

Figure 1.07. The top three problems describe scalar addition as we use
that term in this book. It represents the ordinary addition familiar to
everyone with an accurate checkbook and a viable bank account.

The lower four problems show that vector addition behaves differently
and that 3 + 3 can equal any number between zero and six, or 3 + 4 any
number between −1 and +7 (!). The numerical solutions are only
approximate, a note added in haste lest some purist feel compelled to write
me a note about the accuracy of my slide rule. The drawing simply illustrates a point.

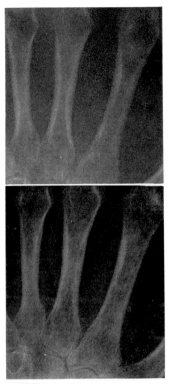

Figure 1.08. Living bone is not just a piece of inactive ivory! But its mysteries and enchantments dance and weave their spells over a much longer time period than that of ordinary conversation, and only when one's mind prepares itself for that fact does one really begin to see and understand this stuff.

Top: Metacarpal x-rays of an adult female patient of Dr. Howard Duncan, taken (in B.E.C. Nordin and/or S. Garn fashion) before she began treatment with an adrenalcorticosteroid hormone analog, for a problem not involving this hand.

Bottom: After some six months of treatment the marrow cavities have expanded significantly (i.e., the *endosteal envelope* has enlarged because of a sudden, strongly negative bone balance arising on it) but no other locus of bone loss appears. *Conclusions:* Bone is dynamic even in adults; hormones acting primarily upon the soft tissues in the marrow cavity can secondarily affect bone in contact with it, here to cause an early case of the osteoporosis of Cushing's syndrome; when you want to understand what something does to this stuff you must wait long enough, as discussions in Volume III brought out, and whether your concerns focus upon hormonal effects or biomechanical ones.

as we do ordinary numbers in scalar arithmetic. Thus 5 mph plus 10 mph equals 15 mph.

Velocity on the other hand signifies a *speed plus its direction* in the engineering world, and so it constitutes a vectorial quantity which one must add vectorially according to the parallelogram laws. Thus 5 mph east plus 15 mph west equals, not 15 mph, but 10 mph west.

Now refer to Figure 1.08 and its brief message, and then try the quiz that follows immediately next.

QUESTIONS: CHAPTER 1

1) Define: a) force; b) load; c) energy; d) power.
2) A fly expends a trivial amount of energy in flying from a chair to a window. a) Could one drill a hole in a diamond with that energy? b) or break the window with it? Explain and defend your answer.
3) List several subcategories of forces.
4) A man seated on one ischial tuberosity places 50 lb upon it and its load-bearing cross section area equals 1.5 square inches. State or compute the following:
   a) total load; b) unit load; c) the power involved; d) the work involved; e) the energy involved.
5) List some forces.
6) Refer to the metacarpal bone x-rays in Figure 1.08 and then characterize the following as scalar or vectorial properties.
   a) metacarpal diameter
   b) velocity of expansion of the marrow cavity
   c) cortical thickness
   d) mean cortical thickness
   e) bone turnover in %/year, and in $mm^3/mm^3/year$.
   f) bone turnover on the marrow cavity wall (endosteal envelope) and outer cortical surface (periosteal envelope)
   g) the bone loss which thinned the cortices.

A PHORISM: Let us ask a question. To do so we must set a stage. Thus: Some regard teaching orthopaedic residents as primarily a problem of making available to them the proper rotations, the proper clinical material and lectures, the proper journals and books—and name figures.

But not so. While such matters do provide part of the stuffing of any creditable orthopaedic residency, they constitute only its lawn, upon which one treads daily and as a matter of course. A good teacher exposes his residents to something less tangible, yet far, far more potent in its effects upon the resident's future patients, effects that will stretch over all his later years until he finally puts down for the last time the scalpel, the orthopaedic "antennae", and the living ideals that mark the practicing physician.

Such a teacher conveys to his students (by his every-day manner of living, conduct, and reactions to varied challenges) his values, the dimensions of his moral life, his ability to perceive the facts that do not fit, to recognize those nuances beneath bare words and stark facts which may point to the hidden disease or complication, the abused child, the inner man struggling to find himself in a chaotic and too-often deaf and uncaring world. Residents admire and emulate a teacher's living honesty and guts, his capacity to doubt, to find fault in his own work, his struggles to preserve his ideals (not the same thing as his illusions) before the gambits of the urban life maelstrom and seductress. They forgive him the clay on his shoes, as they find in hard and earnest confrontation with life "as it really is, brother," that some sticks to their own shoes too.

I have been fortunate to have known some teachers whose inner life possessed such extra depth and dimensionality. For one, Prof. Atsuhiro Miyazaki of Kagoshima City, Kyushu, Japan; for another, C. L. Mitchell, now of La Jolla, California; for a third, Prof. S. Kono, formerly of Niigata, Japan and

31

now retired; for fourth and fifth, Drs. F. N. Potts, deceased, and S. Stanisavljevic, still very much with us.

Now ponder a moment: how can an IBM machine recognize such qualities in the little black-rimmed squares of a sheet of examination paper? or in a curriculum vitae? or how can another man, not endowed by nature or experience with similar attributes, perceive them in his colleague? And if machines or some men cannot perceive them, how can they possibly value them?

Now the question: What kind of man will teach your son or daughter? Who will select him? What (and whose) yardstick will measure his qualities and potential? What yardstick would *you* use? To what lengths would you (and should you) go to realize your wishes?

Chapter 2

Stress and Strain

T HIS CHAPTER WILL introduce the reader to two effects generated in structural materials by loads applied to and sustained by them. One represents a subcategory of forces generally, the other a category of dimensional changes in the structure. And as in the previous as well as succeeding chapters we will use some of the opportunities presented to review some matters of basic physics and algebraic conventions. While any clinician totally and resolutely dedicated to not using or learning any kind of math may take some offense thereby, the text verbalizes things in such a way that he too can still come away with the basically useful ideas stuffed in his head, uncontaminated by algebra, trigonometry or logarithms!

I: STRESS

Support a weight at the end of a rubber band. The band will stretch as the weight falls toward the floor, but at some point it will stretch no further and will hold the weight suspended in midair, provided the band does not break (see "C" in Figure 2.01). The force of gravity pulling the weight to the floor (with a force equal to its weight, not its mass) now opposes another force arising within the rubber band and acting in the opposite sense, directionally speaking (i.e., we really now discuss a vectorial situation). This force, pretty evenly distributed throughout the length and over the cross sectional area of the band, represents a *tension stress*. It actually arises in the form of the elastic resistance of the chemical bonds in and between the rubber molecules to uncoiling, to stretching, and sliding past each other. In general, unruptured chemical bonds between various atoms and molecules remain nearly perfectly elastic and resilient in character.

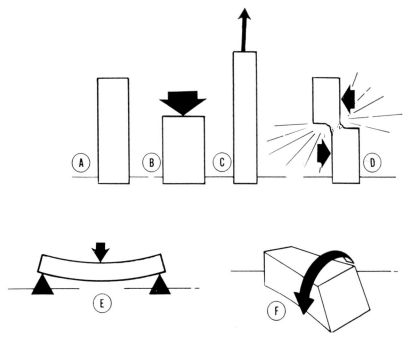

Figure 2.01. This figure illustrates diagrammatically five major types of strain one can cause matter to undergo: uniaxial compression at B; uniaxial tension at C; shear at D; flexure at E, and torque at F. The top three figures also illustrate the three principal stresses, signifying forces within the matter of the structures which act to resist the deformations shown. And the figures also illustrate the meaning of various kinds of loads (see Chapter I), as those causing the actual deformations shown.

Broadly speaking, we call those forces generated within the substance of a material in response to any external loads it carries *mechanical stresses.**

DEFINITION: *Stress: The resistance of the intermolecular bonds in a substance to physical deformation by externally applied loads.*

1) KINDS OF STRESS: We recognize three principal stresses, so-called because any kind of physical load applied to any form of matter generates within it forces (i.e., stresses)

---

* We talk about mechanical stress, quite different from the physiological stress written of by H. Selye.

that one can always resolve into some particular combination of only these three principal stresses. These principal stresses include:

(a) *Tension Stress*: That force in matter which resists pulling or stretching its substance apart. In the rubber band example above, tension stress in the band developed which resisted and finally equalled (and so in a manner of speaking, cancelled) the downward pull of the earth on the weight. Similarly, tension stress develops in a tendon when its muscle contracts, and exactly this stress constitutes the mechanical pull or load on the attachment of that tendon to a bone. Note that gaseous matter cannot develop an effective tension stress (it remains incapable of rigidity in tension); consequently it will expand indefinitely in volume unless confined by some means.

(b) *Compression Stress*: That force in matter which resists pushing it together or squashing it. The legs of the chair you probably sit on at this very moment have developed compression stresses from the action of your body's weight, which tries to "fall" towards the earth's center (which to repeat, equals your body's mass multiplied by the earth's gravatational attraction for all masses of similar magnitude). That compression stress resists the action of the load of your body's weight on the chair legs, and because its sum total in the chair legs exactly equals your weight, it holds you suspended above the floor. Equally, when a man stands up compression stresses arise in his tibias in response to his superimposed body weight. This stress resists or opposes the force of his weight, thereby holding him up.

(c) *Shear Stress*: When a pair of scissors cut paper, the resistance of the paper to this action at the point where the scissor blades meet and overlap forms a force within its substance called a shear stress (see D in Fig. 2.01, right). Likewise the sliding resistance of the coarse adjustment ways of a medical microscope represents a shearing stress arising in the heavy lubricant lying between the slide ways. The brakes in a car convert to equivalent amounts of heat the mechanical work (i.e., shearing load times distance, or W =

FL) done by the brake shoe as it rubs on the moving brake drum or disc. The resistance to that motion, which develops when one applies the brakes, forms a shearing stress, here a particular subcategory of all shearing stresses named friction in this and analogous situations in which motion of one mass of matter occurs on another. (79)   When one runs liquids through glass tubes of small bore, those liquids will run only so fast under the action of the earth's gravitational pull on their matter. That arises because shearing stresses develop within the fluids (and align parallel to the inner wall of the tube) which act to resist acceleration of the rate of flow by gravity. This represents a kind of "fluid friction" named viscosity. Note that both the gaseous and liquid states of matter display the property of a lack of rigidity under shear, while the solid state of matter does possess rigidity in shear.

2) SPECIFICATION OF STRESSES: As with loads, we may choose to express stress in either or both of two ways: as total stress, or unit stress.

(a) *Total Stress*: The entire weight hanging from the rubber band above (i.e., in grams or pounds) equalled the total tension stress at any cross sectional level in the rubber band. We could express it in pounds, grams, or dynes (which in this context one conventionally considers as scalar quantities). Thus the total compression load applied across a football player's femoral neck in the heat of a game may exceed 1000 kg, and this therefore must also equal the total compression stress developed within its substance at any cross section perpendicular to the line of action of that load.

(b) *Unit Stress*: In engineering work, one often needs some idea or index of the amount of stress on the average intermolecular bond in the material, for that then allows one to compare one material to another in a meaningful way, or to decide how much material a given structure requires at some point to perform its assigned task reliably and effectively. In such cases we use unit stress, and express it for example in pounds per square inch, written psi or (lb/in^2) on cross section, or grams per square centimeter, written gm/cm^2; or kilograms per square millimeter, written kg/mm^2, all still considered to represent scalar quantities. Remember that unit stress does not constitute the actual stress on one intermolecular bond; it simply provides a useful index of it. For the football player in the above paragraph, if the bony tissue in his femoral neck which actually carries the 1000 kg total load has a cross section area of some 8 cm², the unit compression stress in his femoral neck would then equal some 1000 ÷ 8 or 125 kg/cm². Now, if we examine the same player's eleventh rib, we find that it carries a total compression or "hoop" load during the same game of some 31 kg. But on cross section area only some 25 mm² (.25 cm²) of compacta carry this load, leading to a unit loading figure of—again—some 125 kg/cm², a striking similarity which immediately suggests some interesting properties of living skeletons.*

Let us again call upon Greek lower case sigma (σ), now to signify mechanical stress in the unit stress context, and write the algebraic expression which relates it to total load (P) and total cross section area (A). We have already seen it:

$$\sigma = \frac{P}{A} \qquad\qquad\qquad Equation\ 2.01$$

3) METHODS OF MEASURING STRESS: Note two things: We do not measure stress directly in materials or structures; we always infer or compute it from other information. Perhaps confusingly, every-day engineering jargon and conversation often makes no distinction between unit loads and unit stresses, a practice which can easily confuse a tyro trying to learn to swim these waters.

(a) *The Load-Area Relation.* In a testing machine for example, the total amount of tension or compression or other load applied to a test structure of known dimensions can appear on a dial. But regardless of how we do it, we know the actual value of the total load on the test structure. That, therefore, must also equal the total stress within the structure. And if we use test structures of known and regular dimensions

---

* We shall find in a later chapter in Part II that some truth lies in such suggestions.

we then can always obtain accurate measurements of A, the total cross section area of structure carrying the load. So we fit these numbers into the above equation, do the necessary division and come up with σ, the unit stress. But the total load P, and total stress σ, relate as follows, given uniaxial conditions:

$$P = \sigma \qquad\qquad \textit{Equation 2.02}$$

As with any other kind of force, mechanical stresses can have both the scalar and vectorial properties but for the particular needs of some problem or purpose one may choose to ignore, or not to ignore, either. And to repeat, customarily in engineering work the lower case Greek letter sigma (σ) signifies stress. Thus, for a tendon loaded in tension, or a muscle contracting, or an elephant standing on one limb (!), the total stress becomes that shown in equation 2.02. (281)

(b) *The Stress-Deformation Relation*: When we know how much a particular material (such as bone or tendon or a given metal) must stretch or squeeze to produce some particular level of internal stress, then by measuring the actual amount of deformation (i.e., stretch or squeeze) of some part of an experimental structure made of this material, we can deduce with sufficient accuracy the stresses generated in it under various loading conditions. (273) We will produce some algebraic expressions that can do this in the next chapter.

(c) *Photoelasticity*: A method exists for inferring stress patterns with the aid of the polarized light. Called photoelastic analysis, it involves the production of fringe patterns in transmitted light by means of crossed polars in transparent, birefringent plastic models of an experimental structure, using scale loads acting on the model in the same way as in the real structure when in actual use. (145)

Now consult Figure 2.02 for a practical example of some of these and the upcoming ideas.

II: STRAIN

Stretch a rubber band; pour water out of a glass; bend a wire (or an elbow); stand on and so squash a tennis ball;

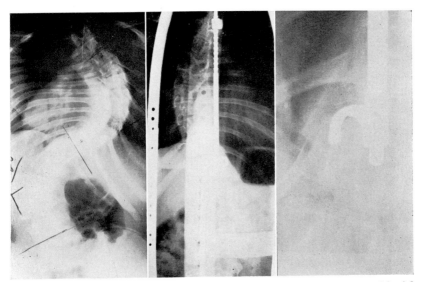

Figure 2.02. *Left:* X-rays taken from the rear aspect of a 15 year old girl who has a severe idiopathic scoliosis, a disorder of the growing spine in which lateral curvatures develop, as shown.

Middle: Nearly two years after I did a two-stage spinal fusion, employing two Harrington distraction rods, the lower one partly hidden behind one of the alloy bars of the Milwaukee brace she wears. As the heart shadow reveals, this film was reversed by the photographer; it's the same patient.

Right: This hook, at the lower end of the upper rod, fits over a spinal lamina to secure mechanical fixation so that the rod can prop apart the concave side of this curve during the time required for the fusion to consolidate and take over this mechanical function. The small area of bone actually in contact with the metal of this hook can cause large enough unit loads on, unit strains of, and unit stresses in, the bone, to damage it and cause it to crumble. This can cause failure of the fixation, and even allow migration and protrusion of the implant into the spinal canal where the spinal cord and nerve roots lie.

Consequently, one prepares the patient for such an operation by stretching the soft tissues on the concave side before the operation, with a Risser-type wedging cast. And so that the fixation may function long enough to fulfill its purpose, one limits the amount of force used to "jack" the curves open further during the operation (better a partial, permanent and assured correction than a complete one that—assuredly if one fully corrected these curves at the table—will fail soon after surgery); and one keeps the patient in bed in a body cast for 6 months after the operation to protect the fragile *bone*—not the metal—until the accompanying fusion consolidates. It helps in such endeavors to have available a high order of skill and craftsmanship in the people who provide the back-up necessary to any such work, such as Mr. Harold Brady and Dr. L. Z. Shifrin, two remarkable men indeed, provided in this case.

compress a femoral artery to arrest hemorrhage; perform closed chest massage; scramble an egg; compress a spring. In all of these examples, an object or a mass of matter becomes deformed by a mechanical load, and because it took or accepted it. Technically, this deformation represents a strain.* A strain occurs whenever a load, no matter how small, acts on a material object, no matter how strong. Grossly visible and obvious strain may arise as in the examples given above, or one may need special and very sensitive apparatus to detect it, for example to detect the strain in a steel beam caused by a mouse walking over it. But the strain always occurs.

DEFINITION: *Strain: Any physical deformation of matter caused by any kind of load acting on it.*

1) KINDS OF STRAIN: All deformations of matter can resolve into combinations of three principal strains, closely analogous to the three principal stresses already described and so readily learned (provided one learned the three principal stresses). They include tension, compression, and shear strains, as shown in Figure 2.01.

(a) *Tension Strain*: This signifies physical elongation or stretch, for example of the earlier-mentioned rubber band with its ends pulled apart. A similar although smaller elongation occurs in steel rope each time it takes a pull, and in a tendon each time a muscle pulls on it.

(b) *Compression Strain*: This means shortening or "squashing," as occurs when one stands on a tennis ball or a rubber eraser, or as develops in a vertebral body when one rises from the prone to the erect position. Compression strains also occur in the legs of a chair when one sits down in it, in the long bones of our lower extremities while we stand, and in the ribs each time we breath in or inspire.

(c) *Shear Strain*: The cutting action of scissors on paper causes a shearing displacement (i.e., strain) of the paper at

---

* People unacquainted with mechanics widely misunderstand, confuse and misuse mechanical stress and strain as terms. And this applies to first year orthopaedic residents who seemingly need approximately a year to get them properly entrenched in their gyri, and to shed the notion that they have anything to do with family tensions or venereal disease.

the juncture of the blades. When this displacement exceeds the elasticity and strength of the paper, the latter tears apart, which we arbitrarily term "cutting" by the shears. Also, a table dragged over a rug to a new place in the room, causes to move slightly sideways those parts of the rug under its legs, because of friction between them. This represents a shearing displacement or strain of the top layer of the rug with respect to its bottom layer. Or, take a magazine lying flat on a table; now roll it up. Where the plane formed by the cut pages at their free edges originally lay perpendicular to the plane of these pages, it has now become oblique as each page moves sideways on its neighbors, another shearing displacement. A similar displacement occurs between that layer of a flowing liquid in immediate contact with the wall of a pipe, and the much faster moving column lying in the middle of the lumen. When this motion represents elastic deformation of a solid substance (i.e., one which exhibits rigidity in shear) we call it a *shearing strain*. When it represents a sliding movement of one solid object on another separate one (as in the case of the magazine pages) we call it a *shearing displacement*; and when it occurs in a fluid material we call it *flow*. Chapter X has a few remarks on these matters but they will probably keep until then.

Note: All real deformations of matter can reduce to some combination of these three principal strains. In addition to the pure deformations already described, these deformations would include bending and twisting shown at the bottom of Figure 2.01 and all combinations of these strains, plus the flow of liquids and gasses and the compression and expansion of gasses such as air. These matters will come up again in a later chapter.

2) SPECIFICATION OF STRAIN: We can express the strain in some object in two ways, analogous to the ways of specifying loads and stresses: as total strain, or unit strain. Both represent scalar expressions.

(a) *Total Strain:* Assume the femur of a man has a total length of 300 mm, and when he stands on it his weight shortens it by one millimeter. Then the total strain in compression equals one millimeter. A rubber band stretched two inches develops a total tension strain of two inches. Commonly, one expresses strain in shear in solids in trigonometric measure as the tangent, but the reader need not go into that because the writer, while convinced the time has come in orthopaedics when every orthopaedic resident must know how to handle elementary algebra, remains equally convinced that only some future generation of residents must also know how to use elementary trigonometry.

But for those who feel they must jump the gun or who disagree, Appendix 4 in Part III provides an elementary introduction to trigonometry. It contains the background needed to wade successfully through this text.

(b) *Unit strain:* In the case of the femur above, if we divide the total strain by the total length of the bone we obtain the result 1/300 or .0033. In words, this means that the strain in compression over a distance equal to the unit of measurement (here, one mm) equalled $\frac{.0033}{1}$ or .0033 of that unit, or equally, .33 per cent of it, as well as of the total length of the femur. Furthermore, this means that any short length of that bone, expressed in any linear measure (such as inches, millimeters, rods or even degrees of geographic latitude), decreased by the same fraction or ratio or per cent. We cannot convert the two-inch total strain of the aforementioned rubber band in tension to unit strain until we also know its original resting length. Its stretched length divided by its resting length gives the unit strain (i.e., change in length) as a decimal proportion of the original length, which, given that its resting length equalled one inch, would equal $2 \div 1$, or 2.00. To express it, or any other decimal fraction of something, in per cent simply multiply by 100 to obtain in this case 200 per cent.

Like the unit stress method of expression, the unit strain method has certain advantages over the total strain method when one analyses the strength of structures at different parts of irregular geometry. For example, if a 70 kg compression load acts on top of an erect human femur, and we find that the unit compression strain just above the femoral condyles at the knee becomes 1.3x that at midshaft, one would infer (correctly) that at midshaft that femur had 1.3x the total compression srength that it had at the lower level. It implies further that probably 1.3x as much bone lay in a complete cross section at the higher level as at the lower, given homogeneous (i.e., equal) materials properties at both levels. Measuring total strain over the whole bone would simply reveal the total shortening between its two ends without yielding any information on the distribution of its structural strength along its length.

Customarily, engineers signify strain in their mathematical calculations by the lower case Greek letter epsilon* (ϵ) ; also they use lower case Greek letter delta (Δ) to signify some change in a measureable parameter. Thus they would write changes in a length, or in a time, or in a stress, or in a strain, as ΔL, Δt, $\Delta\sigma$ and $\Delta\epsilon$ respectively.

Then the equations for strain become, for the case of total strain shown in Figure 2.03:

$$\epsilon = \Delta L \qquad\qquad\qquad \textit{Equation 2.03}$$

and for the case of *unit strain*:

$$\epsilon = \frac{\Delta L}{L} \qquad\qquad\qquad \textit{Equation 2.04}$$

Note: A necessary convention concerning plus and minus signs crops up here. When one stands on his femur, the shortening it occasions subtracts from its resting length and so represents a negative quantity. In other words, here delta L equals $-\Delta L$.

But for elongation of the rubber band, ΔL signifies a positive quantity, so ΔL in equations 2.03–2.04 for this case means $+\Delta L$.

Watch those signs!

3) STRAIN ENERGY: When one strains a material by applying to it a load which deforms it, the deforming force acts over the distance of the actual strain. Accordingly this rep-

---

* Special Table 16 in Part III lists the Greek alphabet.

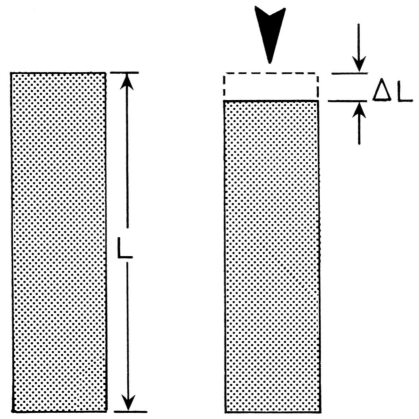

Figure 2.03. When the column on the left of length L accepts a compression load it will shorten slightly as shown on the right. Signified there and in the text as ΔL, this equals the total compression strain. To obtain the unit strain, i.e., the amount of shortening per unit of length, simply divide ΔL by L as shown in equation 2.04.

resents mechanical work done on the intermolecular bonds of the material, since mechanical work or energy simply equals a force acting over some distance. The work usually stores elastically and temporarily within its substance as potential energy.

Or:

work = force × distance
and, in symbols:

$$W = FL$$

Equation 1.07

We will call the work done in straining a material by applying a load to it (against the resistance of its internal stresses) the *strain energy*. Several things might happen to that strain energy. For example, if the material breaks, at least part of that energy represents the work required to break or disrupt the intermolecular bonds holding its matter together. Or, if the material has perfect elastic resilience (i.e., if it has the Hookean property, described in a later chapter) then it simply stores that energy temporarily, and returns all of it as mechanical work (one form of kinetic energy) following deloading. Thus one function of high quality springs in machinery: to store energy temporarily. If the spring material lacks good resilience, it will dissipate or waste some of that energy stored in it as heat, or as a change in chemical or physical state, or in other ways, so it can never return as much energy in the form of mechanical work as was done upon it originally by deforming it. Carried to an extreme degree, we call this dissipation of strain energy into other forms than mechanical resilience the *damping* property. Note that the property of the conservation of energy applies here. That is, only as much work comes out of any system as one puts into it and/or as it originally contained. Note, however: *it need not come out in the same form as it went in.* Sometimes we like this. For example, we put potential heat in our automobile gas tanks and in exchange accelerate and move against gravity and various mechanical resistances a ton or so of metal—plus our own bodies. And some other times we do not like it; for example, less than 30 per cent of the total potential heat we paid to put in the gas tank actually appears as mechanical work at the driving wheels; the rest dissipates as heat and—transportationwise—useless chemical reactions. We will explore some of these matters further shortly, and later on will discuss how the rate of application of strain energy can affect structural materials.

4) METHODS OF MEASURING STRAIN:

(a) *Direct Measurement*: One can measure change in some dimension of a structure by direct means, such as with rulers, micrometers or calipers. Or an optical device, such as a cathetometer or filar micrometer focussed on a mark made on the structure, by means of calibrated scales and mechanical adjustments can reveal the movement of the mark after applying a known load, and with suitable equipment one can measure that movement. The strain can also appear as an electrical current generated by the motion of a coil in a magnetic field (or conversely), or as a change in electrical capacitance caused by the relative motion of two condenser plates. (Appendix 7 in Part III reviews some of these electrical fundamentals).

(b) *Strain Gauges*: These special devices, looking somewhat like postage stamps, when glued firmly to the surface of an object will change their electrical characteristics (usually electrical ohmic resistance) in accurately known ways when elongated or compressed. One can measure a change in ohmic resistance very accurately with the aid of a Wheatstone bridge circuit. Any device which changes one form of physical behavior or energy into another constitutes a *transducer*. Therefore a strain gauge forms a transducer. So too does the ear, which converts sound waves (i.e., variations in air pressure) to electrical pulses in nerves. Bone, cartilage and other collagen-containing tissues (all biological structural materials) form transducers too, for they can convert mechanical strain patterns into meaningful and very important patterns of cellular behavior. More of this in Part II of this book and in Volumes II and IV of this series.

(c) *Stresscoat*: In this method, a very brittle lacquer painted or sprayed onto the surface of the structure under study, has the property that when dry, it cracks when stretched (i.e., strained in tension) beyond a certain percentage of its resting dimensions. One can make the cracks visible by several means (a colored dye caught in the crack crevices forms one) after deloading the part. The number of cracks per linear centimeter, and their orientation on the surface, reveal the relative amounts of tension strain and its direction of greatest action. This method has practical usefulness in testing a wide variety of experimental devices, and when at Yale University School of Medicine some years ago I observed

Dr. C. O. Bechtol using this method to identify some of the design weaknesses in bone plates, hip nails and hip endoprostheses. Using this method F. G. Evans did some quite interesting studies some years ago of stress patterns developed in skulls and bony pelvises following impacts, such as might occur in automobile collisions and during aircraft seat ejection.

(d) *Photoelasticity*: The photoelastic method already mentioned actually measures physical strain rather than stress, but given a knowledge of how much stress equates to a given amount of strain in the particular plastic material used to construct the structural model, and one can then infer the lines of action and magnitudes of stress from the fringe pattern orientations and spacing. One applies the method by constructing an accurate model of the real structure out of a transparent plastic of accurately known physical and optical properties which one determines from measurements made in a materials testing laboratory. One can also mold a layer of birefringent plastic over the surfaces of some optically opaque actual structure, and with suitable equipment then read strain off as a displacement of fringes in reflected light. It has recently become possible to make three dimensional stress-strain analyses by the photoelastic means.

Remember (the arrow below signifying "cause") :

loads⟶*strain*⟶*stress*

QUESTIONS: CHAPTER 2

1) Define mechanical stress and strain.

2) a) In those terms, which does the pressure represent inside an exploding cartridge? b) Given that pressure acting on the enveloping barrel and chamber, and that you as a designer wish to design the barrel for ample strength, what does that pressure then represent to you?

3) A 100 kg man stands on one heel, forefoot off the floor. His tuber os calcis with a mean length of 7.0 cm shortens in compression by .01 mm. State and/or calculate the following with respect to the tuber:

a) ΔL; b) total load; c) total stress; d) the kind of stress; e) total strain; f) kind of strain; g) unit strain.

4) A column, made of an elastic material having a Young's modulus of 2.5 x 10⁶ psi/in, has a total compression strength of 1500 lb, and fails at 2 per cent shortening. How could you fashion the column to retain its total strength but to fail only after 4 per cent shortening? In other words, how might you increase its bulk compliance two-fold without sacrificing its total compression strength?

Chapter 3

Basic Stress-Strain Relationships
in Solids

Relationships appear between stresses and strain in real
materials and structures which become important in understanding their bulk behavior, whether we consider and/or
study the intact structures, or the materials composing them,
or any liquids used—or serving as—lubricants. This holds
as true for living structures and materials as it does for those
inanimate ones known to engineers and mechanics. Many of
these relationships have received special names, and one can
illustrate many of them by plotting mechanical stress graphically on one axis, against strain on the other, as shown a bit
later in Figure 3.02. We will describe some of these properties
briefly next, for solids first and for liquids second. We will
follow the conventional practice of plotting stress (i.e., σ)
on the vertical axis, and strain (i.e., ϵ) on the horizontal axis
on all such graphs.

I: STATIC PARAMETERS

1) Elasticity: In an elastic material the strain arising
as it takes a load disappears completely following removal
of the load. In other words, an elastic material returns to its
original dimensions and shape following a deformation. The
tennis ball in Figure 3.01 illustrates one case: it squashes if
you stand on it, but resumes its spherical shape when you release it. A number of important properties of materials center
around their elastic behavior.

Note: In engineering work the term elasticity does not
define or mean how quickly a structure returns to its original
dimensions after deloading; elasticity defines the fact that
it does so, regardless of how readily. This of course differs

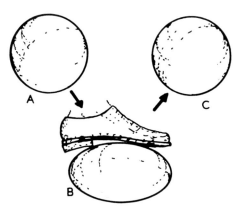

Figure 3.01. When one stands upon a tennis ball it deforms, decreasing in vertical height (a compression strain) and increasing in horizontal diameter (a tension strain). Because it returns to its original shape and dimensions when you deload it, it behaves elastically. But as the text makes clear later, that need not also mean it has good resilience. While all resilient materials behave elastically, not all elastic materials have good resilience.

from the lay usage of that term. Thus the highly resilient tennis ball, and poorly resilient nylon thread, and moist, live bone, each constitutes an elastic material, because each returns faithfully to its original shape and dimensions following a deformation or strain.

2) Hook's Law: When as one increases the strain of a material, its internal stress increases proportionally, then we say the material obeys Hook's Law, and we call it a "Hookean solid." If one doubles the strain in a Hookean solid, one doubles the stress; or if he lowers the stress to a third, likewise the strain, as shown in the straight region of the curves in Figure 3.02. A perfect Hookean material would form the perfect spring (but see *resilience* below), and the one most nearly so known to us constitutes air. In defining the Hookean property we assume that we change the loads on the material under test so slowly that special time-dependent properties appearing under circumstances of very rapid changes in loading do not enter into the problem in any way of practical significance. (133) When we consider resilience and compliance, time dependent phenomena will become quite important. We

can write the above relationship algebraically, using k to signify a constant of proportionality (or scaling factor) :

$$\epsilon = k\sigma \qquad\qquad\qquad Equation\ 3.01$$

Note on the left hand curve in Figure 3.02 that above point
(A) the stress (vertical axis) no longer increases in proportion to strain (on the horizontal axis) . The curving trajectory
of that graph line shows that strain now increases faster than
stress above that point. Thus above point (A) the material
no longer acts as a Hookean solid. But if it returns faithfully
and completely to its orginal dimensions following removal of
the load (i.e., deloading) then it still behaves perfectly elastically. Steel, glass, bone and tendon all have the Hookean
property in that within some stress-strain range, stress and
strain remain essentially proportional to each other.

3) YOUNG'S MODULUS: In any structure carrying a load
which stresses it within its Hookean limit, the actual value of
the stress divided by the actual elastic strain* represents
Young's Modulus, usually signified by the letter E, and in
effect it signifies the amount of stress one would find generated in a unit cross section area of the substance if first, one
strained it a unit amount (i.e., 100 percent) and if, second, it
didn't break or enter into a nonHookean range of behavior,
an untrue assumption for most materials of course but, none-
theless, a highly useful one. This follows then:
Young's modulus defines the stiffness of a material, i.e.,
its resistance to deformation by a load.

The larger the modulus, the stiffer the material. Thus, a
rubber band would have a low modulus as in the straight,
only slightly slanted right hand line in Figure 3.02, while
steel would have the higher one on the left. As a result the
same total load causing identical unit stresses in each material
can cause a large strain in a rubber band (which has a low
Young's modulus) , an intermediate one in bone or pine wood,
and a very small one in steel wire (which has a high modu-

---

* One must use consistent units of measure. Young's modulus is also known
as the *elastic modulus,* and *Young's modulus of elasticity.*

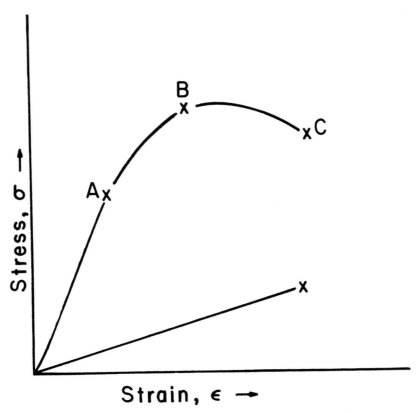

Figure 3.02. A stress-strain graph or plot, in which one plots the strain on the horizontal axis, against the stress on the vertical one. Since Young's modulus measures stiffness as the amount of stress required to "cause" (actually to *resist*) 100% deformation, high values indicate stiff materials and low ones the opposite: compliant ones. The left curve shows a constant proportionality between stress and strain up to a point A, and this, therefore, represents the "Hookean range" of this material and the stress at point A constitutes its proportional limit. Between A and B no constant stress-strain proportionality exists, so the material no longer exhibits Hookean behavior. But if it still returns to its original dimensions and shape after deloading it remains within its elastic range. At B it reaches its yield point and begins to deform *plastically* (i.e., permanently), and at C it finally ruptures. Note that its ultimate strength (the highest part of the curve) exceeds its breaking strength; many (but not all) metals exhibit this property.

The right hand curve illustrates a rubber band, which proves far less stiff (or if you prefer, more compliant).

TABLE 3.01
YOUNG'S MODULUS (E)

Substance	lb./f/in²		10^{11} Dynes/cm²		Tensile Strength, Ultimate, psi
Aluminum	10	$\times 10^6$	7	$\times 10^{11}$	9,000
Lead	.7	$\times 10^6$	.5	$\times 10^{11}$	2,000
Tungsten	60	$\times 10^6$	40	$\times 10^{11}$	215,000
Titanium	17	$\times 10^6$	12	$\times 10^{11}$	100,000
Iron (cast)	20	$\times 10^6$	14	$\times 10^{11}$	40,000
Tool Steel	28	$\times 10^6$	19	$\times 10^{11}$	75,000
Stainless Steel	25	$\times 10^6$	17	$\times 10^{11}$	160,000
Vitallium	30	$\times 10^6$	21	$\times 10^{11}$	85,000
Spruce (dry)	1.2	$\times 10^6$	.8	$\times 10^{11}$	5,000
Bone (wet)	2.5	$\times 10^6$	10.5	$\times 10^{11}$	12,000
316 stainless (annealed)	28	$\times 10^6$	19	$\times 10^{11}$	85,000
Nylon	.4	$\times 10^6$	.3	$\times 10^{11}$	8,000
Rubber	.005	$\times 10^6$	.0035	$\times 10^{11}$	2,000
Sapphire	50	$\times 10^6$	35	$\times 10^{11}$	
Glass	10	$\times 10^6$	7	$\times 10^{11}$	5,000

This table lists for a variety of materials their Young's moduli in tension or E, in English units (left) and in cgs units (right), as well as their ultimate tensile strengths in psi (pounds per square inch of cross section). Note that E signifies that stress computed or extrapolated to cause 100 per cent elongation in tension based upon tests made within its breaking stress (which involves elongations for various materials on the order of 0.5%–30%). Taken from references (4, 39, 111, 123, 173, 280).

lus), all of the same diameter. Table 3.01 lists some values of Young's modulus for a few materials, along with their ultimate strengths in tension.

We can write the above relationship algebraically in this manner, E signifying Young's modulus:

$$E = \sigma/\epsilon \qquad\qquad \textit{Equation 3.02}$$

Note: Strength and stiffness do not represent the same quantities, another matter where lay usage of terms could cause some communication difficulty. A material can have an impressively large Young's modulus, and still prove at the same time easily broken or weak (ex: chalk), or very strong (ex: hardened steel).

While real solids strain simultaneously in tension, compression and shear, the amount of strain corresponding to a unit amount of stress does not always remain equal for each kind of strain. Consequently one uses separate moduli to define each of those properties, called the tension modulus, compression modulus and shear modulus (the latter also sometimes—but improperly—called the bulk modulus) respectively. Usually calculated from values measured in the materials testing laboratory for the corresponding unit stress and unit strain, some homogeneous materials do have essentially the same moduli in compression and tension (i.e., strain isotropy). This characteristic appears in many solids, such as many metals and plastics.

Note: *Strain isotropy* does not characterize biological structural materials such as bone, tendon, cartilage, muscle and tooth, nor most other materials that have a physical grain. In such materials the Young's modulus not only may differ considerably in tension and compression, each may change according to the direction in which one tests it. This property, in which a material (*note:* not a finished structure) develops different unit strains under equal unit loadings when one changes the direction or line of action of the load, constitutes *strain anisotropy* (the reader occasionally may find it less properly termed stress anisotropy). It follows then that strain-anisotropic materials have different moduli or stiffness in different directions. Further examples of grained materials would include wood, prestressed concrete, and forged steel parts.

Materials lacking the elastic property constitute anelastic materials, and possess the property of *anelasticity*.

II: DYNAMIC PARAMETERS

1) RESILIENCE: A new tennis ball dropped onto a concrete floor rebounds nearly to the height from which you dropped it. The better the quality of the ball, the more nearly its bounce approaches the height it fell from. This illustrates the property of resilience, often confused in lay language with the property of elasticity. But where elasticity refers solely to the *dimensional changes* of a material regardless of the forces involved (in a perfectly elastic material net $\Delta L =$ zero), resilience refers to the *mechanical work* done in deforming an elastic material, i.e., to $W = FL$. In a perfectly

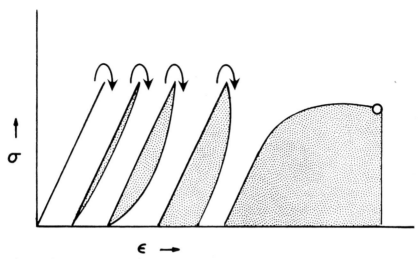

Figure 3.03. Each of these stress-strain curves shows on its left hand ascending limb the stress-strain relationship as a load is applied to the material, and on its right or descending limb the same relationship following and during deloading. On the left hand curve a single line results, signifying perfect resilience. On the second curve the deloading curve does not coincide, and the shaded area between the ascending and descending limbs represents the mechanical energy lost (as heat usually), and so signifies less than perfect—but still good—resilience. The third curve carries this further, and in fact more than 60% of the strain energy present at its peak dissipates in forms other than mechanical work returned to the system.

Note that all of the three left hand curves return ultimately to their origins, signifying perfect elasticity. But the fourth curve does not do this; some permanent deformation remains. This material has undergone *Plastic flow,* and taken a permanent set. The ascending right curve soon departs from its proportional limit, and then from its elastic limit, and finally breaks at a stress level below the other curves. But it absorbed much more energy or work before it broke than the other curve, and so it forms by far the toughest of these five specimens.

resilient material net ΔW equals zero, that is, the material returns as much mechanical work in regaining its original shape and dimensions as was done upon it in straining it originally, as shown in curve #1, Figure 3.03. Most of the tennis ball's resilience arises from air under pressure inside it; air constitutes one of the most resilient materials known.* Were this air let out before the ball dropped, it would then bounce

---

* Another example, a solid: the ivory used in making billiard balls.

less than a quarter of the height it fell from, because now it lacks the resilience due to air and depends for its bounce upon the much lesser resilience of its rubber casing. *Yet note*: in both instances the ball behaved perfectly elastically, because the dent made in it by the floor disappeared on the bounce. Nylon, and the foamed plastics used to pack delicate instruments, both lack resilience. Yet nylon remains elastic (it behaves similarly to curve #3 in Figure 3.03), because after a deformation it will return to its original shape, although slowly. However, the crushing produced by an impact on a foamed plastic remains permanently; i.e., it possesses neither elasticity nor resilience so that a ball of such material does not bounce when dropped on the floor; it stays there as though glued to it. At the point of that impact with the floor the ball becomes slightly flattened. The mechanical work required to make this flattening equals that work done in lifting the ball to the height from which it fell, and expends in breaking the bonds between its molecules (to deform it permanently) and in generating some heat. A lead ball—another substance essentially neither elastic nor resilient—behaves in much the same way.

DEFINITION: *resilience: a perfectly resilient material returns in the form of mechanical work all of the mechanical work done in deforming it.*

To the extent that some of the work done in deforming a material disappears or dissipates by other means (such as heat, or breakage of the material) it lacks resilience. One can thus define a *modulus of resilience* representing the mechanical work returned during deloading divided by that initially put into it. Thus:

$$R = \frac{W - \Delta W}{W} \qquad \textit{Equation 3.03}$$

This expression can range in numerical value from 1.0 (perfect resilience as in curve #1, Fig. 3.03, to zero (total lack of resilience as in curve #5, Fig. 3.03). The smaller ΔW, the more resilient the material. And the more resilient a spring for example, the better its quality as a temporary energy storage device.

Note: No perfectly resilient real materials have been found.

2) DAMPING: This, the opposite of resilience, signifies a material which does not return to its original shape with the same vigor with which it was deformed, i.e., it dissipates in other forms of energy some or most of the mechanical work done in straining it. So we say, "it damps out the force of impact." Figure 3.03 compares a representative damping stress-strain curve (#5) with that of more resilient materials (#1, #2). Compressed air forms a bad damping material because it returns most of the energy taken to deform it.* On the other hand, the foamed plastics make good ones because most of the work done in deforming them converts instead into both heat and the energy required to rupture the intermolecular bonds that hold it together, and so becomes permanently lost as mechanical work (curve #5, shaded region). Wet bone forms a better damping material than dry bone, which proves quite resilient, and this remains true even though in both states bone remains perfectly elastic over most of its useful stress-strain curve range. Wet tendon and cartilage also form good damping materials as do nylon, polyethylene (and bureaucrats). Curve #4 in Figure 3.03 shows the stress-strain curve of a fairly good damping material, one which takes a permanent set, i.e., deforms permanently, like a bent paper clip.

We can define a modulus of damping in terms analogous to those used to define the modulus of resilience, again using ΔW to signify that part of the mechanical work done in deforming a material which dissipates in forms not returned to the system as mechanical work.

---

* *But this depends on time:* When loading and unloading occur quickly, the resilience of air remains high but when the loading and unloading occur slowly its resilience becomes less perfect because enough time arises to allow some of the heat caused by compressing the air to dissipate into the environment. And it cannot return in the form of mechanical work the energy represented by that heat loss. Resilience in general proves time dependent in most real materials.

Thus:

$$D = \frac{\Delta W}{W} \qquad\qquad Equation\ 3.04$$

You may increase your facility with such equations by noting that the proper substitutions reveal that the damping modulus also equals:

$$D = 1 - R.$$

3) TOUGHNESS: This means resistance to fracture or mechanical failure. Drop a glass ball or an egg on a concrete floor, and they will probably break. Drop a steel ball, or a ball of the same size made of wet bone, on the floor repeatedly and they will not break. The steel and bone balls exhibit toughness.

In a more rigorous sense, a tough material constitutes one that will absorb a large amount of energy in the form of mechanical work before it breaks, and so toughness measures the amount of work one has to do on a unit amount of the material to fracture it. It relates only distantly to the phenomenon we term sttrength, another area where common language usage departs from engineering practice. Strength signifies breaking load or stress (a force), while toughness signifies breaking energy (work). Thus a high carbon steel drill may have great breaking strength (unit stress to cause fracture in tension may easily exceed 150,000 psi), and a stainless steel bone drill may have less than half of that (65,000 psi). But when you attempt to break the two, either by pulling them apart or simply by clamping one end in a vise and bending the other until it breaks, you discover that the much larger force needed to break the carbon steel drill needs to act over a rather small distance to do so, while the stainless steel one, requiring less than half that force to bend it, must bend back and forth more than 10 times before breaking. Thus the toughness of stainless steel exceeds that of the carbon steel drill at least five-fold, although the latter's breaking strength exceeds the former by at least two-fold.

DEFINITION: *toughness: The total mechanical work (in the form of strain energy) required to break a solid material.*

A tough material therefore can absorb a lot of such work or punishment, and curve #5 in Figure 3.03 illustrates this characteristic in the form of a stress-strain curve.

Then why make drills out of high-carbon steel? Simple: because they have another more necessary property: great hardness of the cutting edges. That hardness (described at the end of Chapter X) allows them to hold their cutting edge well, and in fact to cut into and drill holes in softer but much tougher materials. The loss of toughness accompanying the desirable hardness simply represents a penalty or trade necessitated by the basic materials properties of solid matter.

One can define a modulus of toughness in terms such as the work done (in terms of kg-M or ft-lb) per unit area of fracture surface, or per unit volume of a fractured test sample. In testing laboratories, such moduli often are determined by impact loading so arranged as to cause breakage in flexure.

4) FRAGILITY: This serves as the antonym to toughness and so means that a substance will absorb relatively little strain energy or mechanical work before it breaks. Chalk forms one good example and eggshell another.

5) BRITTLENESS: This term signifies a solid material that breaks after only small total strains have arisen as a consequence of some form of loading. In addition to fragility relative to stainless steel, the carbon steel drill above possessed the property of brittleness. Note that brittle materials may come either as weak ones (i.e., chalk) or as strong ones (the carbon steel drill again). To put this in different words, brittle materials do not strain greatly nor do they flow or bend to new shapes; they break or fracture instead. Independently of that however they can prove weak or strong.

6) DUCTILITY: This signifies the ability of material to deform or strain progressively in tension without breaking, and it represents a fluid-like flow of its atomic planes or crystals upon each other (we will do better with explaining this problem in Chapters V, VI). Thus it represents a function in part the opposite of brittleness, but not exactly so. One sees this property utilized in industry where wires of progressively

smaller diameter arise by drawing them through circular reducing holes in very hard dies.

7) MALLEABILITY: This property, related to ductility,
signifies the ability of a solid material to flow under hammer
blows. At room temperature gold forms one of the most
malleable solids known. In industry and manufacture a
tough and/ brittle material may convert temporarily to a
malleable state for shaping purposes, simply by heating it.
This constitutes the essence of the hot forging process. Copper and gold represent highly malleable solids at room temperature.

8) COMPLIANCE: Orthopaedists may expect to hear this
term with increasing frequency in coming years. In ordinary
words, it signifies the readiness with which a material (or a
structure) yields or gives way or strains before some dynamic
load applied to it. Because it can include the time element,
it can differ from Young's modulus; the latter usually expresses the stiffness of a material under conditions of such
leisurely changes in static loading that any peculiar effects
related to the time factor do not show up. Thus one way to
specify compliance as static compliance or C, consists simply
of using the reciprocal of Young's modulus (defined earlier
in this Chapter) or:

$$C = \frac{1}{E} \qquad\qquad Equation\ 3.05$$

In more rigorous, time-dependent terms, dynamic compliance (again signified by C here) equals the acceleration
produced per unit of applied loading force, or:

$$C = a/F \qquad\qquad Equation\ 3.06$$

and since acceleration equals speed (i.e., distance per
second) achieved per second, we can express c in units of

$$C = L/sec/sec/F.$$

Thus one finds the compliance of a phonograph needle
expressed in units (in the c.g.s. system) of cm/sec/sec/dyne.
A high number signifies a good needle, one which will track

faithfully the wiggling grooves in the record while so little resisting that sideways motion that wear of the sides of the record grooves becomes negligible.

How does this behavior differ from Young's modulus? In this way: consider a test sample of bone which, under very leisurely made changes in loading that allow plenty of time after each change for the instruments to stop quivering and attain steady readings, has a stiffness or Young's modulus of 2×10^6 psi (i.e., stress units to cause a unit amount of strain). Now retest it but with a dynamic load which builds up very rapidly (exactly as would occur during the impact upon it of a steel bar). Of course, one will need different kinds of measuring, recording and display apparatus to catch these fast changes; oscilloscopes abound in laboratories working in such furrows. Such testing machines may now show the bone's ratio of stress strain now equals 3×10^6; in other words, under those rapidly changing dynamic loading conditions it displayed half again the stiffness it did under static conditions. And a further increase in the speed of loading would probably reveal an even further increase in its apparent stiffness (i.e., a *decrease* in its compliance).

Note: If it still took the same total amount of strain to break this bone under high speed loading as it did under leisurely conditions, then the decreased compliance (or effectively increased Young's modulus) associated with it means that it would take half again as much mechanical work to break it. Accordingly under rapidly changing loading conditions—impacts—bone would (and does) exhibit significantly greater toughness than under static conditions. We do not yet have much actual testing data about this for biological structural materials, so we do not know the real numerical value of that relationship at present.

Since some endoprotheses (such as total hip replacements) function largely under conditions of dynamic loading, and since as we put them into younger and more vigorous people we will bring to the forefront any time-dependent phenomena even more than we have in the recent past, the match between the dynamic compliances of the bone and the device at their mechanical interface should become even more important in determining durability (both mechanical and temporal) than matching their statically determined Young's moduli. A good match of dynamic compliance will prove of the essence in achieving a long-lasting mechanical acceptance by the living of the inanimate. As yet the designers of such appliances have paid little attention to compliance (to repeat we do not even have good, time-dependent figures for fresh wet bone at this writing), but the patterns of our device failures will compel investigators in this field to turn in that direction in the near future. Examples of poorly compliant every day materials would include steel, vitallium, glass, bone and wood, in order of increasing compliance. Examples of high compliance materials would include all objects of small total mass, such as pins, phonograph needles, cells and free molecules (given in order of increasing compliance), plus art gum rubber erasers and cold jello.

Of some biological interest, note that fresh and normally hydrated bone, tendon and cartilage have significantly greater compliance than they exhibit in the dried state. Among other things this affords them improved protection from impact damage, by augmenting their toughness.

9) IMPACT: To understand what occurs to the mechanical stresses within solid objects during an impact, i.e., a blow of one rapidly moving object on another, we must (again) review some elementary college physics. Begin by recalling that force equals mass times acceleration, or:

$$F = m\ a$$

Now during the collision of two bodies, the total *momentum* in both remains conserved, another way of saying that we end up with as much energy in the system after the impact as we began with before it. Momentum (M) represents mass times velocity (v), or

$$M = mv \qquad\qquad Equation\ 3.07$$

Observe that the momentum of a moving mass does not equal the kinetic energy, which one usually writes as $1/2\ mv^2$.

Typically one finds the muzzle energy of bullets given in the latter form, but the recoil energy of the weapon appears as the momentum defined above.

When a hammer with mass m_1, moves with velocity v_1, to strike a man's tibia and then come to rest, it transfers to the tibia with mass m_2, a velocity v_2. Since momentum remains conserved, this relationship holds, the superscripts referring to time one before collision, and time two after collision; the subscripts to the tibia (one) and the hammer (two).

$$^1(m_1v_1) + {}^1(m_2v_2) = {}^2(m_1v_1) + {}^2(m_2v_2)$$

Equation 3.08

which merely says the sum of the momentums of the leg plus that of the hammer before the collision, equals their sum after the collision. Now the change in momentum of the tibia before and after the hammer struck it (ΔM), represents the change in its velocity times its mass. Since its mass does not change, only the velocity will change. The change in its velocity (Δv) represents its original velocity ($^1v_1$, here equal to zero) plus the speed the hammer imparted to it. Recall that speed or velocity equals acceleration times time, or $v = at$. Thus its change in speed, Δv, equals:

$$\Delta v = a\,t \qquad\qquad\text{\textit{Equation 3.09}}$$

where t signifies how long the acceleration acted or lasted. Since $F = m\,a$, and so $a = F/m$, then the force (F) exerted to produce a given change in momentum (m v) equals that change divided by the time period over which it occurred, or

$$F = \frac{m\,\Delta v}{t} \qquad\qquad\text{\textit{Equation 3.10}}$$

Note: The shorter the time during the impact over which the momentum transfer occurs, the greater the force.

Consider now two specific examples. You start swinging a hammer weighing 0.5 kg, imparting to it a velocity of 10 m/sec over a one-second swing. The force you exerted on it to accelerate it equals:

$$F = \frac{0.5\ (10)}{1} = 5 \text{ Newtons (roughly 0.49 kg, or one lb)}.$$

But as it strikes the tibia the hammer's velocity changes
again, decreasing now to zero, and furthermore in only one
one-thousandth of a second of time, or one millisecond. What
loading or acceleratory force does it apply to the tibia? The
mass remains the same here, and the change in velocity likewise (it changes from 10 m/sec to zero), but t, the time over
which that change occurs, now equals .001 sec. Thus:

$$F = \frac{0.5\ (10)}{.001} = 5000 \text{ Newtons, or more than } 500$$

kg f, or 1100 lb f. No wonder the tibia might break as a
consequence.

Note that physicists define a quantity termed *impulse*
as the force acting on a body times its duration of action, or

$$I = F\ t \qquad\qquad Equation\ 3.11$$

But you can see from equation 3.10 that F t simply equals
the change in the momentum of one body after a collision
with another, or after any other momentum—exchanging
process. Thus the mechanical arrangement we call impact
represents in a literal and rigorous sense, the physicist's impulse, and it signifies a change in momentum in a particular
body.

Note: One decreases the time over which momentum
transfer occurs by making the impacting materials stiffer.
But simultaneously that raises the acceleratory forces involved, which raises equally the internal stresses within any
material, and rather easily can raise them past the point at
which it fractures. On the other hand, increasing the duration of the momentum transfer process decreases the acceleratory force—and resultant internal stresses—involved, and
thus tends to protect the material from breakage. Hence
damping materials constitute those which can spread out
the temporal duration of the momentum transfer process,
*and to achieve that with real matter one increases the dis-
tance over which the momentum transfer occurs.* Note in
the hammer—on—tibia example above that the soft tissues
(skin and fat) over the tibia could easily do this, so that the
momentum transfer might require 5 milliseconds instead of

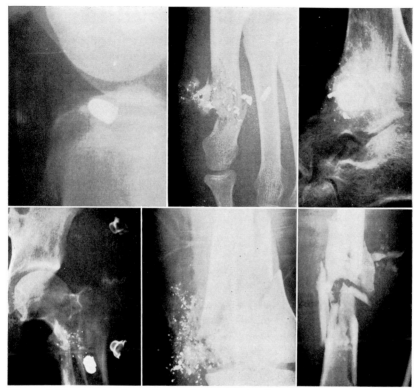

Figure 3.04. A selection of gun shot wounds the author has encountered in orthopaedic practice, which exemplify some problems of exterior ballistics, impulse and the materials properties of our body tissues.

Top left: A .32 ACP handgun cartridge. Muzzle velocity about 900 fps., kinetic energy around 130 ft-lb, mass ± 4.9 grams or 77 grains, and a tough gilding metal jacket encases the lead bullet. This slug dissipated its momentum in the soft tissues of the victim's knee without undergoing significant deformation and without shedding any lead in the tissues.

Top middle: "Jes' walkin' down the street man, an' this cat he leans outta this car window an' 'bam'." Unjacketed .22 long rifle slug fired from a small handgun. Bullet velocity around 1100 fps., kinetic energy ± 130 ft-lb, mass 3.4 grams or 50 grains. Because the lead bullet lacked any protection, when it struck bone it yielded up a large fraction of its momentum thereto and in a quite short time period. That generated large internal stresses within the lead bullet which exceeded its strength, and so disrupted it.

Top right: An unjacketed .38 special revolver bullet (left twist rifling so probably fired from a Colt) entered this ankle and came to rest in the talus. Bullet velocity about 750 fps., kinetic energy about 200 ft-lb, mass 150 grains or 9.6 grams. It deformed markedly and shed lead particles in the soft tissue. That it came to rest within the tissues still essentially in one major piece indicates that from the ballistic standpoint it travelled fairly slowly, and so its deceleration was not very violent as one rates such matters in ballistic problems.

Bottom left: This young man took two .380 ACP handgun slugs (same story as top middle!) in this region. Bullet velocity around 900 fps., kinetic energy some 180 ft-lb, bullet mass 95 grains or 6.0 grams. Most ammunition made for semi-automatic pistols has gilding metal jackets enveloping the lead bullet to facilitate reliable function of the arm's action. Here we see that in traversing the intertrochanteric region of this femur the jackets "shed" from the lead cores, practically intact. One lead bullet core came to rest within the femur (complete transfer of its momentum to the victim) while the other emerged through a soft tissue wound of exit.

Bottom middle: This young drug addict took a .30-30 rifle slug through the medial femoral condyle. Travelling at approximately 2200 fps., kinetic energy about 1800 ft-lb, and bullet mass some 150 grains or 9.4 grams, and designed to expand on impact in order to improve momentum transfer to the target, in doing just that this slug simply blew out nearly all of his medial condyle (and femoral artery), left some lead particles behind and still had enough kinetic energy left over to continue on through the limb and out the far side.

Bottom right: In line of duty, this young police officer's thigh took a fully jacketed military rifle bullet, velocity probably 2700 fps or so, kinetic energy some 2400 ft-lb, bullet weight 180 grains or 11.5 grams. Its impact on the femur literally exploded it and also did great damage to the enveloping soft tissues but not a particle of lead remained; the tough jacket protected the lead core. Bullet never found of course; it went right on through.

one. That would reduce the stresses in the tibia to one-fifth the previous value, so that while the victim of such an assault might well yelp, his tibia probably wouldn't break.

QUESTIONS: CHAPTER 3

1) Define: a) elasticity; b) resilience; c) Hook's law; d) tough; e) fragile.

2) In plotting on a graph the stretch of some spring against the force it exerts on the clamps restraining it, what would Hookean behavior predict of the line plotted from such points?

3) A tennis player, testing a ball by dropping it on a hard surface and observing its bounce, remarks that it has "lost its elasticity." Evaluate the scientific accuracy of that characterization.

4) How can one expend a given amount of energy so that on one occasion it does not the slightest damage to a baby

guppy, yet on another occasion it pushes a hole through a quarter-inch thick vanadium steel plate?

5) Define: a) momentum; b) impulse; c) work; d) stress, e) $1/2$ m v^2.

6) In Figure 3.04 top middle, given a bullet velocity of 850 fps, a metatarsal thickness along the bullet's path of 7mm, and the assumed fact that the bullet imparted two-thirds of its momentum to the metatarsal, then compute: the approximate time of the impulse or momentum transfer; and the foot pounds of that transfer, given a bullet weight of 800 mg (you must convert all numerical data to a common system of units to solve this one. See the special conversion tables in Part III).

Chapter 4

Basic Stress-Strain Relationships in Fluids

1) HYDROSTATICS. Let us describe first several phenomena that characterize motionless fluid systems.

(a) *Bulk pressure phenomena*: As to pressure behavior in fluid in bulk (as opposed to behavior peculiar to its surfaces), the total hydrostatic pressure of force F, on the walls of a fluid-filled container with total area A, sums up over that area a unit pressure P, of

$$P = \frac{F}{A} \qquad \qquad \textit{Equation 4.01}$$

The density, d, of the fluid in that container equals its mass divided by its volume, or

$$d = \frac{m}{v} \qquad \qquad \textit{Equation 4.02}$$

Note that the closely similar *specific gravity* expresses the mass of a given volume of a substance compared to the mass of an equal volume of water. Thus the specific gravity of iron equals 7.91, in any system of units. But while its density in cgs units likewise equals 7.91 gm/cc, in English measure its density equals 493.8 lb/ft³, while that of water equals 62.4 lb/ft³.

Then given a graduated cylinder in a chemistry lab filled with fluid, the lateral pressure on its walls will vary with depth h, according to this relation (using cgs units):

$$P = hdg \qquad \qquad \textit{Equation 4.03}$$

One might typically use cgs units which would give answers in dynes/cm². Observe that P signifies unit pressure at depth h, d represents the density of the fluid, and g the gravitational constant. To express the answer in grams force/cm², divide through by g to obtain:

$$P = hd. \hspace{3cm} Equation\ 4.04$$

Since in a container at rest the fluid within does not move about (let us ignore thermal expansion and convection effects), yet the pressure P must exist at all points within it at a given depth, that pressure must act equally from all directions to allow a static equilibrium to exist. Hence we have:

Pascal's principle: pressure applied to a fluid at one point within a closed, fluid filled container transmits equally throughout the fluid.

This principle holds true until the rate of change or movement of the piston or other device applying rapidly changing pressures begins to approach the speed of sound in the fluid (which equals ≈ 4000 fps in water). Pascal's principle operates in our car brakes every day, for a relatively small foot-pedal pressure on a small piston in the brake fluid cylinder converts to equal unit pressures on much larger sized pistons at the brake shoes, multiplying on the brake drums the total load of the foot many-fold. This provides a hydraulically achieved mechanical force advantage, analogous to that one can achieve mechanically with a crowbar. While such hydraulic systems can provide enormous multiplication of force, the do not—and cannot—augment the mechanical work put into them.

Or; work in = work out; input force × distance = output force × distance; FL in = FL out.

Observe an example in action. Given the mean diameter of a skull as 6.5 inches, and a mean intraarterial pulse pressure above external atmospheric pressure of 20mm of mercury: find the total load tending to explode the skull, and which the bones of the cranial vault must carry.

Ans: One atmosphere, or 15 lb/in² of air pressure (we will use the ordinary lb ft units throughout the answer), equals 760mm of mercury, so the mean intracranial unit pressure in lb/in² equals:

$$P = \frac{20}{760} \times 15, \text{ or } 0.4 \text{ lb/in}^2.$$

A section through the middle of a sphere (we can easily afford to idealize thus a real skull) of diameter 6.5 inches constitutes a circle with area:

$$\tfrac{1}{4}\pi D^2 = \tfrac{1}{4}\pi 6.5^2 = 28.5 \text{ in}^2$$

Each of those 28.5 square inches carries a mean hydrostatic pressure of 0.4 lb/in² or psi, so the total tension load (i.e., bursting load carried by the bone surface lying on the plane of a hemisection of the skull) carried by the skull bones equals:

$$28.5 \times 0.4 = 11.4 \text{ lb.}$$

If more than 4 in² of the bone present along the line of hemisection of the skull, then its unit tension stress will fall well below 3 psi, a trivial value indeed for a structural material whose mean ultimate tension strength equals some 12,000 psi.

(b) *Surface Tension*: Here we deal with a phenomenon peculiar to a fluid's surface. When a liquid has an interface with air (or with any other material), its surface contains a localized, planar tension force called surface tension. One may see it in action by lowering a dry capillary tube into it; the water will rise within the bore of the tube to a height determined by a) the value of the surface tension of water, a constant at a given temperature, b) the diameter of the bore of the capillary tube, which simultaneously determines the total circumference of the fluid-glass interface (which determines the total upward attraction of surface tension on the fluid column) and the total mass of water beneath the surface area per millimeter of height of the fluid column

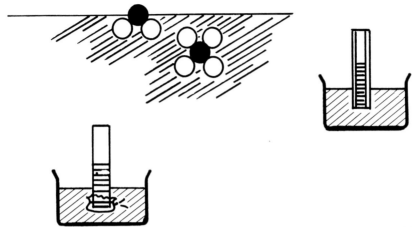

Figure 4.01. *Right:* A capillary tube introduced as shown into a fluid causes the fluid to rise within it to a height lying somewhere above the fluid level in the main vessel. This represents a visible effect of a force called surface tension which arises at the surface of all liquids.

Upper left: The surface molecule (the one shaded in) attracts weakly and is similarly attracted by all those similar ones near it. But since none lie above it, a net force exists tending to pull it downwards, and since all molecules at the surface experience the same phenomenon one may say that a "film of force" exists at the surface. Molecules below the surface, completely surrounded and so attracted equally upwards as well as downwards, do no reveal this phenomenon.

Lower left: A semipermeable membrane (impermeable to sucrose molecules but permeable to water) closes off the bottom of the small glass tube. Originally sucrose solution was poured into its top until the level equalled that in the surrounding main vessel containing pure water. Unequal diffusion of water molecules across the membrane, more upwards than down, gradually raises the height of the sucrose solution (an effect called *osmosis,* and measured as *osmolality*) until the increased height of the fluid column adds a mechanical water pressure to bring the total partial pressure of water in the sucrose column up to that of the pure water in the main vessel.

above the main body of the solution,* as shown in Figure 4.01.

---

* Because the surface tension varies directly as the radius of the capillary, but the mass below the water surface in the capillary varies as the square of the radius, doubling the diameter of the capillary would double the upward pulling surface tension force (which relates directly to the perimeter of the fluid-glass interface) but would increase *four-fold* the mass of water held up by that tension force. And so it would not rise as high by "capillary attraction" in the larger tube as in the smaller one.

One may explain the genesis of this force by the following analogy, illustrated on the upper left side of Figure 4.01. Thus: all molecules have a mutually attractive force, one different from gravity because it decays much more rapidly with distance than gravity. The right hand of the two blacked-in molecules lies surrounded by others like it which pull it equally in all directions, so no net excess of force of that type in any one direction arises. But the left hand one lying at the surface of the fluid has no such attraction above it, for other molecules lie only beside and below it. This creates a net downward-pulling force acting across the whole surface, one which *causes the surface to seek the minimum area consistent with any other forces acting upon it.* Since the minimum surface area of any solid body consists of a spherical surface enclosing a spherical volume, one would expect liquids free of other large forces to assume spherical shapes because of the surface tension which, like a diaphanous balloon, tries to shrink their surface to a minimum area. And indeed raindrops and even molten steel and lead drops, do tend to assume spherical shapes when in free fall because of their surface tension. In fact manufacturers use that property to make lead shot and BB's by allowing drops of molten metal to fall from a high tower into cold water.

One can measure surface tension in a variety of ways but it acts as though it constitutes—and one can measure it as—a force tending to prevent sideways disruption of a unit length

TABLE 4.01
SURFACE TENSION

Substance	T (dynes/cm)		Substance	T (dynes/cm)	
Water:	15°C	73	Ether	20°C	17
	100°C	59	Ethanol	20°C	23
Mercury	20°C	465	Olive Oil	20°C	32
Soapy water	20°C	26	Paraffin Oil	20°C	26
Iron	1535°C	1800	Lead	330°C	450
Nickle	1735°C	1470	Tungsten	2500°C	3410

A brief list of the surface tensions T of some fluids, given in cgs units, or dynes per centimeter. Convert to grams force by dividing by g (i.e., by 980 cm/sec^2). Observe that increasing the temperature of a fluid lowers T, as does the common detergent, soap, and that little correlation exists between a liquid's surface tension and its viscosity, as comparison with values in Table 4.02 will reveal.

of the fluid surface. Thus one may express it in dynes/cm. The accompanying Table 4.01 lists some examples. Note that surface tension (T) usually decreases with rising temperature. A simple instrument for making such measurements constitutes the "du Nouy tensiometer."

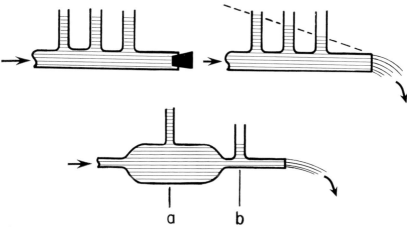

a   b

Figure 4.02. *Top left:* As long as the stopper in the right end prevents any flow of liquid through this system, all of the vertical manometers register the same height, and thus identical transverse pressure (Pascal's principle).

Top right: But when one permits flow to occur one finds a pressure gradient to arise, the transverse pressure decreasing towards the open orifice at the right. This arises because of fluid friction or viscosity, against which the pumping force must work.

Bottom: Now make the fluid move through lumenal cross sections of differing cross section areas. At section *a* the fluid moves quite slowly while at *b* it moves rapidly. In this system equal volumes of fluid must move past *a* and *b* in equal times. And under that circumstance the transverse pressure—seemingly paradoxically—proves greatest in the slow moving region and lowest in the fast! This forms the *Bernouilli effect,* and it really arises because of the inertia of the fluid. In effect, in the fast moving regions it has less time to push laterally against the container walls than it does in the slow moving regions. Thus this effect becomes the larger as the density or specific gravity of the fluid increases. Reversing the direction of flow through this system would not change the fact that the pressure at *a* exceeds that at *b*; it would only change the amount of difference by a factor depending upon the viscosity of the liquid.

Mechanical engineers also call this principle the *Venturi effect,* and rather than use it to measure pressure directly they often use it to measure velocity of flow, for example in aircraft air-speed indicators, or in fluid pumping systems.

2) HYDRODYNAMICS:

Now we shall deal with some phenomena of fluid motion, one at the gross level of observation and one at the molecular-level.

(*a*) *Pressure in flowing systems*: When fluids begin to move some unexpected behavioral things begin to show up. Let us begin with *Bernouilli's principle*. Thus in Figure 4.02, top left, the fluid-filled column or pipe system, given zero flow through the system, displays equal heads of pressure in all of its upwards projecting tubes. But if one pulls the plug to allow the fluid to move, as on the right, a pressure gradient appears, and the upwards pressure decreases from left towards the right as shown (a general surgeon named George Rennaker and I once observed this effect in a woman's femoral artery but, needless to say, not for long). This reflects the effects of fluid friction or the viscosity of the fluid which tends to resist its flow and so to "back it up."

Now examine events when the moving fluid column changes in its cross sectional diameter, as in the lower drawing. The mass of fluid flowing past point *a* in a given period of time equals $V_a A_a d$, where V stands for the velocity of flow, A the cross section area of the column, and *d* the density of the fluid. That flowing past point *b* then equals $V_b A_b d$.

As the physical arrangement illustrates, equal masses (and volumes) must flow past both points of observation in equal times. We may write it thus:

$$V_a A_a d = V_b A_b d \qquad \textit{Equation 4.05}$$

Consequently the velocity of flow must vary in inverse proportion to the fluid column's cross section area. Now in the same figure this relation applies to the transverse pressure, P:

$$P_a + \tfrac{1}{2} d V_a^2 = P_b + \tfrac{1}{2} d V_b^2 \qquad \textit{Equation 4.06}$$

Clearly in the smaller diameter tube the V_b^2 term exceeds the V_a^2 term for the large diameter region, and for the relation to balance the P_a term (unit transverse hydrostatic pressure at *a*) must exceed the P_b one. Thus one of Bernouilli's principles:

In fluid columns moving in parallel lines, lateral pressure in slowly moving regions exceeds that in faster moving ones.

We will find a possible minor application of this particular effect in Part II when we discuss fluid flow in moving joints. Both vascular surgeons and anesthesiologists deal with physiological manifestations of this effect in their own flowing fluid and gas systems every day.

(*b*) *Diffusion*: When one opens a perfume bottle in one corner of a room full of air (but free of convection currents), other persons in the far corner will soon smell it, for the molecules of the perfume gradually move through or diffuse through the air during their thermally driven, ping-pong ball-like motions between, and random collisions with, the air molecules. Equally, molecules of a gas (or liquid) can diffuse through other liquids or solids. For example hydrogen gas diffuses through even the thick walls of the steel pressure tank containing it. Atoms of solids can even diffuse through other solids, even if slowly, a phenomenon finding very good use in the manufacture of some types of electronic semiconductor components, as well as in ordinary metallurgical practice.

Diffusion under special restrictions in fact serves as the basis for osmosis, without which no known form of cellular life can exist. In the lower drawing in Figure 4.01, the two vessels shown originally were filled to equal height, but the external one with pure water, the inner one with a sucrose solution. A cellophane membrane closes off the bottom of the inner vessel, and we call it semipermeable because water molecules can diffuse easily through its ultramicroscopic pores in either direction but sucrose molecules in aqueous solution have too large a molecular radius to diffuse readily through them. In other words, it forms a kind of "molecular sieve." As a consequence of the lower partial pressure of water in the inner vessel, more water molecules diffuse across the membrane upwards than downwards and this continues hourly until at the stable fluid height shown, the added mechanical partial pressure of water in the small tube brings the total partial pressure of water within it (remember this reflects the number of molecules colliding with the membrane per second) up to the partial pressure level in the main vessel, i.e., that of pure water.

Note: To repeat, diffusion can occur in gasses, liquids and solids. It occurs most readily in the former and least in the latter. It also depends upon the size of the diffusing molecule, larger ones exhibiting greater impedence or resistance to motion by diffusion than small ones. It also depends upon temperature, elevated temperatures facilitating it and lowered ones reducing it.

(c) *Viscosity*: The chief property of fluids that interests us here, viscosity, represents the resistance of any liquid to flow, a resistance often called fluid friction. Flow itself simply constitutes a form of shearing strain. Thus their different viscosities cause alcohol and acetone to run out of a glass tube quickly (low viscosity creating low resistance to shearing deformation) , but glycerine or heavy machine oil to run out slowly (high viscosity, high resistance to shearing deformations) . High viscosity fluids usually lubricate slow moving bearing surfaces (which includes animal joint surfaces) better than low viscosity fluids because the former, by viscously resisting expression from between the two bearing surfaces, can keep slowly moving bearing surfaces (or joint surfaces) from touching, i.e., can "float" them and so better protect them from wear and seizure.

We express viscosity in a unit called the *Poise,* but in practice use a more practical unit, the *centipose,* or one one-hundredth of a poise. This measure indicates how these fluids resist flow under controlled conditions of temperature, pressure and shearing rate. Table 4.02 shows some viscosities of ordinary fluids. The bulk modulus of the fluids stated therein measures their volume compressibility.

The Poise and Centipoise: We may express viscosity as follows: it equals the frictional forces arising per unit area (or $\frac{F}{A}$) of a thin layer, which one expresses as the resistance of one cm^2 surface to shearing displacement on

TABLE 4.02
SOME TYPICAL VISCOSITIES

Fluid	Temperature °C	Viscosity (absolute) Centipoises
Water	+25	.89
Water	+100	.29
Synovial fluid	+25	10–1,000
Acetone	+25	.32
Carbon tetrachloride	+15	1.04
Ether	+25	.222
Alcohol, ethyl	+25	1.10
Glycerine	−20	134,000
Glycerine	+20	1,490
Iron	+1,400	2.25
Mercury	+20	1.55
Oil, castor	+20	986
Oil, machine	+37	127
Air	+25	.000182
Hydrogen	+20	.000087
Steam	+100	.000125

The table lists viscosities in centipoises of a variety of fluids, some at two different temperatures. Note the drastic drop in viscosity when water transforms to the gaseous state (steam); that glycerine at room temperature has over 600 times greater resistance to flow than liquid (i.e., melted) iron; and that glycerine at 20°C above zero has only one-tenth its viscosity at 20° below zero. Thus increasing temperature lowers viscosity.

the next adjacent layer at uniform unit speed. Thus in any fluid flowing at velocity V, parallel to a more stationary and equal area or layer of fluid or container wall, but separated from it by distance *d*, using Greek lower case eta (η) to signify the *coefficient of viscosity*:

$$\eta = \frac{\frac{F}{A}}{\frac{V}{d}} = \frac{Fd}{Av} \text{ dyne-sec/cm}^2 \text{ (i.e., Poises)}$$

Equation 4.07

The answer in other words comes out in dynes per "the rest of it," which you may or may not wish to memorize.

Since Poiseuille first defined such matters, eta has become expressed in units called the Poise or, as mentioned above, in hundredths or a Poise or *centipoise*.

One may measure viscosity eta in Poise by allowing a liquid to flow through a tube under constant pressure with a pressure difference P at its two ends separated by length

L, and with a lumen of radius r, through which the fluid
flows at v cm³/sec.

$$\eta = \frac{II \ r^4 p}{8Lv} \qquad \qquad Equation \ 4.08$$

To convert to *Stokes* (another numerical measure of
viscosity) divide the absolute viscosity eta (η) by the density of the fluid. This has also become known as the kine-
matic viscosity.*

(d) Flow and Shear of Fluids: When a fluid moves inside
a stationary tubular container, a shearing motion or strain
occurs parallel to the walls of the container, which we call
flow. In essence this shearing strain represents the fact that
the layer of fluid molecules immediately next to the walls of
the container tends to stick to it and not flow at all. Those
layers in the fluid farther away from the wall move by sliding
over those layers closer to the walls. Thus the column of
fluid in the middle of the lumen of the tube moves along
much faster than the layers close to its walls. Exactly that
relative movement forms the shearing displacement or strain
which we name flow. The resistance of a fluid to such flow
arises in the resistance of each of those layers to moving on
its neighbors, and equals the fluid shearing stress (i.e., the
fluid friction or viscosity). Liquids with high viscosity display greater resistance to a given speed of flow than low
viscosity liquids. Because moving a fluid against its shearing
stress does work on the fluid, it generates heat in it. In oil
lubricated machine bearings which operate at high speeds
this work-engendered heat can reach large enough amounts
as to require special equipment to cool the lubricant in order
to prevent thermal damage to both it and the machinery.

(e) Laminar and turbulent flow: Fluids flow in two basically different ways: laminar, and turbulent.

In *laminar flow* (which one might characterize as smooth,
even flow), a given molecule and/or layer of fluid moves in
an essentially straight line and parallel to the wall of the

---

* To repeat: Work means a force pushing something over a distance, and
one specifies it in units such as foot-pounds, or kilogram-centimeters. Technically,
energy signifies a quantity of work, and power the rate at which one uses energy.

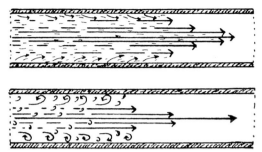

Figure 4.03. *Top:* A longitudinal section through a column of liquid flowing through a tube. The arrows designate flow or stream lines, and their lengths the speeds. Record that the fluid in the middle flows faster than that close to the edges of the tube. Smooth, steady flow such as this represents *laminar flow.*

Bottom: As one raises the flow rate a critical point comes when the fluid near the walls begins to eddy, or move along in helical paths. This phenomenon, called *turbulence,* sharply increases the resistance to flow and so represents a condition to avoid whenever one wishes to obtain efficient transfer of flowing liquids. A figure of merit called the *Reynolds number* serves engineers for purposes of computing the velocity and pressure conditions which will precipitate turbulent flow.

container, and maintains the same distance from the wall of the container (see Fig. 4.03 top). Laminar flow exists at low flow rates and it requires a minimum amount of pumping work and power to maintain. As the flow speed increases a critical point comes when turbulence develops in the fluid, consisting of many small swirling eddies. This turbulence sharply increases the resistance of the fluid to increased pumping and consequently requires a sharply increased amount of pumping force, work and power to maintain the rate of flow (see Fig. 4.03, bottom). When such turbulence arises within an arterial aneurysm, Roger Smith or John Hageman would detect a bruit with their stethoscopes, for that turbulence generates sound.

While maintaining laminar flow has proven of some importance in the physiology and pathophysiology of blood flow in vessels in vascular surgery, it has not appeared (at least yet) on the basis of hard evidence to form a major one in joint physiology. And in the body the rate of heat production in joint and other biological bearings seems to lie well within the capacity of those systems to dissipate it, so that thermal damage has not yet received recognition as a factor in the diseases of such structures. One may suspect however that when bare bone rubs on bare bone in an osteoarthritic hip joint, some local thermal damage of microscopic regions and volumes of living tissue may develop.

(f) Newtonian and Non-Newtonian Fluids: In a particular lubricant lying in a bearing, an increase in the bearing speed (i.e., an increase in the rate of shearing displacement) may cause a proportional increase in the resistance (i.e., shearing stress, or friction) * of the lubricant to shear. Thus, doubling the r.p.m. would double the fluid resistance to the turning of a shaft in a bearing. When the shearing stress remains proportional to the shearing rate in this manner, we call the fluid a Newtonian fluid.

But when such proportionality does not persist, the fluid forms a non-Newtonian one, and in theory and as Figure 4.04 illustrates, it might depart from the Newtonian property by one of two ways: Proportionally speaking, and as one increased the shearing rate, the shearing stress either might increase more than the strain rate, or less. Synovial fluid, the lubricant of our joints, has the non-Newtonian property as does our blood (Dintinfass[57]), and in the sense that the shearing stress does not increase as much as the shearing strain or flow rate. We shall examine some probable reasons for that when we discuss the properties of synovial fluid. But note here that this non-Newtonian aspect of synovial fluid resembles in analogy the property of compliance in the solid state already discussed. At low bearing speeds synovial fluid proves thicker than at high ones, and that forms a biologically useful property.

This and the previous chapters have laid an elementary kind of ground work which prepares us to consider the somewhat complex relationships between real matter and its mo-

---

* Another point of view problem. In the general case of rigid solids, the resistance of the intermolecular bonds to deformation means stress, but in problems of the motion of one solid object on another separate one we give this resistance the special name, friction, and for the case of a liquid, viscosity.

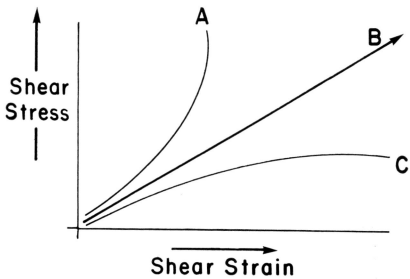

Figure 4.04. A stress-strain graph of three flowing liquids. Curve A characterizes one in which the resistance to flow increases faster than flow speed increases, a nonNewtonian characteristic. Curve B characterizes a Newtonian fluid: Resistance to flow increases proportionally to speed of flow, at least over the range tested. Curve C illustrates another nonNewtonian fluid in which resistance to flow increases more slowly than flow speed. This curve characterizes human synovial fluid, which serves as a natural, aqueous lubricant in all of our gliding joints, tendon sheaths and bursae.

lecular-level organization and properties. Accordingly the next three chapters will discuss some varied properties of matter as a structural material and, in the process, provide some elementary information about certain common and/or orthopaedically important specific materials and classes thereof.

QUESTIONS: CHAPTER 4

1) Define a) viscosity; b) Poise; c) diffusion.
2) What is a) Pascal's principle? b) Bernouilli's principle? c) hydrostatics?
3) Which of the three principal stresses best characterizes the viscosity of fluids?
4) Which of the three principal strains best characterizes the flow of fluids?

5) If synovial fluid has a surface tension of 80 dynes/cm, does that provide an important source of fluid film strength (i.e., preventing its rupture) of the lubricant "floating" a knee joint moving under a 700 kg total load, given a total bearing surface transferring that load (across the fluid film) of 20 cm²?

Chapter 5

Basic Properties of Solid Matter

W<small>HILE ONE MAY</small> say with some truth that the mechanical properties of matter derive from the properties of its component atoms, as for the case of the body and its component cells that statement misleads one badly and grossly, for it suggests it contains the whole truth when in fact it contains only a small fraction of it. New properties appear in matter in bulk form, as atoms assemble into groups of various kinds and sizes and complexity, and as these groups then interact with each other. We therefore will describe in the next few chapters some of the atomistic and, organizationally speaking, higher level phenomena that legitimately relate to the purposes of this text.

I: PROPERTIES OF ATOMS

Atoms (and molecules) attract each other by means of two different overall classes of interatomic and intermolecular forces or bonds. Both, however, arise ultimately from the basic electrostatic attraction of the positively charged atomic nucleus to the negatively charged clouds of electrons whirling around it. In fact we recognize a primary and a secondary class of bonding forces (199).

1) P<small>RIMARY</small> B<small>ONDING</small> F<small>ORCES</small>: Here three subtypes exist. *(a) Ionic bonds* arise when as an example a chlorine atom "steals" an electron from a sodium atom, basically because the chlorine nucleus has a stronger attraction for one of the peripheral sodium atoms than the latter's own nucleus. But a residual attraction of the now electrically unbalanced positive sodium atom for the extra negative charge at the periphery of the chlorine atom binds the two together in an "ionic bond," one which can demonstrate great strength.

When dissolved in water, the ionically bonded atoms break up into charged ions in solution which can conduct electricity quite well. As solids, such materials conduct both heat and electricity poorly.

(b) *Covalent bonds* arise when two atoms "share" one or more of their peripheral electrons, as in the hydrogen (H_2), and oxygen (O_2) molecules, amino acids, carbohydrates and the like. Diamond represents covalently bonded carbon atoms, and as the hardest substance known it reflects the potentially great strength of such bonds. CO_2 also represents a covalently bonded molecule but, unlike the previous examples, one in which the two kinds of atoms do not share equally the bonding electrons. The less completely saturated atom (carbon here) can then devote the remainder of its binding capacity to arrangements with other atoms and elements, one of the reasons for the great variety of carbon compounds found in nature.

When dissolved in water, covalently bound materials do not conduct electricity well, and as solids they conduct both electricity and heat poorly.

(c) *The metallic bond* characterizes metals, representing atoms of those elements which have relatively few electrons in their outer shells. We believe currently that those atoms share *en masse* a sea of highly mobile electrons moving around them. Such materials conduct both electricity and heat well in the solid state, and our electrical and electronics industries depend upon the good electrical conductivities of metallic elements such as copper, silver, gold and aluminum. One may find a clue to the strength of the metallic and covalent bonds in Table 5.01, which reveals the tensile strengths of "whiskers" of several materials compared with bulk materials. Whiskers represent perfect single—and usually very tiny—crystals of an element or compound.

2) SECONDARY BONDING FORCES: These arise between molecules (only), are known as van der Waal's forces, and arise because in many molecules the geometric centers of the positive and negative charges do not coincide. Thus the

TABLE 5.01
MECHANICAL PROPERTIES OF FILAMENTS[199]

Material	Type of Bond	Tensile Strength 1000 psi	Modulus of Elasticity Millions psi	Specific Gravity
Graphite whisker	Covalent	3,000	100	1.7
Quartz whisker	Covalent	3,000	10	2.65
Sapphire whisker	Ionic	2,600	70	4.0
Iron whisker	Metallic	1,800	28	7.8
Steel, fine wire	Metallic	60	30	7.8
Glass fiber	Covalent +	20	11	2.5
Nylon	Covalent +	8	0.7	1.07
Bamboo fiber	Covalent +	5	4.9	—
Quartz, fused	Covalent +	7	10.4	2.2

Small needles of pure single crystals of a material, known as whiskers, can demonstrate phenomenal unit strength in tension, and also in compression and shear. The tension values in the upper four rows range from 1.8 to 3.0 million pounds per square inch, and can demonstrate great stiffness too. This reflects the great strength inherent in covalent, ionic and metallic bonds.

Yet in bulk material, tension strengths may run from 100 to 1000 times less. Metallurgists and physicists had quite a time explaining this discrepancy. Its major (but not sole) cause proved to be the dislocation mechanism. Scientists now try to achieve the obvious: make fiber (or whisker) reenforced materials which take advantage of the great strength of these whiskers. Major problem: producing whiskers in commercial quantities at feasible prices.

more positive end of one molecule can attract weakly the more negative end of another to bind, or join them together. These bonds have much less strength than the primary bonds, and one can easily break them by mechanical loads or by moderate heating. Note that the melting point of a material provides a good clue to the strength of the bonds holding its atoms together. The stronger the bond the higher the melting point. Another and much weaker secondary bonding force constitutes (according to contemporary physical thinking) the gravitational attraction of one atom and any larger body of matter for any other.

3) PROPERTIES OF CRYSTALS: Since metals have great importance in orthopaedic surgery, and since they represent crystalline forms of matter, and since some of the bulk properties of those crystals profoundly affect the bulk mechanical properties of any metal or alloy, let us say a few words about them next. To begin, note that metals and most ceramics routinely and regularly become crystalline in the solid state whereas many organic polymers (compounds of carbon) do

not. The noncrystalline solid state constitutes the amorphous state.

Question: What characterizes the crystalline state?

In a crystalline material the atoms or molecules forming its atomistic components solidify from the melt in definite and stereotyped spatial relationships with each other. The lines connecting their centers then form a lattice and, if more than one kind of atom or molecule is involved, each always takes the same relationship to others throughout the lattice. Thus long range order of atomic and molecular stacking and relationships characterizes the crystalline state.

Three crystal systems (of the more than twenty possible) occur most frequently in metals and alloys: *close-packed hexagonal* (CPH), *face-centered cubic* (FCC) and *body-centered cubic* (BCC). We need learn no more about these systems here other than that they represent different ways of packing or stacking atoms together in a lattice, and that each has a unit cell, or that smallest group of atoms whose spatial arrangement defines the structure of the entire crystal lattice. Also note that the FCC arrangement packs atoms more closely together than the BCC one, and so puts the same amount of matter into a slightly smaller volume of space.

Polymorphism: Many metals can arrange their atom stacking in different ways, i.e., according to different crystal systems, usually as a function of temperature.

Thus, iron exists in the BCC form (called alpha iron or ferrite) below 1183° k and above 1676° k, but in the FCC form (delta iron or austenite), in between those temperatures. Metallurgists also name this ability to change crystal form and habit, or polymorphism in crystal structure, as *allotropy*. Because allotropic changes involve changes in the density of atom packing, they also involve visible changes in the volume of the bulk material, and they usually also require a fair amount of time to occur, often because they occur by atomic diffusion within the solid state and as we noted in an earlier chapter diffusion in solids occurs quite slowly. Fortunately for the present case such diffusion needs to occur only over distances equivalent to one or a few unit cells, usually less than one hundred Ångstroms in steels, so it can occur within reasonable time periods. Its relative lethargy allows one sometimes to freeze into a bulk material a lattice property normally characteristic only of a higher temperature. One achieves this by rapid cooling of the metal or quenching it, a phenomenon and procedure regularly used to harden steels, which we discuss in the next chapter.

Polycrystallinity: When a melted metal cools past its freezing point, innumerable separate tiny seeding regions of solid crystals begin to develop and grow throughout its bulk, and as the liquid phase disappears by enlargement of the seeds, the latter then impinge upon each other. But since their lattices originally arranged randomly in space they rarely align in register with each other in the completely solidified material. Metallurgists call a region within which a homogeneous alignment of the crystal lattice exists a grain; then the interface between different but adjacent grains, at which their malaligned lattices adjoin, constitutes the grain boundary. Figure 5.01 illustrates this situation for a single atomic plane in three adjoining, crystalline grains.

We will now consider several kinds of defects that can occur within single crystalline grains which contribute greatly to the otherwise puzzling phenomenon that, while pure single iron crystals in the form of whiskers may have a tensile strength exceeding 1,800,000 psi, bulk iron may begin to flow or break at only some 30,000 psi, or *less than 2 per cent of the strength of a single crystal.*

4) CRYSTALLINE DEFECTS: Point defects commonly exist in the lattices of real crystals. They include vacant lattice positions, or extra atoms jammed in between atoms that do lie in their proper lattice positions, or substitutions in some lattice position of an atom unusually large or small compared to its neighbors.

Another kind of defect, the line defect, concerns us far more. These line defects have become known as dislocations, several types have become recognized, and metallurgists have even demonstrated them directly by electron microscopic studies. Dislocations locally weaken the bonds

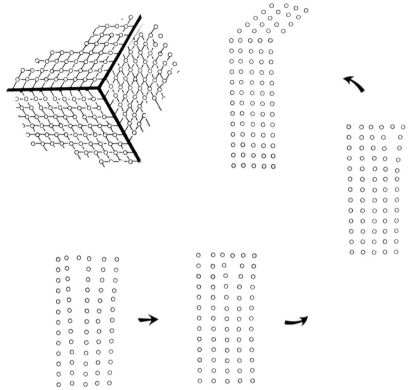

Figure 5.01. *Top:* In this diagram of a flat, polished metal surface, three differing crystalline regions lie adjacent to each other, their lattice planes oriented in differing directions in 3-D space (the small circles represent the atoms in each). Call each separate crystalline region a *grain;* then the heavily lined interface between differing grains constitutes the *grain boundary.*

Bottom: Beginning at the left, this series of drawings illustrates the motion through a crystal of a line type lattice defect or "edge dislocation." It allows the top plane of atoms to shift in step-by-step fashion towards your right on the underlying stacks of atomic planes; in doing so it carrys along with it all the other lattice planes stacked above it but omitted from this drawing for clarity's sake. Thus while the line of the defect lies vertically on the paper, its rightward motion through the lattice, as it jumps from one position to another, proceeds perpendicularly to the defect line. This represents an *edge dislocation,* and it and a related helically progressing or *screw dislocation* account for most of the markedly greater mechanical weakness of bulk metals and alloys as compared to the strengths of perfect, single-crystal whiskers. That weakness arises mostly through shearing motions of atomic planes on each other caused by dislocations (see Figure 5.02).

of a crystal lattice by locally straining or prestressing it. It then requires much less applied load to cause or initiate a shearing slip through such a region because the internal stress already there subtracts from the external load needed to initiate shear. The relative effects of bulk weakening by dislocations in metal crystals appears well (and typically) in the case of aluminum, where line defects reduce approximately two thousand-fold the shearing rigidity and strength of the bulk material compared to perfect single aluminum crystals. Figure 5.01 bottom illustrates for the case of the edge dislocation, how this process would work in a single lattice plane. Note that the vertical defect line on the left drawing, moves towards your right and so *perpendicularly to the defect line*. Note too that the lattice becomes strained because of the partially missing row of atoms, and that strain generates a shearing stress in the lattice oriented horizontally in the drawing. The final result of yielding before an externally applied load forms a gradual, step-by-step shearing displacement of the top row (or plane) of atoms towards your right, and relative to the lower rows of atoms. The top row would then carry with it all other crystal planes stacked above it. Because of this step-by-step displacement process, only one set of atomic bonds at a time need rupture for each step, and it requires much less externally applied load to drive this piecemeal process than it would take to make all of the bonds in a single plane slip simultaneously in shear.

Another important kind of dislocation, the screw dislocation, we need not go into here; it simply extrapolates into the third dimension the basic idea just outlined, so that the slip plane progresses in a helical fashion, somewhat as a screw's thread progresses around its central axis towards a particular direction.

Dislocations appear the rule in metals and other crystalline materials. Even very pure and carefully prepared metallic single crystals present some 10^8 dislocation lines per cm^2 of surface, and this can increase more than one thousand-fold simply by cold-working the metal.

Note bene: Both types of dislocations markedly weaken crystalline and otherwise very strong and stiff materials. *They do so by weakening individual crystals in shear,* which allows them to flow plastically at much lower levels of internal stress than prove required to deform—or break—perfect crystals.

(a) Work hardening: As noted, dislocations of both types greatly reduce the strength in shear of individual crystals as well as of bulk crystalline materials. Also as one strains a metal its initially relatively few dislocation planes, separated from each other by many hundreds of atomic lattice planes, begin to generate large slips and then, in some manner, to cause even greater numbers of new slip planes to arise. In other words, straining a metal tends to *multiply* the number of dislocations within it, and by as much as one thousand times as just noted. In fact these multiplying slip planes can become so numerous that they begin to run into and interfere with each other's motions; and, too, when such planes reach a grain boundary and encounter another grain with its lattice so aligned as to resist effectively the intrusion into it of any great shearing displacements of the former, the dislocations in the former tend to arrest or hang up, making that region more shear-resistant than before. Then it follows that it requires greater external load to overcome that resistance and produce further dislocation - mediated shearing displacement. By this means many metals tend to become stiffer and stronger after undergoing straining (by malleable or ductile means, such as repeated flexure, hammering, twisting, pulling) (111). This phenomenon constitutes strain hardening or, equally, work hardening.

In this regard foreign atoms, if of the right size, can add significant strength to a material simply by blocking the lattice movements required for dislocations to advance. Similarly, decreasing the average grain size can strengthen a material, since grain boundaries provide some resistance to propagation of dislocation planes across from one grain and over into another adjacent one, and decreasing the average grain size increases the grain boundary surface/volume ratio (surface decreases as the square, the volume as the cube, of the change in diameter) so that fine-grained metals have more dislocation-resisting grain boundaries per cubic mm of metal than course-grained ones.

(*b*) *Plastic Flow And Strain Hardening*: In some crystalline materials, for example in many ceramics, the stress level required to fracture the material in tension lies below that required to move and multiply its crystalline dislocations. Hence such materials behave brittley, that is, they break within their Hookean range of deformation rather than develop the kind of flow in shear we have just described (we call it plastic flow).

Those crystalline materials which allow dislocation movement and multiplication at stress levels below the material's breaking point can—and do—behave plastically before they fracture. One aspect of this behavior proves helpful in understanding the strain hardening process.

Figure 5.02 shows a small column carrying a compression load and on one of its faces, the grains and grain boundaries cut across by that face (greatly enlarged to clarify the processes). Note that the major dislocation planes in the top two grains lie, one perpendicular to and the other parallel to the line of action of load. Consequently no great shearing loads can develop on their lattice planes, and so no shearing stress, and so their dislocation systems stay put within them. In effect, to that particular direction of loading, these grains appear immensely strong. But on the right edge of the column lies a grain with its slip planes oblique to the compression load. Accordingly a shearing load component arises acting parallel to the slip planes, and ranging in magnitude from zero when θ equals $0°$ or $90°$ or $180°$, to a maximum value when θ equals $45°$ and/or $135°$.

It follows that a similar kind of shearing component acting on the lower left oblique grain will develop a similar unit shearing stress.

Now, as long as the magnitudes of these shearing force components (arising from an applied load) lie below the minimum stress level required to move any dislocations

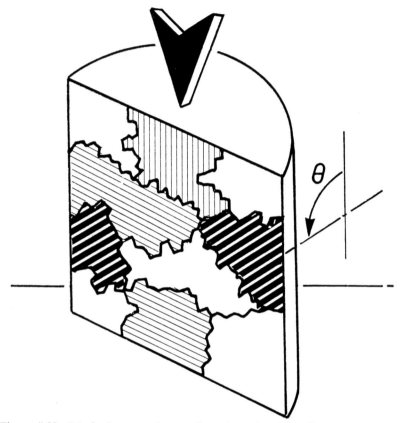

Figure 5.02. We look at a microscopic region of a face of a metal column carrying a superimposed compression load. On its face one sees outlined a number of grains. The parallel lines within each grain indicate its plane of easiest shearing motion, and arise due to lattice defects which generate dislocation systems within its crystalline lattice. Observe that when these slip planes lie either exactly parallel to or exactly perpendicular to the line of action of the load, they display no tendency to shear along those planes and so those grains will demonstrate great mechanical strength. But in other grains these planes lie in varying intermediate inclinations (i.e., the angle θ) and as a consequence a definite component of shearing force arises from the superimposed compression load. It attains its maximum values when θ equals $45°$, which explains why in bulk materials under uniaxial compression or tension loading, the maximum shear resultant stress and strain align at $45°$ to those loads.

Note: Thus when a bulk material deforms plastically in uniaxial compression, on the microscopic scale this arises as oblique shearing displacements of slip planes in millions of individual grains whose lattices align randomly in space. It follows that a plastic tension strain or permanent set really constitutes a summation of shearing strains in numerous individual grains, strains due to dislocation movements within their lattices.

through the bulk material, the bulk will only strain elastically in shear. But when these components rise above that minimum level, those grains most favorably oriented (i.e., when $\theta = 45°$) will begin to flow in shear first (by dislocation movements); after their slip planes have hung up at the edges of less favorably oriented grains, further increases in the superimposed load can then make them begin to flow plastically by the same dislocation—mediated process, and so on.

Hence plastic flow in essence is a shearing phenomenon in which fluid-like behavior arises and occurs within a cold, solid material. Now when all possible slip planes have jammed up and become unable to move any more, further increase of the load on the material will then generate stresses above its breaking strength and cause it to fracture.

As a consequence of such phenomena, strain hardening increases the strength, hardness and stiffness of a metal,* and decreases its ductility and malleability, sometimes useful phenomena in increasing the strength of finished machine and structural parts. One can readily eliminate strain hardening if desired by *annealing* the metal, which means heating it high and long enough to allow its internally stressed lattice regions to rearrange themselves into less distorted arrangements.

Thus in making many devices of metals the manufacturer may elect to shape the nearly finished part by some form of cold working to add to its final strength and stiffness. Or, if too much embrittlement occurs during earlier cold working he may anneal it (for iron the internal lattice and other rearrangements permitting this begin at about 700°k). And if he wishes to deform it plastically by large amounts he may *hot work it,* meaning heat it to a semiplastic temperature (1300–1500°k for steel) so it will flow more easily under the blow of a hammer or a die.

---

* You might wonder then; why not use hard, stiff and strong materials exclusively in making machines and tools? The answer: because of the trade imposed by the materials' properties. Hardness also means brittleness, increased fragility and decreased fatigue resistance.

QUESTIONS: CHAPTER 5

1) Define a) lattice; b) crystalline state; c) van der Waal's forces; d) dislocations in crystals.

2) A mechanic, looking at a broken steering tie rod, says "it crystallized." Evaluate the accuracy of the statement.

3) a) What is allotropy? b) A grain (to a metallurgist)?

4) How could one correct undesirable work hardening present in a finished device or part?

5) Why do bulk structural materials so often prove vastly weaker than perfect, pure, small crystals of the same stuffs?

Chapter 6

Metallic Structural Materials

I: ALLOYS: GENERAL CONSIDERATIONS

ALLOYS REPRESENT METALS which admix two or more metal elements. In *isomorphous alloy systems* the atoms of the two different metals have similar enough properties (i.e., in regard to valence, size and mass) that they can substitute freely for each other in the lattice positions, and an infinite range of percentage compositions of each becomes possible (example: gold-silver and copper-nickle systems). One could call these systems true mixtures, and in them only one phase exists in the solid state, although if one allowed the melted alloy to freeze slowly, several different compositional phases might exist at the liquid-solid interfaces of the numerous "seeding" regions of the freezing and already crystalline solid phase. But by atomic diffusion and remixing processes, these phases usually have equilibrated by the time the whole mass has solidified. For pure metals a definite temperature characterizes the transition between the liquid and solid state (*liquidus* and *solidus* respectively), for example 1356° k for copper and 1123° k for nickle. But for an alloy, solidification or freezing occurs over a range of temperature, called the paste range, and it occurs gradually.

In some *binary systems* of alloys the atoms of the second element may have so small an atomic radius as to fit in between the atoms of the major constituent atoms without greatly straining the crystal lattice. Both carbon and nitrogen atoms can do this in steels.

In *eutectic alloy systems* (and equally, of some nonmetallic solids), the admixture of either of the two elements to the other lowers the freezing temperature of he resuling alloy. In freezing, such an eutectic alloy has three compositional phases. In a zinc-tin system for example, the eutectic phase exists consists of a specific and consistently reproducible compound or crystal containing nine atoms of Zn to ninety-one atoms of Sn; it has a constant and sharp melting point of 473° k, and if the bulk contained these metals in that exact proportion it would solidify at that temperature without a paste range. But if the bulk liquidus had Zn atoms in excess of that ratio, during the beginning of freezing pure Zn crystals would begin to solidify out first at 693° k (the melting point of zinc), thereby decreasing the Zn remaining in the liquidus (towards the eutectic ratio, here of 9:91). On the other hand, if Sn existed in excess of that ratio in the liquidus (because of the composition of the bulk) then tin crystals would begin to solidify out first, but now at 505° k (the melting point of tin), thereby removing Sn from the remaining liquidus and concentrating the Zn in it towards the eutectic ratio of 9:91. Thus any finally solidified alloy belonging to the eutectic system will always have in it crystals of the eutectic phase (of a constant composition or atomic ratio) interleaved with crystals of whichever of the two metals lay in excess of that ratio in the melt. In describing such changes, metallurgists use a kind of graph called a phase diagram which plots allotropic and phase transitions as functions of temperature on the vertical axis, and varying composition of the melt on the horizontal. But it serves little purpose to go into that in this book.

In the above Zn-Sn system the two components solubilized completely in each other in the liquid phase, but remained completely insoluble in the solidus.

Other alloy systems exist in which one or more of the component elements do partially solubilize in the eutectic phase in its solid state (exs: brass, bronze, some aluminum alloys). Thus these solidified alloys also can have three phases but ones now more variable in composition, depending upon the ratios of the two components in the original melt or liquidus: crystals of metal A (usually called the alpha phase), which may have small amounts but only up to some limit of metal B (the component of the beta phase) dissolved in solid solution in it; the eutectic phase* which may have small amounts of A or B—whichever lay in excess in the melt—dissolved in solid solution with it, and crystals of metal B, the beta phase, if that metal lay in excess of the eutectoid proportions in the original melt.

To the above properties of alloys one may add two others encountered in metallurgy, both of theoretical and equally of practical interest. Thus, after complete solidification and usually with a further drop in temperature, one or more of the solid phases in an alloy may then undergo an internal change in its crystal structure without any change in composition, i.e., exhibit allotropy. Metallurgists call these changes which do not alter the composition of a solid phase, *congruent transformations,* and they prove quite important in steel metallurgy. Or, during the solidification and cooling processes (but still within the paste range) the previously deposited solid phase seeds may then begin to interact with the liquidus to produce a new solid phase, or vice versa. Metallurgists call these changes, which do alter the composition of a solid phase, *peritectic transformations.*

Cold and hot working: The above matters bear on the suitability of metals for a variety of manufacturing operations. Thus isomorphous alloy systems usually cold work quite well, and by cold working and then recrystallizing (annealing) one can control to some degree their grain size. But in eutectic alloy systems one of the phases usually tends towards brittleness and hardness, causing the material to tend to fracture upon cold working. This ensues because the brittle phase acts to jam up the dislocations in the more ductile phase until the stress levels needed to move the slip planes through and/or around the harder phase exceeds the breaking strength, and fracture rather than further plastic deformation occurs. Manufacturers may cope with this problem simply by heating the alloy, and/or hot working (i.e., forging or rolling it) .

---

* Which will have a constant ratio of A and B in it.

Age hardening: In most alloys the changes in composition of the solid phase which lead to a uniform composition of the final bulk solid require a fair amount of time to occur; after all many of them involve atomic diffusion through matter in the solid state. Thus, simply by cooling a just-frozen metal rapidly, one can trap or freeze into it chemical combinations normally unstable, and tending inherently to change to more stable configurations and/or compositions if given time. Given time, and occasionally helped by modest heating, these changes will occur and can lead to great improvement in yield strength, creep properties and hardness of the finished product. Metallurgists call this age hardening.

II: SPECIFIC METALS AND ALLOYS

A few words now about particular metals may help to relate the foregoing and possibly rather esoteric material to more practical matters.

1) BRASS: This term designates, not one alloy but a series of alloys of *copper and zinc* which, over the range of Cu-Zn ratios at which brass can exist, can demonstrate three solid phases, called alpha, beta and gamma. Alpha brass (35% Zn) proves soft and malleable, while beta brass (35–50% Zn) exhibits greater hardness and brittleness. Additions of other elements can alter the mechanical and corrosional properties of brasses in a variety of useful ways.

2) BRONZE: One of man's oldest, these alloys (again a series rather than a single one) comprise eutectoid mixtures of *copper and tin* which in solid form combine four distinct phases (alpha, beta, gamma and delta). That, plus the further properties endowed the series by adding small amounts of other metals and elements to it (such as Al, Pb, Zn, or phosphorus) make a versatile and widely used alloy system.

3) ALUMINUM: A large number of alloys of aluminum exist, largely because the pure metal lacks the strength and stiffness we usually need in our structural materials. Some

of its alloys cannot be heat treated (for that does not change their mechanical properties in any useful way), while others can, particularly the duraluminum alloys (Al-Cu eutectoid systems). Magnesium, silicon, nickel and iron may also serve as alloying elements. Because of its light weight it serves widely for the manufacture of orthopaedic braces of varying types. If you look at such devices you will observe that the hinges and locks are made, not of aluminum alloys but of steel. That is because the latter can be hardened effectively by heat treatment (description coming up) so as to provide good wear resistance.

4) STEEL: This signifies the element, iron, mixed with carbon in amounts up to 1.7% (with higher percents we get into cast irons, which we'll mention later). Steels may contain many other elements added for specific purposes, and as a class they constitute one of the most important kinds of materials in our whole industrialized technology.

(a) Composition: Iron has the allotropic property, existing as the face-centered-cubic lattice system (austenite) above 1270° k, and as the body-centered-cubic lattice system (ferrite) below that temperature. Since these transitions depend upon atomic diffusion within individual grains and occur well below the freezing point of the bulk material, they occur slowly, and for practical purposes do not proceed at all at room temperature. Thus by heat treating one can create austenite, and by rapid cooling or quenching, then freeze much of it into the solid at room temperature.

The carbon in steel exists in several forms. Some small proportion of it lies in interstitial positions in the ferrite lattice, meaning stuck in between iron atoms (more on this later). Most of it exists as iron carbide or cementite, $Fe_3 C$, which possesses great hardness and brittleness. Thus, steel, a eutectoid system, has a minimum of the four following solid phases.

(1) alpha, consisting of ferrite, the BCC system.
(2) gamma, consisting of austenite, the FCC system.

(3) Fe_3 C, or cementite.

(4) The eutectoid, composed of a constant-composition mixture of ferrite $+ Fe_3$ C. Metallurgists know this eutectoid as pearlite.

Note these properties of slowly cooled carbon steel, according to its carbon content: at 0.83% C the solid consists entirely of pearlite, the eutectoid. At a higher per cent of C (hypereutectoid steel), cooling ferrite rejects the excess carbon to form free cementite, and often the latter then sequesters at the grain boundaries. At lower per cent of C, (hypoeutectoid steel) the bulk metal contains alpha (ferrite) mixed with the eutectoid. Excess amounts of silicon ($>$ 0.4%), phosphorus ($> .05$%) or sulfur ($> .05$%) embrittle steel (by blocking dislocation systems), and so steel makers usually try to hold these elements down to trivial levels in the finished product.

(b) Hardening by heat treating: Heating a cast steel to a high enough temperature (but still below the melting point) allows both the pearlite and ferrite to transform into austenite, while the carbon then diffuses evenly throughout the bulk. Since each original pearlite grain develops numbers of smaller austenite grains within it during this process, this reduces the grain size, increases the grain boundary surface/ volume ratio, and thereby more effectively jams dislocations. As a result steel treated in such a manner and then cooled usually has improved strength, and the metallurgist calls it fine grained.

Heating such a steel too long allows the austenite grains to grow and coalesce, and since this reverses the above strengthening effect, manufacturers usually avoid such procedures.

But if one cools the heated austenite rapidly, or quenches it (note we do not discuss melted steel, but rather the solid at about 1180° k), the austenite transforms quickly, and by a process not depending upon atomic diffusion of the carbon, to a new phase with a body-centered tetragonal (BCT) lattice, and without accompanying carbide precipitation. This important new phase, named *martensite,* remains supersaturated with interstitially located carbon atoms which endow the material with great resistance to dislocation motion and thus great hardness, as well as brittleness. In fact, this material proves so brittle as to have little use in actual manufacturing practice.

(c) Tempering. By reheating the now martensitic steel between 373–473° k, some of the interstitial carbon atoms can come out to join with iron atoms and form some cementite, while some of the quenched-in mechanical stresses or lattice strains can relieve. This heat treated or tempered material now has gained very significantly in toughness, at the expense of some of its hardness. But enough of the latter still remains to provide good wear resistance.

Upon heating between 473–673° more carbon comes out to form Fe_3C, and some of the BCT lattice martensite then begins to convert to the BCC ferrite. This material still has great strength and even greater toughness, although obviously it has lost some of its previous hardness and brittleness.

Above 673° the material completes transforming to ferrite and pearlite but in addition some of the carbide coalesces into large spheroidal granules which weakens the material considerably and so constitutes the state of overtempering.

(d) Alloying elements: Some elements such as nickel, chromium, and molybdenum in amounts up to four to five per cent can significantly retard the rate at which one must cool the austenitic steel to retain the martensite phase. Since the sudden quenching process can create large, locked in stresses in bulky parts due to differential thermal effects, stresses which can actually cause them to crack apart as they cool, the ability to cool the metal more slowly and still retain the martensite phase allows manufacture of larger parts and members of very tough, strong, steel. Without such elements, large parts cooled rapidly develop different rates of thermal contraction of their outer skin and in their depths. A very extensive and complicated expertise exists in the field of heat treating steel, and other alloys, and those interested in further information on it should refer to a standard metallurgical work.

(e) Corrosion Resistant Steels: Chromium added in amounts over eleven per cent produces (by combining with atmospheric oxygen) an oxide coating of Cr_2O_3 on the surface of the alloy. This coating proves highly resistant both to corrosion and to any further oxidation. Any break in this skin by mechanical abrasion leads to immediate healing by combination of freshly exposed Chromium atoms with further environmental oxygen. Thus one can make steels corrosion resistant (i.e., stainless) by adding Chromium usually in amounts of about seventeen to eighteen per cent. Two types of such steels exist, the hardenable and non-hardenable.

(f) Hardenable stainless steel may contain up to about 0.25 per cent carbon and on heating and quenching can develop and retain considerable amounts of martensite. This makes them suitable metals for making osteotomes, dies, knife blades and the like. The 440 stainless used currently to make surgical osteotomes constitutes such a steel. Less hardenable stainless steels might contain only about 0.1 per cent carbon and will not quench harden. Ferritic completely, they accordingly have considerable ductility and toughness. While they will not quench harden they can work harden.

(g) Nonhardenable stainless steels arise by adding nickle, which preserves the austenitic condition through the cooling process. That explains why metallurgists call them austenitic stainless steels. While they do not produce and retain martensite on heating and quenching, they may do so if severely cold-worked, which then embrittles them, a phenomenon many orthopaedists have encountered in one or another way. Our familiar 316 stainless, used to make a variety of implants for use in orthopaedic surgery, belongs to this type.

5) CAST IRON: When the carbon content in the iron melt exceeds 2%, we obtain cast iron, a relatively cheap and easily cast material, although not equal in strength and toughness to steel. Depending upon its composition and cooling rate,

it consists or (a) pearlite and cementite, or (b) ferrite and graphite (i.e., pure carbon granules), or (c) pearlite and graphite. When lots of cementite occur the resulting hard, brittle product has become known as white cast iron. A graphite phase produces a much softer, grey cast iron.

6) SINTERED FABRICATION: Reduce an alloy to a fine powder, its particules having any mean diameter one chooses (typically in sintered metal parts fabrication, ranging from 5–100 microns). Then fill a mould of a part to be made with this powder and apply great pressure to compact its particles together. Finally, fire it at high temperature to make the various particles fuse with each other. One thereby obtains a porous yet quite strong part which the moulding process can turn out in a large variety of complicated shapes that might prove very expensive to mill out of solid ingot stock. By controlling particle size and moulding pressure one can vary the porosity (termed specific pore volume) within wide limits and also the sizes of individual pores. And by this means one can adjust the bulk stiffness of the part over some range extending below that of the pure solid material. One calls this method of making metal parts sintering.

7) FIBER SINTERING: Here one reduces the metal to fine wire cut into short lengths, then moulds it under pressure and again fuses it under high temperature. Again one can control the pore size and the specific pore volume within wide limits. And, again, this allows one to modify the stiffness of the bulk material over a limited range of values, but never higher than that of the pure solid. Some investigators have used this class of materials to provide pore sizes large enough for bone trabeculae to invade, in an attempt to obtain secure fixation of bone to metal. Of some possible interest to us, controlling the bulk or overall compliance of such materials may make it possible to match that of living bone rather closely, a desirable objective for construction of surgical implants or for replacing parts of a bone with an artificial substitute or endoprosthesis. As will become apparent in later chapters of Part II, this does not constitute the only

problem to solve in making a workable and reliable therapeutic expertise out of such an approach.

While we could say a great deal more about metals and metallurgy, one of man's oldest fields of technology, let us now turn attention to a much newer one, plastics.

QUESTIONS: CHAPTER 6

1) a) Define a eutectic phase; b) an alloy.
2) Can one alter the mechanical properties of some alloys by pounding or stretching or twisting them?
3) a) What is cementite? b) martensite?
4) What constitutes tempering of steel?
5) What role does chromium play in so-called stainless steels?
6) Most osteotomes are made of hardenable and actually hardened steels, whether of the stainless type or not. Should one sharpen them on a power-driven grinding wheel?
7) Why does a hardenable steel in a very hard state hold its cutting edge poorly when used to cut living tissues?
8) Why do manufacturers specify bolts heat treated to a predetermined level of hardness in some critical locations in the construction of machinery?
9) A plain carbon steel hacksaw blade proves incapable of cutting a chrome-cobalt alloy intramedullary nail, although the Brinell hardness of its teeth as it left the retail dealer's shelf considerably exceeds that of the nail. On the other hand, an alloy tool steel blade of slightly lesser hardness does cut the nail. Why?
10) Why should one always sharpen good knife blades by hand rather than on power driven high speed equipment?
11) a) Ductile metals possess that property as a consequence of what phenomenon found at their grain level? b) And in which of the three principal strains does that phenomenon function?

Chapter 7

Polymeric Structural Materials

I: GENERAL PROPERTIES

A POLYMER CONSISTS OF a series of basic molecules called mers which attach to each other to form long chains of molecules. When the attachment represents a chemical reaction in which a broken double bond of one mer molecule combines with that of another, one calls it an addition reaction and no chemical byproducts of the polymerization process arise (examples: polyethylene, polyvinylchloride and polytetrafluorethylene). In condensation reactions a chemical byproduct of the bond arises or condenses. When only one type of mer exists the resulting polymer forms a *homopolymer*. When two (or more) mers exist one has a *copolymer*, analogous to a metal alloy, a situation which seems to offer some promise to orthopaedists in terms of chemically engineering useful mechanical properties into the bulk material. The finished polymer may remain linear, or form a tangled felt work of chemical bonds extending in all directions. Thermosetting polymers usually develop such felt work style bonds, usually of the covalent type, and so tend towards strength and rigidity. Thermoplastic polymers usually bond side-to-side by Van der Waal's forces and so have greater flexibility, and will melt when heated.

1) AMORPHOUS POLYMERS: These materials lack any crystallinity and their molecules interweave randomly (example: polymethylmethacrylate or Perspex®). Such materials do not transform suddenly from the solid to the liquid state as one heats them. Rather a transition zone intervenes known as the glass transition temperature range, within which the material behaves like a rubber. Thus, below this range a material may have good strength and rigidity, but

loses it as it heats up. Increasing the covalent cross linking of adjacent polymer chains (irradiation by neutrons or x-rays can cause this) usually increases both the rigidity and the glass transition temperature of such a material. Deliberately increasing the asymmetry of the mer molecules, and forming increasingly complex bonds between adjacent mers of the same polymer (just like installing increasing numbers of cross braces in a building's walls), have similar effects on the bulk properties.

2) CRYSTALLINE POLYMERS: This represents a partial misnomer for no polymer is truly (or wholly) crystalline. Rather one determines and states their degree of crystallinity, for they have small regions of good crystallinity (which confer strength and hardness on the material) embedded in others of poor crystallinity (which, however, confer toughness and compliance on the material). These crystalline polymers also have a glass transition temperature (examples: polyethylene, polypropylene, Teflon or polytetrafluoroethylene) but their crystallinity rather than that temperature determines the bulk of their mechanical properties.

In general, polymers have the following materials properties of some interest to our needs.

(a) They have lower densities than metals. Thus steel weighs 7.8 gm/cc, aluminum 2.7, polyethylene 1.2 and nylon 1.1.

(b) They have lower thermal conductivities than metals by about five hundred fold, and ten thousand times greater electrical resistance.

(c) They have lower melting points by a factor of ten or so than metals.

(d) They have less strength and rigidity than metals by factors of ten to one hundred.

(e) Many of them demonstrate greater strength and rigidity upon impact than upon static testing, a property deriving in part from the next listed one.

(f) They exhibit viscoelasticity, meaning that under constant load they gradually and progressively deform,

probably because relatively weak Van der Waal's bonds break and slide past each other. Increasing the temperature enhances this effect. When de-loaded such a material will usually return, and equally or even more slowly, nearly but not quite to its original dimensions. Thus it lacks resilience under static testing conditions although some poly-mers (i.e., rubber) may possess good resilience under rapid strain conditions.

(g) They demonstrate considerable creep, meaning pro-gressive permanent deformation under constant loads which stress them well within their yield and frac-ture points. This creep increases greatly as the temperature rises towards the glass transition tem-perature (just as the Young's modulus decreases similarly). In this respect, cross linking (as occurs in vulcanized rubber) greatly reduces creep at tem-peratures well below the glass transition, and in-creasing crystallinity (i.e., 80%) does the same in crystalline polymers. Thus amorphous polymers usually show greater creep than crystalline and cross linked ones, other things remaining equal.

Creep also causes an inverse phenomenon called stress relaxation. For example, stretch a nylon thread a fixed amount, hold it there and continuously monitor the tensile force it exerts on the restraints or clamps holding it. That force will progressively decline with time, implying gradual yielding of elastically deformed bonds within the material. Since the stress relaxation phenomenon does represent a kind of creep under constant strain conditions (whereas we first described variable creep strain under constant load con-ditions) the same temperature, compositional and physical factors affect each in similar ways.

II: SOME PROPERTIES OF PARTICULAR POLYMERS

Let us characterize briefly a selected list of polymers of some contemporary interest in orthopaedic surgery.

1) POLYETHYLENE: The mer of this material, the gas ethylene (often used for gas sterilization of heat-sensitive surgical instruments) combines end-to-end to form long chains, as shown in the top of the accompanying Figure 7.01. Entanglement of the filaments and some branching of the molecular chains provides the bulk properties of this material. As ordinarily made it has a crystallinity of fifty per cent, a melting point of 388° k and a density of .92 gm/cc. But by making it under pressure and by using different catalysts to initiate the polymerization reactions, one obtains so-called high density polyethylene with density .96 gm/cc, melting point of 415° k, and ≈ ninety per cent crystallinity. This material currently finds some use in artificial joint systems for use in human beings, mostly as a straight polymer but to some extent also as a copolymer. Its increased hardness and rigidity associate with some seventy per cent greater strength, better wear resistance and much less creep than one finds in ordinary polyethylene. To shape this material, one heats it close to the melting point and then presses it into dies or moulds.

Note: Since many plastics (including polyethylene) exhibit marked changes in their mechanical properties with rising temperature, those intended for use in the human body should be tested and engineered for its characteristic internal temperature of 37°C or 310° k.

Note: Degrees kelvin equals degrees centigrade plus 273.

2) RUBBER: Also called elastomers, the majority of these represent polymers of the dienes (second row in Fig. 7.01, where R = H = butadiene; R = Cl = chloroprene; R = CH_3 = isoprene) or isoprene, the mer of natural rubber constituting the cis isomer, as at the right in the second row of Figure 7.01.

Natural rubber, at room temperature, lies above its glass transition temperature, and the manufacturer purposely cross linked it (as we find it in ordinary commerce) to increase its strength and resilience; natural rubber or latex does not have good resilience. As natural rubber ages, various agents

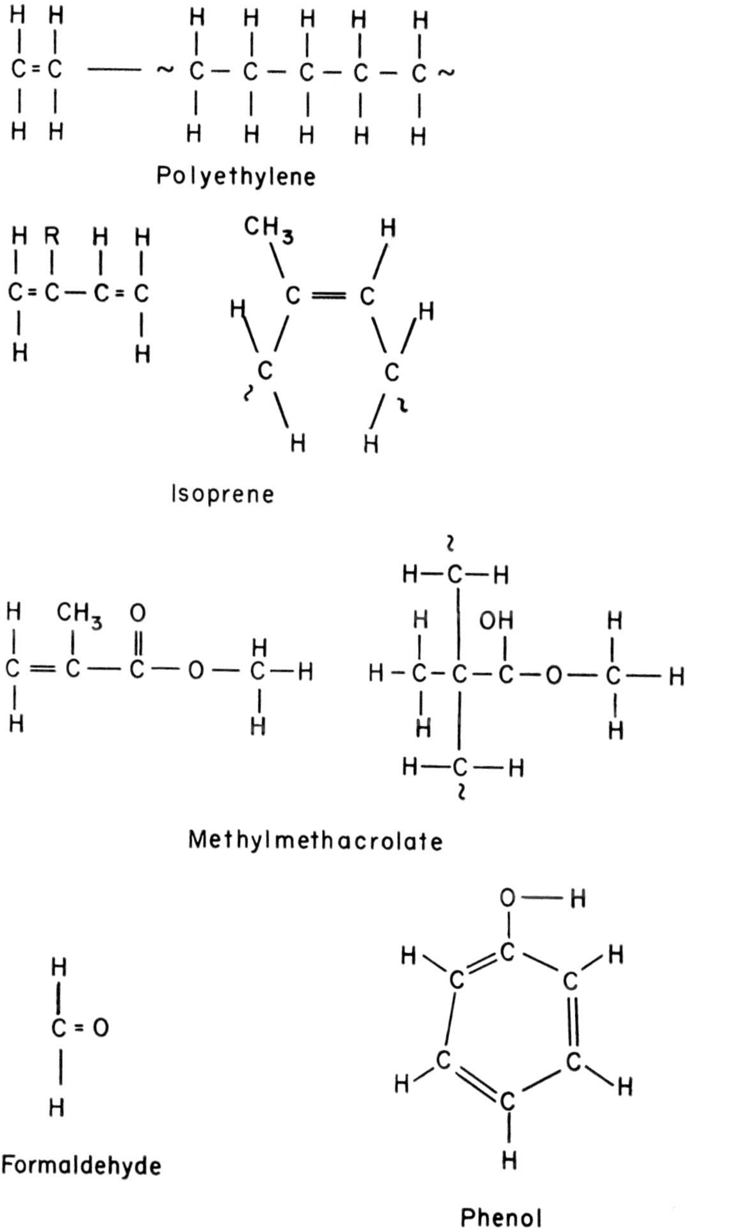

Polyethylene

Isoprene

Methylmethacrolate

Formaldehyde

Phenol

Figure 7.01. In each row, the left side provides the chemical formula for a mer, and on the right the polymer made of it.

such as gamma and light photons and reactive chemical radicals in its environment (smog has many such) increase further the cross linking within it, leading to greater hardness, embrittlement and cracking. The manufacturer often uses small amounts of various chemical additives to retard this aging process, plus others to color it. Amorphous in its unloaded or unstrained state, rubber develops both crystallinity and optical birefringence when strained which, as anyone who has ever tested a rubber band can attest, also increases its rigidity and hardness.

We need say nothing further here about the classes of butadiene, nitrate and butyl rubbers.

3) POLYMETHYLMETHACRYLATE. The left drawing of the third row, Figure 7.01, shows the basic mer, methylmethacrylate. In polymerizing into the amorphous polymer the double bond breaks, the left end carbon atom accepts another hydrogen, while the second one then bonds with similarly positioned carbon atoms of adjacent mer molecules. The resulting material, transparent and colorless and also known as Perspex R, may have average molecular weights running from 60×10^3 to 100×10^3 per chain. Its modulus of elasticity equals about $1/9$ that of steel, its density 1.19 gm/cc. It currently sees some use and success as a bone cement for fixing endoprostheses into the living skeleton. The major technical problems encountered in its use and requiring some past attention arose from the exothermic nature of the polymerization process (the stuff can become hot enough to burn tissue if it polymerizes too quickly), a sometimes erratic speed of hardening which created an operating room problem during a total hip replacement procedure that Dr. Joseph Hohl solved very neatly here two days ago, and a seeming tendency to retard for some months the ability of the living tissues in contact with it to resist bacterial infection.

4) NYLONS. Right: Many nylons exist, not just one. Several different mers serve to build up the polymer chain, and in addition to the carbon atoms in the chain they also have nitrogen atoms, usually in the amino configuration.

Cross linking of the amino (and other) groups can affect the rigidity, strength and melting point of the finished product. Nylon tends to absorb water, and exhibits considerable strain hysteresis, another way of saying that its elastic behavior exceeds considerably its resilience.

5) PHENOLIC RESINS: Bakelite forms a typical example of this group of thermosetting, covalently cross linked polymers. They arise by combining in one of several ways molecules of phenol and formaldehyde (shown in the bottom row of Figure 7.01). The phenol-formaldehyde condensation reaction must occur first, a die or mould is then filled with the resulting material and heating then causes covalent, three-dimensional cross linking to provide a rigid, hard, brittle solid.

QUESTIONS: CHAPTER 7

1) a) What is an amorphous polymer? b) the glass transition temperature?
2) Define a) a mer; b) a polymer.
3) a) What is stress relaxation? b) and an elastomer?

Chapter 8

Some Properties of Ceramic Materials

C ERAMICS FORM COMPOUNDS of metals with nonmetallic elements to form compounds such as oxides, nitrides and carbides. One forms them by firing the basic constituents at a very high temperature until they react chemically, thereby to fuse into one mass. As they cool considerable differential thermal contraction occurs, both in the bulk and within individual grain-like regions. Usually one finds ionic, covalent and van der Waal's bonds occurring all together within them, and they may exist in both crystalline and amorphous forms. The former usually contain MgO, Al_2O_3 and or SiO_4 groups. The amorphous forms (i.e., glasses) physicists consider technically to constitute supercooled liquids with very high viscosity; they lack the long range ordering of atoms that characterizes the crystalline state.

The atoms in ceramics (unlike metals) have greatly differing charges and sizes, factors which create considerable straining of the lattices of their various phases in the bulk, in a manner of speaking prestressing them. These defects inherently tend to block dislocation movement (as interstitial carbon does for martensite in quenched steel). For this among other reasons, ceramics lack malleability and ductility in tension, compression and shear, and behave as brittle solids, with high Young's and shear moduli. While they may also possess respectable compression strength, they usually have much lower tension strengths, perhaps in part because the above mentioned many small regions of locked in stress or prestress, associated with spatial distortions of interatomic bonds, represent regions of inherent tension weakness. Additional tension loads simply further stress these already partly stressed bonds, allowing them to rupture, possibly in a kind of step-by-step fashion. On the other hand, compression loads relieve some of this prestress but do not harm already compressively stressed regions which, with each increment in such strain, simply resist harder.*

Since dislocations characterize the crystalline state in general, and cause most of the plastic flow phenomenon in bulk metals, the amorphous ceramics (ex: glass) do not have dislocation systems and so do not creep or deform plastically by that means. But they may deform viscously (i.e., as a liquid of very high viscosity), and more obviously so when heated close to their melting points.

QUESTIONS: CHAPTER 8

1) Why are ceramics usually much stronger in compression than in tension and shear?

2) How does the step-by-step mode of fracture of a solid mentioned reduce the magnitude of external load required to break it?

3) Define the glassy state of solid matter.

---

* Primary bonds do not break in compression at the level of the atom; they can fail only in tension and/or shear.

Chapter 9

Some Properties of Composite Materials

W<small>E WILL DESCRIBE</small> rather briefly here some of the changes in mechanical properties of a bulk material that can arise by mixing two different materials in different ways. We will deal with four classes of this important group of structural materials.

1) D<small>ISPERSION-</small>S<small>TRENGTHENED</small> M<small>ATERIALS</small>: Here very small particles (i.e.,≈0.3μ diameter) of one material lie embedded in amounts less than fifteen per cent by volume of a second material. The idea has not yet served in making a practical plastic structural material but in metals the fine particles serve to block dislocation movements, and their sizes and average spacings in the bulk must conform to the needs dictated by the actual sizes of dislocations and their separations. By proper selection of the material (s) serving as the dispersed phase, such a composite material can demonstrate great work hardening, and retain its creep resistance and hardness at high temperatures. It can also retain these properties if repeatedly melted and cooled, which many carbon steels often do not.

2) P<small>ARTICLE-</small>S<small>TRENGTHENED</small> M<small>ATERIALS</small>: In these materials, the hard particles have larger size (i.e., $> 1.0\mu$) and compose in excess of twenty-five per cent of the volume of the bulk material. Rather than block dislocation movement, they mechanically restrain deformation or flow around them of the softer embedding matrix. Thus these materials will tend to demonstrate that sensitivity to temperature which characterizes the lower melting point phase.

The same principle also can apply to polymer production, the added particles serving to improve such properties as strength, wear resistance, hardness, creep resistance or resistance to viscoelastic deformation and the like. Thus twenty per cent carbon by volume can make new rubber ten times stronger than the pure material.

3) CERAMETS: These represent porous, ceramic particulate materials which have had their pores infiltrated at high temperature with a metal matrix. They can have very high temperature resistance and so can serve as metal cutting tools in industry, but because of their brittleness and low toughness they have not so far found any wide application as structural materials.

4) FIBER—REENFORCED MATERIALS: This particular and important class of materials concerns us for two good reasons. One, bone, tooth, tendon and cartilage, nature's structural materials, represent exactly such composites. Two, they seem very promising as a class for future use in making implants for use in the body, provided all of the problems associated with that use prove solvable.

Figure 9.01 shows that basic idea, which incorporates the following features. Here much elongated rods of a stiff and very strong material lie embedded in a matrix of more compliant and weaker material. The rods lie aligned in essentially uniform orientation so their directions of greatest tensile and compression strength sum up throughout the material. Of course one pays a price for this because their directions of greatest weakness do likewise but along different resultants. In other words, this material has mechanical grain or strain anisotropy. Furthermore, a chemical union exists between the matrix and the surface atoms of the rods so that they do not readily pull apart or slip in shear on each other.

(a) *Mechanical behavior*: Assume this bulk material now carries a tension load; let's see how it behaves in tension, compression and shear.

1) *Tension parallel to grain*: As the tension load develops the bulk material strains in tension, i.e., it elongates. Because of their union, both phases will elongate essentially equally but, because of its much greater stiffness, the needle

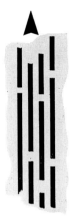

Figure 9.01. A fiber reenforced material, the rods representing fibers of a very strong material, the intervening spaces a softer or more compliant matrix embedding them and adhering to their surfaces. Thus the matrix distributes the applied loads over the relatively large surface area of the fibers, and by its compliance yields mechanically to stress relieve any potentially damaging stress concentration. The fibers carry the major fraction of the load, and in the approximate ratio of their Young's moduli, assuming equal portions of each phase in terms of volume, in the bulk material.

phase material develops much higher tension stress, and therefore carries most of the applied load. The matrix phase, attached to the needles by some form of chemical bond along their whole length, simply serves to apply and distribute the tension load equally over the whole surface of the whole lengths of individual needles.

Thus the numerous fine needles or rods actually carry most of the load, which the softer matrix distributes evenly over the needles to avoid and/or to minimize any tendency to harmful local stress concentration.

In such systems strainability derives from three interrelated factors. If the matrix possesses greater extensibility than the embedded phase, rupture of the latter in tension will govern the manner of its failure (human collagen ruptures at ≈3% elongation in tension). If the chemical bonding or adhesiveness of the matrix to the surfaces of the needles provides less total strength in shear than the load gradient over the length of a given needle, the matrix will simply separate off from the surfaces of the needles, suddenly reducing the tensile strength of the bulk material to that of the matrix. That latter will then elongate until it fails. If the total tensile strength of the needles in the bulk becomes exceeded they will fail in tension in a brittle manner, throwing all the load on the much weaker matrix which, after some additional elongation, will also fail. One can derive some fairly simple equations which express and relate these phenomena more exactly, and which can help in trying to design desirable mechanical properties into such materials in the engineering laboratory. We will leave that to those more competent than we to do so.

Note: In essence, mature human fibrous tissues (exs: tendon, ligament, fascia) contain a crystalline polymeric protein named collagen, quite stiff in tension but flexible or compliant (but still rigid) in shear, embedded in a matrix consisting of a gel (hyaluronic acid-protein complex) in just the above manner. These tissues exist primarily to carry and transfer from one place to another, a variety of pure tension loads.

Now let us examine the case of compression loading.

2) *Compression parallel to the grain*: When the material in question lacks any respectable stiffness in shear, i.e., when it has high compliance in shear, then under an applied uniaxial compression load it will simply buckle exactly as would a shoe string or a short length of rope. But if the particulate dispersed needle phase possesses great stiffness and strength in shear, the bulk material will not buckle easily in uniaxial compression. The following happens.

Again (as when loaded in tension) the bulk material strains as it accepts the load, in compression this time of course. And again the total strains in the matrix and the particulate phases, length for length, remain essentially (but obviously not exactly) equal. But because of its far greater stiffness, the needle phase develops by far the greatest internal stresses (approximately as the ratio of Young's moduli in compression of the needle relative to the matrix phases). Consequently the needle phase carries the bulk of the compression load. And again, the softer matrix phase tends to distribute that load evenly over the surface of each particulate needle or rod, and by local minute elastic deformations to dissipate any tendency towards harmful regions of stress concentration.

Now if the rodlike particles have great length (L) relative to their diameter (D) i.e., for L/D ratio's much above twenty, and also behave in very brittle fashion, the flexural moments generated within them (by any eccentricity of their neutral axes relative to the end loads they carry) will easily break them, even if very strong. But for modest L/D ratios, in the range of five to twenty, the compliant matrix allows the ends of the rods to move laterally just enough to prevent high flexural stresses arising in their midportions (the apatite crystals of bone display this property).*

Now given a bulk fiber reenforced material in which the fiber phase has much greater strength than the matrix, and in addition one in which the grain remains highly uniform over considerable distances so the rods lie accurately parallel to distant as well as close neighbors, then this happens:

Under uniaxial compression load the bulk material tends to shorten but, also, to expand laterally, as shown in the top row of Figure 9.02. This lateral expansion increases the circumference of the structure which forms a tension strain, one which furthermore acts across the grain in its direction of greatest tension weakness, rather than parallel to the grain. With sufficient such strain the matrix at the periphery can then fail in transverse tension, as shown in the overloaded case on the right middle. Certain types of wood do exactly this.

One might offset this bursting tendency in several ways. One of them represents building the bulk up out of separate layers or lamellae in which the fiber grain in any one layer

---

* Since bone apatite crystals have an inherent tendency to grow in length by purely physical chemical processes, while normal mechanical use of the skeleton, by breaking too long apatite needles via this flexural mechanism, tends to limit or shorten the average apatite needle, one suspects that someday we may become able from measurements of mean lengths of apatite crystals to determine how much mechanical usage a skeleton had experienced in the past. Perhaps some future Sherlock Holmes-equivalent will one day solve a criminal case by such means (161).

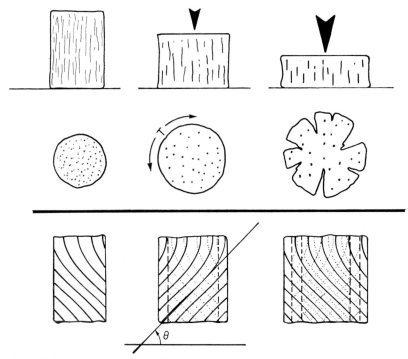

Figure 9.02. *Top:* In these side views of a wood column, as uniaxial compression loads on a structure made of fiber-reenforced material (exs: wood, bone) increase, a tangential tension strain develops circumferentially around the perimeter, shown in the cross sectional views in the middle row. It can ultimately cause a special kind of fracture of the material as shown, i.e., by radial cracking as at right middle.

Bottom: Introducing an overlapping, helically wound series of layers of the material, odd and even layers winding in the opposite way, adds significant tangential tension strength to the structure. One finds exactly such arrangements in some naturally occurring, living structural materials, for example the secondary osteon and tree trunks.

winds helically around the central axis of the structure, and in alternate layers the fiber directions run in opposite directions as shown in bottom row of this figure. In this arrangement, enlargement of the perimeter of the section under load not only strains the matrix in tension; a component of it (equal to P cos θ) now becomes carried as a tension load by the helically winding rods, and since the rods have much greater strength than the matrix, this arrangement very handily prevents the circumferential disruption shown at the right of the middle row of diagrams.

Note: Human bone exhibits exactly this alternating helical, layered orientation of the collagen bundles in its organic, compliant matrix, described in part by the Italian workers, A. Ascenzi and E. Bonucci (16). One may infer, at least in first approximation, that this arrangement serves some purpose such as just described and does not represent a structurally meaningless phenomenon.

(*b*) *Dislocations*: While in principle, plastic flow by propagation of dislocation based slip systems should occur as readily in the rods of the particulate phase as in bulk material made wholly of the same phase, if the rods remain small in diameter (less than the grain diameter in a fine-grained metal) and/or if the lattice depends upon ionic and covalent bonds for its strength, the rods may reach their breaking stress and fracture before the applied loads can free and move dislocations to cause plastic flow. In other words, the rods can possess brittleness plus great strength. Such a phenomenon probably occurs in the mineral phase of mammalian bone and accounts for its high stiffness in shear across the grain.

(*c*) *Fatigue*: Composite materials of the class under discussion can demonstrate much better endurance in fatigue (see next chapter) than bulk materials made wholly of the particulate phase and loaded to similar unit stresses. In essence this comes about because if any fatigue crack does begin in a rod, it rapidly traverses its diameter and then encounters the matrix whose compliance relieves the locally raised level of stress, thereby protecting even closely adjacent rods from crack propagation. In bulk material made wholly of the rod material, any given crack tends to propagate through the whole cross section, and the more brittle the material the faster this will occur.

By way of conclusion then, cartilage, tendon, tooth and bone all represent fiber reenforced structural materials, so some of the interesting properties of this class of man-made materials concern us here. But in addition to that relevance, the writer suspects that future implant materials may become manufactured out of as yet undeveloped composite materials of the fiber reenforced type. They offer the prospect of phenomenal but useable tension and compression strengths in excess of 500,000 psi, which would allow us to fashion much less voluminous and massive implants with better overall strength and durability than we can achieve with currently available materials (see the later chapter in Part II which outlines criteria for implant acceptability).

QUESTIONS: CHAPTER 9

1) a) What is a ceramet? b) a composite material? c) a fiber reenforced composite material?
2) Why do we concern ourselves with the engineering properties of fiber reenforced composite materials?
3) What provides protection from gross fatigue failures in fiber reenforced composite materials?

Chapter 10

Mechanical Properties of Structural Materials (4,25,29)

Next we will describe some further and less basic general properties of real materials and structures, concentrating on some of those that most concern our interests in the life sciences. One group of these properties concerns stress-strain relationships directly, while others deal primarily with chemical or physical-chemical aspects. Before doing so, we might well point out some important and fundamental mechanical differences between the solid, liquid and gaseous states of matter. And you will find if you ponder the matter that to do so we need a useable definition of rigidity, so let's formulate one now.

DEFINITION: *Rigidity: The property of resisting indefinitely a principal strain in the face of an applied external acceleratory force.* As we shall see later, this definition has an unexpected twist or so.

1) GASEOUS STATE: We noted earlier that a gas cannot develop an effective tension stress. In addition, it lacks rigidity in volume (i.e., both tension and compression) and in shear. Or in other words, it lacks rigidity to all three principal strains. As a result it always expands to fill its container, it always adopts the shape of that container, and in a vacuum it will expand without limit.

2) THE LIQUID STATE: Like gasses, liquids remain totally nonrigid in shear, but they do have an inherently fixed or rigid volume, one which will persist in a vacuum. A rigid volume simply means rigidity in both tension and compression, a statement that may appear a little slippery until you envision a graduated cylinder half filled with a liquid, and

acted upon by a piston (like the plunger of a syringe) which can alternately load it in compression and tension. By eliminating the shear factor this situation reveals the truth of our statements: fluids do possess rigidity in both tension and compression. Under external compression or tension loads the volume of a liquid can—and does—change elastically, but in a vacuum it reaches a constant volume, one affected only by evaporation. The lack of rigidity in shear constitutes precisely the mechanical property that allows liquids to flow, and the loss of the shear rigidity of any solid represents precisely the change that converts it to a fluid (187).

3) THE SOLID STATE: Solids remain rigid to all three principal strains, including volume (meaning in both tension and compression) and in shear, too.

Thus we can express the mechanical differences in the three different classical states of matter as simple differences in rigidity under the three principal stresses.

Matter need not necessarily change sharply from one state, say from the liquid to the solid. For example, raising its temperature gradually converts a steel alloy or a wax to a liquid. (This procedure will destroy a composite material such as bone.) In the temperature interval or range separating the obviously solid from the obviously liquid states (the paste range of an earlier chapter) a gradual transition occurs such that while the force of gravity alone may not suffice to make a material flow, at that point additional loads applied by various means (such as a press or a hammer) will make them flow. In metal working, one may deliberately evoke a temporary, controlled conversion from the solid to the liquid state* to aid in shaping or working it. That conversion may arise from heating a metal until it achieves a pasty or semifluid consistency, or by hammering it cold. The impact of each hammer blow generates very large but briefly acting shearing loads and stresses that transcend its shearing strength and permit momentary flow, a process called cold forging when done without preheating. For example, such

---

* This happens in forging metal parts.

combined heating-shear loading happens before the cutting edge of a drill or a lathe tool, which explains why the ability of those tools to maintain their strength, hardness and edge at elevated temperatures becomes of prime importance in determining their service life durability. Note that at room temperature a heavy grease may act like a rigid solid in response to small loads such as the force of gravity, yet like a liquid in response to larger ones such as the pressure of one's thumb or the torque on the gears in a differential.

Now for some solid mechanics.

I: MECHANICAL BEHAVIOR OF SOLIDS

1) THE PROPORTIONAL LIMIT: When a real beam or bone carries a gradually increasing load, the resulting strain will become and remain approximately or accurately proportional to the stress for a while (i.e., it will act like a Hookean solid). But, as the load keeps increasing, a point usually comes on the stress-strain curve when the strain begins to increase faster than the stress (and materials do exist where the stress begins to rise faster than the strain). This point on the stress-strain curve equals the proportional limit, shown at A in Figure 10.01. In designing machines, buildings

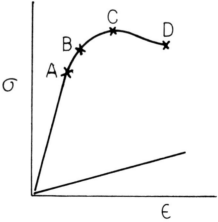

Figure 10.01. This curve demonstrates the meanings of the proportional limit (the most important one in design problems), elastic limit and yield point of metals. See text.

or structures, *it forms one of the most important properties of a material that the engineer must know.* Table 10.01 lists some mechanical properties of several different materials. Not all materials have a true proportional limit; some instead take on some degree of residual deformation after each strain.

2) ELASTIC LIMIT: Even when a material deforms past its proportional limit, it may still return completely to its original shape and dimensions after removing the load. If so, then it still behaves elastically. But with a further increase in load, a point will come when the material no longer returns to its original shape and dimensions after removing the load. Then it has deformed beyond its elastic limit, which lies at B, Figure 10.01, and one says that it has taken a permanent set, and in doing so its substance has undergone some degree of plastic flow. The elastic limit usually lies fairly close to the proportional limit on the stress-strain curve and handbooks often list it because it proves the easier to find in testing samples of a material. (See Table 10.01.) When something strains beyond its elastic limit, it takes a permanent set because its material has flowed plastically and it remains partially deformed after removing the load. In a manner

TABLE 10.01*
SOME MECHANICAL PROPERTIES OF SELECTED MATERIALS

Substance	Proportional limit PSI	Elastic limit PSI	Yield Point or Rupture Strength	Allowable Unit Stress
Douglas Fir (compression)	5,000	9,000	10,000	1,200
Cast iron (compression)	—	—	25,000	15,000
Structural steel	36,000	39,000	43,000	20,000
316 stainless	—	—	30,000	20,000
Vitallium	—	—	70,000	30,000
Bone (compression)	14,000	15,000	16,000	?

* I am grateful to the Zimmer Corporation for supplying some of this information.

While the breaking strength of fir equals some 10,000 psi in compression, that lies 11 per cent above its elastic limit and 100 per cent above its proportional limit of 5,000 psi. Given a safety factor of four, then the maximum allowable stress in a structure becomes only 1200 psi, or about ⅛ its breaking strength. Similar kinds of relationships exist for all structural materials, their major differences lying in the varying magnitudes of these effects in different materials.

Keep in mind that our two best alloy systems, the 316 stainless and the chrome-cobalt series, do not have either true proportional or true elastic limits.

of speaking, the loads inducing such plastic flow cause the material temporarily to transform partially to the liquid state (i.e., to lose shear rigidity) which allows them to flow, even if they demonstrate very large viscosities in the process. One readily sees plastic flow in a cold metal by bending a paper clip. A remotely analogous thing can occur in a greenstick fracture of a child's forearm bones, in which the intact cortex usually takes a kind of permanent set.

The ability to flow plastically under a tension load without breaking forms ductility, and under a compression load, malleability; obviously each represents a temporary change from the solid to the liquid state within the affected material, such that shearing displacements can occur.

3) YIELD POINT: Some materials including some steels (but not the biological structural materials), at a critical point of internal stress begin to stretch steadily (i.e., undergo plastic flow) without further increasing the load. This, called the yield point and representing a form of ductility, lies at C in Figure 10.01. Materials having a yield point usually take impact well and display greater toughness than those that lack this property. Such latter materials usually take impact poorly and we call them brittle (also fragile).

4) ULTIMATE STRENGTH: The maximum stress a material, or the maximum load a particular structure, will sustain before actually fracturing or breaking constitutes its ultimate strength. This lies at the highest part of the stress-strain curve in Figure 10.01.

5) RUPTURE STRENGTH: When a material reaches its yield point it begins to elongate (if loaded in tension) and to become narrower sideways, so that one needs less and less total external load to produce further strain. Elongation continues with progressively decreasing total loads until the material finally breaks; this point represents the rupture strength. In brittle materials, the ultimate and rupture strengths prove equal but in ductile solids the rupture strength often lies well below the ultimate strength. Table 10.02 lists some rupture strengths.

TABLE 10.02
TYPICAL RUPTURE STRENGTHS

Substance	Tension PSI	Compression PSI	Shear PSI
Cement	320	3,000	500
Birch	4,400	2,640	
Ash	7,200	4,520	
Walnut	10,500	16,400	
Wrought iron	51,000		
Bone	12,000	15,000	8,000
316 stainless (annealed)	85,000	85,000	40,000
Vitallium	100,000	85,000	40,000

This lists for varying principal stress some rupture strengths for bulk materials as defined in the text. Note that for brittle materials compression rupture strength usually exceeds tensile strength, and that most all materials demonstrate greater strengths in tension and compression than in shear. In the grained materials such as wood and bone, shear strength across the grain considerably exceeds that parallel to it, and this difference becomes even greater when one considers the fatigue resistance of the material.

Pay attention to concrete for a moment: A brittle material, as a later chapter will point out for ceramics, it has far more strength in compression than in tension, and for that reason engineers often reenforce it with steel rods to boost its total tension (and shear) strengths.

You can see then that rupture strength does not provide a very useful measure of a ductile material's strength when designing structures or appliances for manufacture out of it.

6) THE APPARENT ELASTIC LIMIT (OF JOHNSON) : Many materials prove neither Hookean nor truly elastic in their behavior so that no matter how small the load they carry, they always take some amount of permanent set, i.e., they stay bent slightly when bent by outside forces, or they elongate permanently (although slightly) when stretched. It becomes necessary to establish some arbitrary stress limit to use in designing structures for manufacture with such materials. One such limit forms Johnson's apparent elastic limit.

7) THE YIELD STRENGTH: Another measure of the design tolerable stresses in a material which either has no yield point, or no fixed proportionality between stress and strain in any range of loading, consists of the yield strength, sometimes also called the offset stress. This simply describes the limiting stress that will produce an arbitrarily acceptable amount of permanent set or strain. The amount of allowable strain

chosen in practice usually runs between 0.1 and 0.5 per cent. The stress at this point forms the offset stress.

8) SAFETY FACTOR: An engineer estimates the largest load a structure would conceivably ever have to bear, multiplies it by a number called the safety factor, and then designs the structure to carry this augmented load. Saftey factors in common use range from two to over ten and vary with the particular circumstances (178). We do not yet know enough about the actual loads applied to living bones to allow reliable estimates of the safety factors evolved in nature (nor in cartilage or tendon). But to some extent the self repair capacity demonstrated by living structural materials should have allowed significant reduction of that safety factor.

Table 10.03 provides some data on allowable unit stresses for wood used in construction, and the safety factor here ranges from five to over ten.

9) CREEP: (We use the mechanical rather than sociological meaning of this word.) The steel beams in any bridge gradually sag in service, so the engineer who designed the bridge usually made them slightly convex on top to compensate for this. This very gradual give or plasticity of some

TABLE 10.03
MECHANICAL PROPERTIES OF WOOD
(2 × 4 section)
ALLOWABLE STRESS, PSI

Type	Surface fibers in bending	Uniaxial Tension	Uniaxial Compression	Shear parallel to grain psi	Young's Modulus, psi
Ponderosa pine	850	500	1000	95	$.95 \times 10^6$
Douglas fir	1810	1190	1190	95	1.8×10^6
Western Cedar	850	500	1150	180	$.86 \times 10^6$
Redwood	1640	1100	1190	125	1.2×10^6
Hickory	2200	2000	2100	260	2.0×10^6

This table of *allowable stresses* (not of breaking strengths) provdes good illustrations of how materals properties may vary according to method of test-loading (observe the greater allowable tension stress in flexure than in uniaxial loading, first two columns), and according to the particular principal stress at issue. While we remain uncertain at this time due to lack of data, comparable values for living bone would probably run twice those of hickory.

You can see from such data that our structural steels and alloys in bulk form run some ten to twenty times stronger than wood, and five to ten times stronger than bone.

materials we call creep. (In the days when manila served for the standing rigging in ships, considerable creep in the shrouds required providing an adjustment at one end. Hence the lanyard and dead-eye set up). Probably bone, cartilage and tendon all exhibit creep. Teflon® (a fluorine-containing plastic) has a low coefficient of sliding friction and very low chemical reactivity in the body so artificial joint surfaces were once made of it. But they showed so much creep in actual service life that most of them failed and required removal. In effect, when given the time to do it they flowed like warm wax under combined compression and shearing loads.

10) SURFACE PROPERTIES: The stresses in most machinery and in surgical implants usually reach their greatest values at their surfaces because in addition to unaxial loads they carry combinations of flexural and torque loads which typically create maximum unit stresses on a structure's surfaces. *Accordingly, structural failures of our surgical implants, braces and similar devices usually begin at their surfaces.* For this reason impurities, cracks, scratches, gas holes, compositional separations and other defects that can develop during manufacture, the marks made by tools, and sharp changes in contour, all prove most deleterious to the performance of a structure when they lie on its surface, and least likely to cause trouble if they lie buried inside the material. The shape and treatment of the surfaces of machine parts and orthopaedic implants have become of great importance in their design and manufacture. More on this next.

II: FATIGUE

Of this mechanical materials property of great practical importance, second in importance only to chemical corrosion, note, and *note bene: Fatigue has proven the most often ignored and/or misunderstood cause of implant failures since man first began to put artificial devices into the human body.*

The failures that arise in fatigue arise from a group of phenomena, as follows:

Design features which predispose to it.

Manufacturing procedures and materials usage which predispose to it.

Usage in the body which predisposes to it.

Just as fatigue of inanimate objects can arise, so it does also in the natural, living skeletal tissues but with one important difference in terms of their effects: the living structural materials have built into them the capacity to repair fatigue damage while still microscopic—and thus trivial—in extent. We will have more to say of this in later chapters.

Now, what the devil is this fatigue?

Take an engine crankshaft, or a nail designed to pin a broken hip, each designed to withstand a maximum unit stress of 50,000 psi in tension or compression. Assume the actual loads (i.e., service loads) never exceed 30,000 psi. One might think that under those circumstances these structures would never break.

But not so: *Both would surely break if subjected to enough cycles of load-deload.* In the case of the hip pin (see Fig. 10.02) , the bone will usually heal before the pin breaks, but if the bone did not heal, the pin inevitably would break, or extrude, or work a large enough hole in the enveloping bone as to effectively deload it permanently.

Breakage caused by repeated loading and unloading within the overall stress design limits of the structural material, has become known as fatigue.*

As far as we know, *all* solids exhibit susceptibility to fatigue failure, and this includes the kinds of biological structural solids of animal musculoskeletal systems: bone, fibrous tissue, cartilage and teeth. Many major design and manufacturing problems which arose as machinery became important in our technology proved due to fatigue. Thus, fatigue failures of air frames have made aircraft crash, ships' propellor shafts snap at sea, piston rods break in internal combustion engines, and household appliances break after enough usage. Much of the breakage of the plates, pins,

---

* And bears no similarity whatsoever to the general condition of college students at 8:00 AM on Monday.

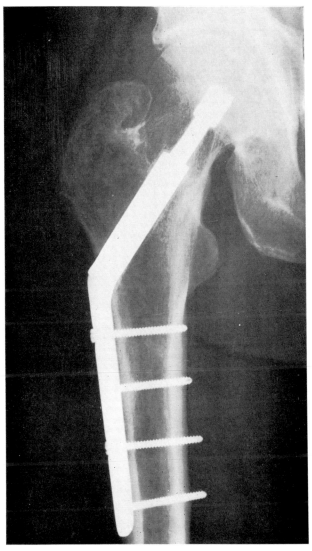

Figure 10.02. A Ken nail, used here to internally fix or hold together the ball and the neck of the femur below it after a fracture. I "set" or reduced the fracture first, and then instructed the patient (an intelligent and cooperative one) not to bear any weight on it or to kneel on it until we told her the fracture had healed (which in some four months time it did). The upper end of the nail has a triflanged cross section to provide a large bone-metal interface with minimum volume of metal, and it slides in the hollow lower piece, so it protects the fracture against shearing, torque and

screws, nails, plastic arterial grafts, sutures, wires to electronic pacemakers, heart valves and other devices implanted in the human body arises from fatigue or fatigue-like failures. Keep in mind that usually these implant failures do not signify or derive from manufacturing flaws. Rather, they arise from compromises imposed on design by the conflicting needs of mechanical factors on one side, and of biological ones on the other. Sometimes they reflect man's inability to foresee or to understand all the guises of fatigue, all the limitations of appliances and tissues, all the problems and challenges a device may have to meet. Hence the need where possible to use such devices only as temporary substitutes, rather than as permanent ones. While living structural materials rarely fail in fatigue, this almost certainly occurs because they have the self repairing property, not because they have any inherent immunity to fatigue.† When they do occasionally fail by fatigue, this usually means their self repairing ability has become impaired in some manner.

A later chapter will consider this.

Fatigue damage takes time to develop, and it may prove impossible to find any detectable evidence of its early stages by any presently practicable means. Therefore, once they

---

† We have learned a great deal about this kind of thing in bone as a consequence of the *in vivo* tetracycline bone labeling technique, which has given us the time dimension in bone turnover, as well as allowed us to study its patterns and causal associations. We haven't even begun to exploit this technique however. Volume III provides pertinent references.

---

flexural displacements but allows the upper fragment to slide down on the axis of the nail until the two bony surfaces lay in direct and intimate contact.

The side plate and the four self-threading transfixion screws running horizontally through it, affix the lower two-thirds of the nail to the lower bone piece, or *distal fragment,* a necessary feature because the middle of the nail part lies inside the marrow cavity of the neck ("Ward's triangle") almost totally out of contact with any bone.

The restrictions of loading described, plus the limited but finite fatigue endurance of the metallic implant and the bone in contact with it held the parts together until bone healing occurred, whereupon the device became a useless—but inert—foreign body in the tissues.

have served in a patient one should not reuse biological implants.

Note Bene: Time-dependent fatigue constitutes the factor most often underestimated or misunderstood in biomechanical design and service problems.

1) THE THEORY OF FATIGUE: STRESS RISERS: Surface scratches (even or especially microscopic ones), tooling marks, sharp angles, grooves, chemical discontinuities and the like, probably weaken structures by locally concentrating mechanical stresses within a small region or volume of the structure so they rise to values lying both above the material's proportional or elastic limit, and respectably above the average unit stress over the whole cross section of the structure. Such discontinuities have become known as stress risers (see Figure 10.03) because they locally raise the value of the surface unit stresses. These local and often microscopic increases in stress levels can then start and/or cause the gradual propagation of surface cracks through the cross section. Thus such a crack grows a little bit at each load-deload cycle, and finally becomes big enough that a normal load can exceed the normal strength of the remaining intact material, causing it suddenly to fail. Of some interest, the crack propagates because as soon as a minute extension of it exposes fresh metal, that metal reacts with oxygen and other compounds always present here on earth to prevent spontaneous healing of the crack. In the vacuum of extraterrestrial space, however, two exposed pure metal surfaces usually weld together upon contact, for no oxide coating exists to protect them. Consequently metal fatigue has not proven as serious a problem in artificial satellites as it has in earthbound machinery.

The ability of a surface scratch or groove, or a sharp change in external contour, to locally increase the average surface stresses represents the notch effect, and the smaller the radius of curvature at the root of such a notch or crack, the greater the local augmentation of mechanical stresses. Such notches can multiply local unit stress levels by factors ranging from 1.1 to greater than 5.0 times the average unit stress over the whole, larger region. Usually one can partially

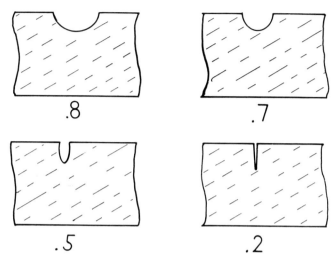

.8   .7

.5   .2

Figure 10.03. The diagrams illustrate a series of notches in the surface of some mechanical structure, as one might observe them in sections sawed through it. Upon flexural or uniaxial tension loading, the upper left one fails at .8 or 80% of the load required to break it if it had a perfectly smooth surface, while the lower right one fails at only 20% of that load. In other words, notches locally concentrate mechanical stress above the average value across the section, and the sharper the curvature at the root of the notch the greater this stress enhancement effect.

A manufacturer's representative recently showed us a new design for the stem of a hip prosthesis, one which contained innumerable fine pits on its surface intended to secure it firmly—and irrevocably—to an embedding polymethylmethacrylate cement. But on the tension loaded side of this stem these constitute stress risers and should certainly cause fatigue fractures in actual use.

offset the stress concentrating effect of sharp changes in contour by rounding off the sharp edges of any holes, or by creating a smooth fillet where one section meets another (the machinist would say, by radiusing them) thereby increasing the radius of curvature at the root of the notch, which reduces the stress concentrating effect. See Figure 10.04. Any sharp or sudden changes in the external contour of a device with a small radius of curvature at its root will raise the local stress levels and create the likelihood of a structural fatigue failure beginning in its root. Or, a small region of a very hard and rigid carbide phase exposed at a device's surface and surrounded by more easily strained material may act as a

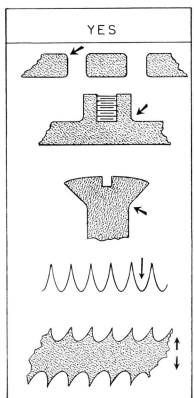 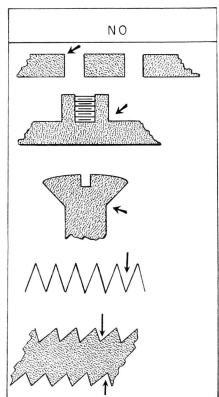

Figure 10.04. These drawings illustrate several of the commoner sources of stress risers which can arise through the choice of design of the shape of various parts, as sudden changes in contour. From top to bottom they illustrate holes in a plate (seen from the side); a contour change at a lug which secures a bolt; a contour change under a screw head; and the root of a screw thread.

By smoothing or "radiusing" as shown on the left, the undesirable sharp changes in contours shown on the right, the local stress concentrations present on the right markedly reduce, and the devices gain very considerable endurance in mechanical fatigue. Because of the disproportionately greater stresses in the thread roots compared to those at their outer edges (in cylindrical cross sections, surface flexural stresses *increase* as the fourth power of the decrease in diameter), the thread root represents by far the weakest part of the screw and so one need not radius the threads' outer edges. Engineers can improve screw strength in part by the means shown and in part by increasing the diameter across the thread roots.

local stress riser, starting a crack in the surrounding substance which then can propagate steadily throughout the
whole cross section.

Some important further aspects of fatigue include the
following:

(a) *Condition of the Surface*: For reasons by now apparent, this has proven of extreme importance in determining
the fatigue susceptibility of the devices used by orthopaedists. Even microscopic scratches on the surface of some
materials can pronouncedly increase susceptibility to a fatigue failure. For example, under laboratory conditions a
hardened, polished steel shaft that would take ten million
cycles of torque at fifty thousand psi unit stress level in its
surface fibers, can fail at only one hundred thousand similar
cycles after dragging a file once across its surface. Or a carefully prepared glass rod might withstand a constant load
generating two hundred thousand psi indefinitely, but fail
at only five thousand psi after a thimbleful of sand grains
fall on it from a height of one foot!

Chemical corrosion of metallic surfaces can produce comparable declines of fatigue resistance in structures, by un-
equally etching microscopic regions of varying chemical
composition.

(b) *Changes in Surface Contour*: As already noted,
sharp changes in the external surface contour of a structure
or device make it more likely to fail in fatigue. For example,
sharp "V" shaped grooves at the thread roots of bone screws
increase their susceptibility to fatigue (28). A surface notch
may weaken a structure, in a static test as well as during
cycles of load-deload, by factors of less than two to over five.
A one-eighth inch hole drilled on the tension side in wet
bone decreases its net flexural strength by twenty to thirty
per cent in a dog. As C. O. Bechtol demonstrated many years
ago it takes a healthy, live bone about eight to ten weeks to
recover from this weakness. The sharper the change in contour, the more this weakens the structure.

(c) *Endurance Limit*: Many materials which have a
propotional limit also have the following property: when

stressed cyclically below some given level of unit stress, and provided the surface stays undamaged, they can seemingly indefinitely resist developing a fatigue failure (52). We say of such materials that they have an endurance limit, even though we have good reason to think that, if cyclically stressed often enough, any real solid will eventually fail in fatigue. Other things remaining equal and in general, this statement applies: tough, ductile and malleable materials resist fatigue better than brittle and fragile ones.

(d) *Materials which lack a proportional limit usually also lack an endurance limit.* Many aluminum and magnesium alloys lack endurance limits, as do also the usual stainless steels and chrome—cobalt—tungsten alloys used to make bone implants. For this reason, it has become common practice in safety oriented aircraft maintenance to replace some parts after a certain number of hours of service life, a necessary stratagem because fatigue damage may remain undetectable right up to the moment of structural failure.

Living bone, tendon and cartilage exhibit operational endurance limits with respect to fatigue but almost certainly because of their self-repairing property (which we discuss in Part II). Probably fatigue damage in them becomes detected by some means while still microscopic in size and then repaired. Dead bone and tendon on the other hand become prone to gross fatigue failure if repeatedly loaded, both *ex vivo* and *in vivo*. Note that although living bone represents a brittle material, it does not prove as fatigue prone as manmade or inorganic natural materials of comparable brittleness.

All substances usually put in the body as implants (at least at this writing) usually lack endurance and proportional limits.* We use them because they have more immediately necessary properties: biologically and chemically they remain relatively inert in living tissue. They do not exhibit absolute inertness however; nothing made of real

---

* It seems that currently available artificial materials with the most desirable mechanical properties prove chemically unacceptable to mammalian tissue fluids, while materials that possess the greatest chemical and electrical inertness in tissues have some undesirable physical properties.

matter does. And unpredictable iodiosyncrasies in people may cause one person to reject or react unfavorably to an implant material that the next thousand others will tolerate.

III: CORROSION

Metals in the body present at least two major problems aside from those of strength and fatigue, because of effects that can arise when their surfaces interact chemically with the body fluids and the ions in these fluids, and because of their electrical properties.

With respect to composition, our metallic surgical implants divide into two types: those made of pure elements, and those of mixtures of two or more elements called alloys. While occasionally we may use pure elements such as gold, tantalum and titanium in the body for special purposes, the bulk of the implants of concern in musculoskeletal surgery at present form either chrome-cobalt or chrome-cobalt-tungsten alloys, or a type 316 stainless steel. Both of these alloys comprise mixtures of two or more elements in carefully controlled proportions. Table 10.04 lists the composition of five alloys currently used to make metallic biological implants. Many elements such as iron, aluminum and magnesium, or alloys and mixtures such as carbon steel and aluminum alloys, all corrode severely in body fluids, in the process also harming healthy tissues and often impeding the healing and adaptive processes. Consequently, we may state this rule:

A primal requirement of any implant material forms resistance to corrosive or other forms of chemical reactivity with the living tissue environment.

Now, as for corrosion of metals:

1) CAUSE OF CORROSION: This has proven primarily electrochemical. Metals and alloys can react chemically with the ions invariably present in the body fluids which, remember, have a normal pH of about 7.39, distinctly on the alkaline side of the neutral point at 7.00. Most metals and alloys possess greater chemical reactivity in acidic aqueous environments than in alkaline ones. When the electromotive

TABLE 10.04
COMPOSITION OF IMPLANT ALLOYS

Element	316 Stainless	18/8 SMO	316L Stainless	Wrought Vitallium	Cast Vitallium	Zimalite
Chromium	17	17	17	20	28	20
Tungsten	0	0	0	15	0	0
Molybdenum	2.5	2.4	2.5	0	6	0
Nickle	12	10	12	10	2.5	10
Manganese	2.0	0	2.0	2.0	1.0	2
Iron	65	70.6	65.	3.0	.7	3
Cobalt	0	0	0	53	64	65
Carbon	.08	0	.03	.1	.25	.15
Silicon	0	.05	0	0	0	0

This lists the chemical compositions in weight per cent of five alloy systems in use for making orthopaedic implants throughout the world. All contain chromium in amounts over seventeen per cent. This element combines with oxygen atoms in the ambient atmosphere—whether air or body fluids—to form a tough, chemically impervious skin over it of chromium oxide, Cr_2O_3. This skin can heal itself almost instantly if mechanically disrupted by fretting, or the tools used to install the implant. But such healing ability requires thorough mixing of the alloying elements, for if a small region—say of cementite or of phosphate or silicate inclusion—presents to the surface, it may lack enough Cr for healing and provide the metal direct access to the body fluids.

The nickle in the steels serves to retain the austenitic state as they cool, and to minimize the production (by allotropic changes) of cementite and ferrite during that time. As a result these do not constitute steels hardenable by heat treating, although they work-harden by repeated straining. One seeks to avoid such hardening for it associates with the precipitation of cementite and high stress-energy regions due to jammed up dislocations, which increases the material's sensitivity to fatigue failure.

potential of the atoms at the surface of the metal implant has a sufficiently negative value with respect to the surrounding body fluids, the surface metal atoms yield up their electrons to become positive ions and, hence, to enter into solution. This removes metal from the implant (i.e., corrodes it) and furthermore can lead to local changes in acidity, and locally high concentrations of metal ions around the implant, which can harm the local cells and/or lead to tissue inflammation. Both of these effects, singly or in combination, can cause the body to reject an implant, matters we deal further with at the end of Part II. In addition, surface corrosion markedly increases the chance of a fatigue failure in an implant by introducing small pits and crevices that act as stress risers. This becomes particularly likely if chemically highly reactive phases of the alloy have moved to the grain boundaries, a situation which can in turn lead to intergranular corrosion (i.e., corrosion between grains or in the grain boundaries, a particular nuisance for those who collect antique machinery containing leaf springs).

2) DIFFERENT METALS: When two different metals co-exist in the same body such as silver and iron (or even two different alloy systems), a voltage difference or potential exists between them. As a result, one acts like the positive or cathodic pole of a battery (here silver), the other the negative or anodic one (iron), while the body fluids serve as an electrolyte or salt bridge that connects them. The electronegative metal then corrodes, meaning it gives up some of its electrons to the electrically more positive metal. In so doing its own atoms, having lost electrons, become positively charged ions which dissolve in the surrounding tissue fluids. The loss of surface metal atoms occasioned by having them enter in solution and move away constitutes the corrosion of an implant, and in principle it need not remain confined to metallic substances.

For the above reason one would seldom implant devices made of different metals in the same body. Table 10.05 lists some elements according to their location in the electromotive series. Elements on the left and above will donate some of their electrons to those below and to the right, and therefore will corrode if connected by an electron conducting medium (such as the body fluids).

3) PERFECTION OF SURFACE COMPOSITION OF APPLIANCES: Even in a single device such as an intramedullary nail, the surface has a complicated physical and chemical structure and composition, involving a series of oxides of its elements, plus the other microscopic impurities (compounds of silica, phosphorus and sulfur) that always exist. As a result, one part of the nail's surface may become and remain electrically positive with respect to another, to set up a battery thereby which leads to corrosion at the electronegative part or region. The quality control of modern appliance manufacturers has become excellent, so that this kind of corrosion seldom arises nowadays. However if it did occur at

TABLE 10.05
ELECTROMOTIVE SERIES

Metal	Potential, volts	Metal	Potential, volts
Anodic (corroded) end		Iron	—0.4
Lithium	—3.04	Titanium	—0.33
Potassium	—2.92	Cobalt	—0.28
Strontium	—2.89	Nickle	—0.23
Calcium	—2.8	Lead	—0.12
Sodium	—2.71	Hydrogen	0.00
Magnesium	—2.37	Copper	+ .52
Aluminum	—1.7	Silver	+ .80
Manganese	—1.04	Platinum	+1.2
Chromium	—0.6	Gold	+1.5
		Cathodic (noble) end	

In this partial list of the electromotive series, the more negative of any two metals can yield up its electrons to the more positive (i.e., less negative) ones, creating soluble ions in the region of the more negative element which enter into solution in the body fluids. There these ions can react chemically with the constituents of body fluids and cells and cause harmful effects of various kinds discussed in Part II. Also, loss of the ionized atoms from the surface of the metal thereby corrodes, or progressively removes metal from the more anodic material. Since the cathodic metal merely accepts these ions and passes them on without less of its atoms, it does not corrode, or tend to react with its environment. However, the electrons it passes on can reduce hydrogen ions to form molecular hydrogen.

a critical part of a device, a corrosion fatigue failure might ensue.

4) Fretting Corrosion: When separate metallic devices touch each other, such as the screws which hold a plate attached to a bone, the microscopic working or strains caused by muscle action and body weight cause tiny but real rubbing motions of the two metal parts on each other. This minute working or strain displacement, termed fretting, breaks up the oxide coating which normally covers and chemically protects the surfaces of the implants from the ions in the body fluids, giving these ions access to the pure and usually much more highly reactive metal atoms under the oxide coating. Since the metal atoms can ionize by yielding up electrons, fretting corrosion can follow and lead to a corrosion fatigue failure of the part.

While man-made structures demonstrate proneness to corrosion in aqueous solutions of electrolytes, biological structural materials show a nearly complete chemical inertness in the fluid environment inside the body. Corrosion and corrosion fatigue have not become known or recognized in these materials, although mechanical fatigue has.

5) CREVICE CORROSION: In very thin cracks or crevices abnormal chemical environments can arise because the ionic diffusion processes that would normally allow rapid equilibration of a region on an implant surface with the extracellular fluid may become markedly retarded. Thus, in very small cracks on the surfaces of an implant, or in the crevice between a well fitting screw head and a plate, two things may happen. The oxygen dissolved in the local fluids may combine chemically with the surface atoms of the implant material, leading to an oxygen-poor fluid region in which ionization and solubilization of the implant atoms can occur, aided by some fretting. Or, the local chloride ion concentration may increase many fold and solubilize the oxide coating on the metal surface, and then solubilize the underlying metal atoms themselves. Such processes can lead to the development in these crevices of HCl and a local acid pH well below 3.5.

6) STRESS CORROSION: During the manufacturing processes internal stresses may become frozen into the substance of an implant, for example as a consequence of work hardening, age hardening or differential thermal expansion and contraction effects during cooling. The affected regions contain locked in energy and that potential energy makes them more reactive chemically in normal body fluids than stress relieved materials. Such regions can then undergo corrosive attack and, particularly if the corrosion tends to follow intergranular pathways (leading to what metallurgists call integranular corrosion) this can then serve as the starting point for a fatigue crack.

7) pH CORROSION: The pH of normal human extracellular fluid lies at about 7.39, or slightly on the alkaline side, and most metals used for implants dissolve in and tend to react chemically at slow rates in alkaline solutions. But in

a region of active infection the local pH may become as low as 5.2, or somewhat on the acid side of 7.0. In such an environment many metals corrode readily.

IV: HARDNESS

To a geologist or mineralogist this term usually signifies Moh's scale which rates the hardness of minerals and rocks on a scale of ten (diamond, the hardest substance known with a Moh hardness of 10) according to whether a given substance will scratch a known one, or vice versa. Moh's scale, and his system of determining hardness, functions most satisfactorily with nearly completely brittle, nonmalleable solids such as the crystalline forms of matter found in rocks, minerals and gemstones. In materials which possess some degree of malleability and/or ductility other bases for measurement can supply useful information.

Thus, an analogous property concerns metallurgists and manufacturers, but they measure it by different and much more accurate means. Typically, either a ball or a point serves to make an impression or dent in a material under a known and constant load applied at a constant and accurately controlled rate. One then measures the diameter of that impression under suitable magnification, and converts it to a numerical measure of the material's hardness by consulting the tables or scales provided with such instruments. One can obtain hardness testing equipment which provides fairly gross impressions, and other types which provide truly microscopic and accurately placed indentations that require testing and measuring under the high power compound microscope (called microhardness testing).

Given regular geometry of the testing ball or point used to make the impression, then it becomes clear that the diameter of a hardness testing impression provides a measure of the volume of metal (or other substance) displaced in making the impression. Equally it becomes clear that to displace such material one must make it flow in shear locally, and also distort it elastically in the region around the impression but not directly in contact with it. Thus hardness testing does not directly measure any single mechanical property of a material.

But other things remaining equal, by the hardness criteria a hard material as compared to a softer one will possess:

(a) *Greater resistance to wear and abrasion;* thus, for making the lockwork of firearms, the gears in many types of machinery, for knife edges and other cutting tools, and for bearing surfaces of most types, engineers choose hard materials. A high quality alloy knife blade will have a hardness (of the metal in its edge or cutting element) on the Rockwell "C" scale of 55–60, or even higher. The alloy in the blade usually was chosen to combat chemical corrosion by tissues. A carbon steel blade may have an even greater hardness of 60–65 but it will prove too brittle for most purposes, and it will rust quickly in most environments.

(b) *Greater strength in tension and compression;* true on the average but with exceptions. For example, some ceramic materials have considerable hardness yet prove quite weak in tension for reasons referred to briefly in the chapter on ceramics.

(c) *Greater toughness.* Here too one must qualify the statement. Thus steel of hardness 50 on the Rockwell "C" scale will prove much tougher than steel of hardness 65, for at the latter value the steel has become as brittle as glass, and excessively fragile. Note that the tensile strength of the steel at Rockwell 65 exceeds that at 50, which in turn exceeds that at 30.

In manufacture it often proves desirable to have great surface hardness to resist wear of moving parts, and simultaneously great toughness to resist impact and otherwise to take a great deal of mechanical punishment without breakage. Since hardness implies brittleness (antithetical to toughness) a manufacturer may make a part out of a very tough bulk material and then specially treat its surfaces with heat and chemicals to create a very hard but quite thin wear resistant skin. Such treatments include case hardening and nitriding, or work hardening the surface by peening it with hard metal balls, either blown against it by some form of air gun, or perhaps by tumbling in a rotating container.

Special Table 15 in Part III compares the numerical values of several hardness testing systems currently in use in industry.

With all of its problems, investigators such as Amprino in Italy (5) ; Carlstrom in Sweden (48) , and Blaimont in Belgium (32) have shown by microhardness testing that the hardness of old bone exceeds that of young (which makes the latter tougher) , and the hardness of subperiosteal bone falls below that of deeper layers (which stress relieves the surface fibers in flexural loading) , and that microhardness correlates well and directly with microradiographic estimates of bone density and mineral content per unit volume.

And, now, some test questions.

QUESTIONS: CHAPTER 10

1) In mechanical terms what distinguishes the liquid from the solid state?

2) a) Can fluids behave elastically in shear? b) can solids? c) can gasses?

3) a) Can a material's breaking strength lie below its greatest (i.e., ultimate) strength? b) Can a highly elastic material provide good damping of mechanical vibration or impact?

4) True or false: a) Brittleness means fragility. b) Resilience implies elasticity. c) Elasticity implies resilience. d) The proportional limit defines a shape factor that determines the strength of a structure. e) Mechanical fretting consists of internal damage to a structure.

5) Define mechanical fatigue.

Chapter 11

Statics

Having described some (and only some) of the basic stress-strain and other properties of matter serving as structural materials, let us now turn to a few basic situations we encounter in which real structures made of such matter, both artificial and biological, serve in buildings and machines. The shapes we construct with materials and the manner in which we use them impose their own demands upon matter, and upon the problems of design and analysis of the behavioral properties of intact structures and machines.

The branch of engineering called statics deals with stresses and strains in structures in which the external loads balance out so the structure does not exhibit acceleration. It may remain stationary as we view it (ex: a building, or a man standing still on the same ground as we stand on), or it may exist in a state of uniform and unchanging motion. Because such structures stay still or static, i.e., remain motionless, hence the term, statics.

Clearly these things form relative matters, because to an observer on Mars (to illustrate the point) both the building and the man would seem to gyrate madly around both the sun and the center of the earth-moon system, and the earth's center of daily rotation on its own axis. Examples of nonstatic structures (in our own frame of reference) would include a bow just after the archer let go of its string, or teenagers performing the latest dance, or the legs of a running man. Kinematics forms the study of moving structures, and will not receive formal consideration in this monograph. We will outline the distribution of stresses and strains in a few idealized beams, bones and tendons which carry various kinds of loads, and mention a few phenomena which deal with unbalanced forces and which also affect our grasp of clinically important phenomena.

For our present needs, two primary classes of loads on solids, and a combined class, arise.

I: PRIMARY LOADS

Of the primary loads we will consider two subgroups: the two uniaxial loads, plus the flexural and torque ones.

The *uniaxial loads* (to use conventional terminology) ideally generate corresponding stresses of only one kind, stresses furthermore distributed perfectly evenly throughout the material in the structure. On the other hand, *bending and torque* each generate unequal combinations of all three principal stresses in a material, and distribute the greatest stresses at the external surfaces and the least at some region inside the structure.

Combined loads generate stress distributions whose directions may prove difficult to deduce intuitively and whose amounts and orientations may prove hard to calculate, particularly in strain anisotropic materials such as bone, cartilage, tendon, fascia, ligament and teeth. In real structures, whether animate or inanimate, combined loads frequently arise and we will have a fair amount to say later about one particular widespread combination.

We will describe the stress-strain distributions caused by these loads in idealized form. One should understand that probably no real examples of these ideals exist, for imperfections in materials and our machines always lead to complex combinations of loading and stresses (and recall here how metals produce bulk plastic uniaxial compression strain by obliquely oriented shearing motion of microscopic dislocation systems). But since the artifice of considering the ideal has served quite satisfactorily the needs of clear communication, understanding and effective teaching for generations, we will continue to use it. The loading situations or arrangements we discuss below will include: uniaxial compression; uniaxial tension; static bending; cantilever bending; torque; combined loads; and hydraulic pressure in closed containers.

1) UNIAXIAL LOADS

(*a*) *Uniaxial compression*: On a solid cylinder made of a homogeneous material, as in Figure 11.01, the word uniaxial means exact centration of the load over the top of the cylinder so that it acts exactly in line with the geometric central axis of the cylinder.

Note: Structural members intended to carry primarily uniaxial compression loads constitute *columns* in engineering language. We say a bit more about columns and some of their problems in Appendix 9.

The following patterns of the three principal stresses arise in columns.

(1) *Compression*: In response to its superimposed load, a compression stress and strain develop, aligned parallel to the line of action of the superimposed load. Consequently

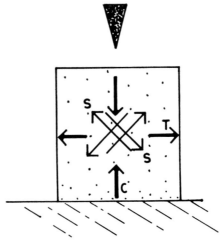

Figure 11.01. This diagram shows a homogeneous cylinder carrying a superimposed uniaxial compression load (black arrow above). This shortens it—a compression strain—which generates a compression stress within its matter (vertical arrow labelled C), one which actually supports the load and which distributes uniformly throughout it. At 90° to that, there arises a tension strain, associated with a comparable stress and also uniformly distributed. Finally, shearing stresses arise and have their maximum magnitude along a line of action lying at 45° from both the compression tension stresses. We omit here the tangential tension strain and stress shown in Figure 9.02.

the cylinder shortens somewhat, which constitutes a longitudinal compression strain (and one large enough to generate a total stress equal in magnitude to the value of the load).

(2) *Tension*: It also expands sideways, representing a transverse tension strain which reflects a transverse tension stress greatest in magnitude in a direction perpendicular to the line of action of the greatest compression stress and strain. Given a homogeneous solid (i.e., one possessing the property of stress-strain isotropy, or absence of any grain), then the unit tension stress equals the unit compression stress in this situation.

(3) *Shear*: Shear stress and strain also develop in this cylinder, and as we see it in the two-dimensional plane of the paper they reach their maximal magnitude along lines of action lying at 45 degrees to the line of action of the greatest compression and tension stress and strain. The unit shear stress equals half the magnitude of the unit compression or unit tension stresses. Note that when we include the third dimension in this consideration the shear distribution actually represents an infinite series of overlapping conical surfaces, each arising at the apex of some point within the material which interest us.

Note: In uniaxial compression loading, the stresses of each kind distribute evenly and equally throughout all the matter in the structure.

(b) *Uniaxial tension*: The typical example here constitutes a wire or rod holding up a suspended weight, as the figure illustrates. The following distribution of the three principal stresses arises in response to that load.

(1) *Tension*: The wire stretches or elongates, so it strains in tension and develops a corresponding internal tension stress, as shown in Figure 11.02.

Note: If the unit tension stress lies somewhere below the ultimate strength of the material in the wire or rod it will not break, but if the stress exceeds that limit it will then either fracture by pulling apart if made of a brittle substance,

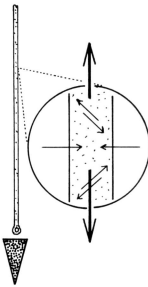

Figure 11.02. This homogeneous wire suspends a weight (below) from a support above, so that the earth's gravitational attraction for the weight applies a tension load on the wire. It develops the vertically aligned tension stress, horizontally aligned compression stress and obliquely aligned shearing stresses shown. As held true for the case of uniaxial compression, these stresses distribute uniformly through the matter in the wire. And note that no matter along what diameter one might choose to section the wire longitudinally to study the orientation of these stresses on the exposed cut faces, they would exactly duplicate this one.

or begin progressively to elongate and reduce simultaneously in diameter if made of a ductile substance, much like pulled taffy.

(2) *Compression*: Accompanying the elongation of the wire, it decreases in its outside diameter. This forms a transverse compression strain perpendicular to the tension strain, which implies a corresponding transverse compression stress. And in living tendon, exactly that transverse compression strain probably fires the so-called tension-sensitive nerve endings within it which help the central nervous system to monitor the dynamic mechanical forces that control musculoskeletal function. At the moment of rupture caused by overloading to failure in tension, the ratio of the decrease

in the outside diameter to the elongation of the wire would form Poisson's ratio, which in most metals usually approximates 0.3.

(3) *Shear*: In addition to the above described tension and compression stresses and strains, shear stresses also arise in this wire or rod. The shear stresses arise from shearing strains, and both achieve their greatest magnitude in a direction lying at 45 degrees from the directions of maximum tension. The unit shear stresses attain a value half that of the unit tension stress and strain.

Note: In uniaxial tension loading, the stresses of each kind distribute evenly and regularly throughout all of the material in the structure.

Note too: No uniaxial case of loading a rigid solid in shear exists.

2) FLEXURE AND TORQUE

In this and the following section we will consider two mechanical arrangements for causing flexure, and we will do so less out of respect for any engineering needs than because of an analytical situation encountered later on when we discuss the relationship between the mechanical loads applied to a growing bone and its gross structure or architecture. These two mechanical arrangements represent the static bending and the cantilever bending ones. Either bending arrangement can associate with either balanced (static) or unbalanced (dynamic) forces.

Note too: Engineers name a *beam* any structure designed to withstand flexure, and henceforth the term flexure will signify any kind of bending deformation.

(*a*) *Static bending arrangement*: Consider the beam in Figure 11.03, supported at each end and having a regular, rectangular cross section. A weight or any other equivalent load such as a tendon pull or muscle pull, applied at its middle and acting downwards, will make it sag slightly. In other words, it bends, or strains in flexure. Tension, compression and shear stresses and strains arise in this beam in the following pattern.

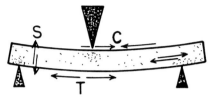

Figure 11.03. The distribution of stresses in a beam loaded in flexure by what this and the previous volume call the *static bending arrangement*. C: Compression, T: Tension, S: Shear.

(1) *Tension Stresses and Strain*: These appear in the bottom half of the beam, align parallel to the direction of its length, attain their largest values at the beam's bottom surface fibers, and in the horizontal plane that divides the beam into upper and lower halves, called the neutral plane, attain zero values.

(2) *Compression Stress and Strain*: These appear in the upper half of the beam, which shortens in overall length as the beam bends. This stress and strain also align parallel to the length of the beam, reach their largest values at the beam's uppermost surface fibers and at the neutral plane attain zero value.

(3) *Shear Stress and Strain*: Two directions of maximum shear arise in this beam. A vertically aligned shearing load (with a corresponding resisting stress) acts to displace downwards the middle parts of the beam relative to the outer parts which tend to move upwards. The resulting shearing strain added up over the whole length of the beam forms its gradual bend or curvature, seen on the upper and lower surfaces, as shown in Figure 11.04. Also, a horizontally aligned shearing stress and strain arise, visualized more clearly by visualizing the beam as actually made of vertically stacked loose boards (174). When a beam made in this way develops flexure, the ends of its boards displace as shown in the lower part of this figure. In a solid beam or bone, this slippage cannot occur but it tries to, and the internal resistance of the material to this form of strain or shearing displacement constitutes the horizontal shearing stress. The vertical shear

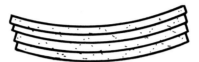

Figure 11.04. *Top:* A beam not carrying any load and made of stacked boards not glued or otherwise attached to each other, and so free to slide horizontally on each other.

Bottom: Upon accepting a load the beam develops flexural strain as shown. And in doing so the ends of the boards slide or shear-displace on each other in the manner shown; one sees the same thing in rolling up a magazine. In a solid beam of course this would not occur but only because an internal shearing stress arises which parallels the plane of these boards and resists that shearing displacement. That shearing stress makes the solid beam much stiffer in flexure than the layered or laminated type shown here.

stress and strain remain essentially equal at all vertical points on a given cross section, and this holds true along the whole length of a beam loaded in bending. However the horizontal shearing stress and strain vary, reaching their greatest values in the neutral plane and becoming zero at the top and bottom surface fibers.

Note: Maximal tension and compression stress and strain levels in structures loaded in flexure occur at their surface fibers, unlike the uniaxial loading cases where those stresses distribute evenly throughout the structure's substance.

(b) *Bending Moments:* At this juncture let us take time out to review in slightly more detail the forces just referred to and described verbally. When one applies a load sideways on the end of any lever (or lever arm) a tendency to rotate arises around the fulcrum, pivot, joint, bearing or whatever, a tendency called a *torque,* and one expresses it in terms such as inch-lb or kg-M or the like. In the drawing shown in Figure 11.05 the torque acting around the support would equal d times P inch-lb for example, whether it acted

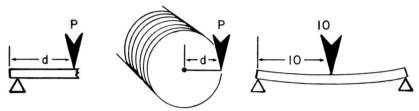

Figure 11.05. *Left:* A beam, supported by a fulcrum beneath its left hand end, carries a load P, located a distance d to the right of that fulcrum. Then the load generates a torque around the fulcrum, one of $d \times$ P length/weight units. Now any arrangement of the magnitude of the load and the distance (called the lever arm) which when multiplied has the identical numerical value will cause an identical torque, and any direct measuring device would register them all as equal.

Middle: That relationship applies equally to a shaft on the outer surface of which any force (or component of another force) acts tangential to (that means parallel to) the shaft's surface. So the torque here, again, equals $d \times$ P length/weight units.

Right: Here a clockwise torque equalling 10×10 length/weight units arises around the fulcrum on the left. But it does not actually rotate this beam because now an upwards reaction arises at the right hand fulcrum, an additional force which acts to neutralize that torque.

on the beam at the left, or on the outer surface of the pulley shaft at the middle. Thus exactly equal torques arise in the following combinations, randomly chosen from all possible ones just to illustrate the point, expressing d in feet and P in pounds for the moment:

$$d \times p = T \text{ in-lb}$$
$$1 \times 10 = 10 \text{ in-lb}$$
$$10 \times 1 = 10 \text{ in-lb}$$
$$2 \times 5 = 10 \text{ in-lb}$$
$$0.1 \times 100 = 10 \text{ in-lb}$$

Whenever anything restrains the ability of a whole beam or shaft to accelerate or to rotate uniformly in response to such a load, a system of forces will arise within the matter of the structure called moments which resist that acceleration. Those forces represent a special distribution of stresses in the beam's fibers accompanied by corresponding strains. To explain them let us define two conditions of static equilibrium:

(c) Laws of Static Equilibrium:

If two or more forces known to act on a body, and which meet or diverge from a common point in it (the coplanar condition), do not accelerate it, then the sums of all their resultants along two mutually perpendicular axes must equal zero. Equally, their vectorial sums must equal zero. Figure 11.06 illustrates an example.

If two or more torques act on a body but do not accelerate it, their sums must equal zero. Recall that a torque or moment equals a force multiplied by its lever arm.

Note: These two conditions remain true whether the body remains stationary or in a state of uniform motion relative to an outside observer.

Figure 11.06 illustrates at the top right a lever on which three forces act, labelled P, Q and W. If the lever lies in static equilibrium then the sums of the torques or moments, around any axis, must equal zero. If we take the moment sums around point *a*, then we have, using the small letters to specify the lever arms and capitals the loads:

$$\text{(ab)} \ Q - \text{(ac)} \ W = 0$$

Note that we omit (a) P. We do so for a simple reason: *a* equals zero, so (*a*) P must equal zero, and including a zero term in the above relation only clutters it up without changing the value of its numerical solution. Note too that we arbitrarily (but quite legitimately) designate a tendency to clockwise rotation as a negative torque, and the opposite as a positive one. Or, if we take moments around point *c*:

$$- \text{(ac)} \ P + \text{(bc)} \ Q = 0$$

Note now the missing (c) W term, for reasons just given. As for the magnitudes of the loads, in the situation diagrammed it seems clear that in order for equilibrium to exist the following must hold true:

$$Q = P + W; \text{ and so } P = Q - W;$$
$$\text{and } W = Q - P$$

Couples: Consider now the loads Q and W acting alone

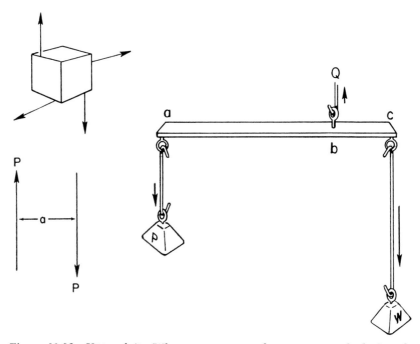

Figure 11.06. *Upper left:* When two or more forces act on a body but do not accelerate it, then first it exists in static equilibrium, and second the vectorial sums of those forces must equal zero, i.e., they must all neutralize, whether one determines this by simple vectorial addition using the parallelogram laws, or by summing up all of their components parallel to orthogonal coordinates (one may locate those coordinates *anywhere* in the plane of the paper and it still holds true).

Upper right: A lever carrying the loads P, Q and W applied at points *a, b* and *c* respectively. See the text.

Bottom: When two equal forces parallel in line of action but antiparallel in direction and separated by any distance *a* arise, we call it a *couple,* and it creates a torque equal to *a* P length/weight units.

on the lever. They act parallel to each other but in opposite directions, and obviously tend to rotate the lever clockwise around any point between *b* and *c*. Thus at point *a* they will exert a reaction upwards (R), opposite in direction but equal in magnitude to load P, given the earlier condition that with all three loads applied it exists in static equilibrium.

When two such parallel forces opposite in direction also have equal magnitudes we say they form a couple. Figure

11.06 at its lower left shows a couple acting on a lever of length *a*. The torque value of such a couple always conforms to this relation:

$$T = Pa \qquad\qquad \textit{Equation 11.01}$$

Where *a* signifies the perpendicular distance between the lines of action of the two forces. Let us now analyze a few specific situations to illustrate how the above material works. The following formula relates the stress in the uppermost and lowermost surface fibers of a beam (σ), the vertical distance of those fibers from the beam's neutral axis (y), and the flexural moments (M) at a given cross sectional plane:

$$\sigma = \frac{My}{I} \qquad\qquad \textit{Equation 11.02}$$

The "I" term signifies the rectangular moment of inertia or "I_0", and constitutes a figure of merit expressing how effectively a given cross sectional shape resists bending forces. The larger the value, the more effectively a given shape utilizes structural material to carry flexural loads. The accompanying figure (Fig. 11.07) illustrates I_0 for two cross sectional shapes of prominent concern in human skeletal biomechanics. Special Table 17 in Part III provides some formulas for I_0, J_0 (the polar moment of inertia used in computing torque stresses) and the radius of gyration used in computing column stresses at the point of buckling. For hollow cross sections (that is, box sections for the left one), simply compute I_0 for the inner or hollow part, and then subtract it from I_0 for the entire outer part. The equations accompanying those two figures make the following important points clear:

As one increases the vertical height of the cross section of a beam of rectangular cross section one increases by the cubed power of that increase its flexural strength and by the fourth power that of a cylinder or hollow tube. And equation 11.02 also means that one decreases by equally large and comparable amounts the maximum stresses at the surface fibers. Thus simply by doubling its depth one increases 8

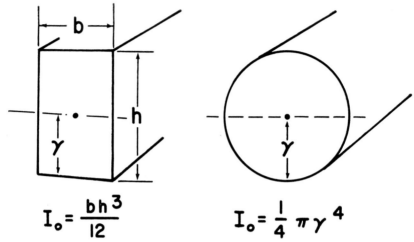

$$I_o = \frac{bh^3}{12} \qquad\qquad I_o = \frac{1}{4}\pi\gamma^4$$

Figure 11.07. The formulas for computing I_o, the rectangular moments of inertia, for purposes of calculating a beam's flexural stresses with the aid of the beam-flexure formulas.

Left: For any rectangular cross section, where b equals the horizontal width, y the vertical depth above or below the neutral plane, and h the total vertical depth. Note that the answer comes out as a length to the fourth power.

Right: For circular cross sections, where y equals the radius. Note again that the answer comes out as a length raised to the fourth power (i.e., in⁴, cm⁴, ft⁴, etc.).

We might point out here that when the material of a beam has different Young's moduli in compression and tension the neutral plane no longer lies in the middle of the beam's cross section. It lies closer to the side of the greater modulus. But this phenomenon forms a minor concern in this text's objectives and we need say no more of it.

fold the flexural strength of a rectangular beam, and 16 fold the strength of a cylinder.

Now let us compute surface stress for a particular case to illustrate roughly how this business works, and then drop the matter, for more detailed explanations appear in introductory texts in mechanics and engineering and this text intends not to make an engineer out of its readers but simply to give them some useable idea or feel for how these matters work.

Assume then on the right of Figure 11.05 that the beam actually represents a cylindrical and solid bone (not accounting for the marrow cavity introduces only a trivial error in the computed result, averaging less than one part in ten for the midshaft of most long bones) with an outside diameter of two inches. Thus I_0 equals $\frac{1}{4} \pi$ (y = one, and one raised to the fourth power still equals one). Thus substitute that value of I_0 in equation 11.02. As for the "y" term in its denominator, that—still—equals one. The M stands for the moments within the beam, which must equal that applied to it. Under the load of ten lb, acting on a lever arm of ten inches, that equals one hundred inch-lb. So we now have $\sigma = \dfrac{100 \times 1}{\frac{1}{4} \pi} =$ approximately 120 psi of tension stress in the bottom fibers, and of compression stress in the top fibers. Given that live bone has a compression strength of 12,000 psi, and a tension strength of 10,000 psi, and no great danger of breakage appears inherent in this situation. Note that if the bone's outside diameter were only one inch, the surface stresses would rise to some 1900 psi, yet still lie well within safe limits.

(*d*) *Cantilever bending arrangement*: Figure 11.08 shows a special flexural situation or arrangement in which a bending load develops on an erect beam by setting a compression load on an arm jutting off to one side of the structure's neutral plane. This eccentric load gives rise to stresses which we can conveniently consider as the sum of the two separate following parts.

(1) A uniaxial compression load lying on top of the beam equal to the load. It causes compression stress and strain exactly like that previously described for uniaxial compression loading which distributes evenly throughout the substance of the column-beam (i.e., along its length and throughout any cross section), as shown by the arrows inside the beam.

(2) Plus a separate bending load or torque which tries to rotate the beam clockwise in the manner and particular example shown. This torque creates tension stress and strain

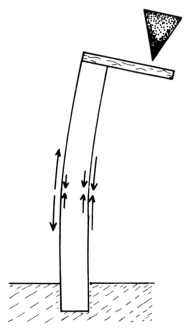

Figure 11.08. This illustrates a *cantilever bending arrangement,* constituting an eccentric (i.e., to the side of the beam's center or neutral plane) application of a compression load. One may obtain the actual distribution of stresses in its surface fibers by the following simple analytical artifice.

First, determine the unit compression stresses caused by considering it a uniaxial load.

Second, to those surface stresses add those arising from the torque the load generates around its lever arm, which equals its distance from the beam's center line, here termed the *eccentricity.* As the arrows illustrate these will constitute a tension stress on the left side and a compression on the right. Their arithmetic sums with the uniaxial compression stress on each side (noting that tensions equal minus values), will then essentially correctly describe the total surface-fiber stresses in any real beam loaded in this manner.

(negative quantities here) on the left side of the beam which therefore subtract from the uniaxial compression stress and strain (positive quantities) already there from (*a*) above. It also adds compression stress and strain to the right side. For each side the remaining or actual total stress will then represent the arithmetic summation of the two components.

The bending or rotating tendency increases when the sideways distance from the beam's center axis to the point of application of the load (i.e., the eccentricity) increases.

Usually flexural moments can generate rather large surface flexural stresses in comparison to the magnitude of the load actually causing the flexure. We recognize this intuitively when we elect to break a stick by bending it to failure, rather than by trying to pull it apart in pure, brute tension. In flexure it still fails in tension on the convex tending side but now as a consequence of flexurally induced stresses. Recall the example computed in the previous section in which a total load of 10 lb could generate more than half a ton of flexural stress in the surface fibers of a one inch diameter bone, if made of homogeneous material. In Part II we will discover one of nature's subtle design changes which reduces maximum surface flexural stresses (but not strains) in living bone, and so makes it actually (and significantly, to the extent of some 30%–40%) stronger in flexure than any manmade structure of identical shape, dimensions and homogeneous material.

(*e*) *Torque*: This, meaning a twist like that arising in a shaft turned by a motor to drive a machine, generates the stress and strain patterns shown in Figure 11.09.

(1) *Tension Stress and Strain*: These become greatest in degree in a direction lying at 45 degrees to the longitudinal axis of the shaft. Furthermore, they reach their greatest values at the shaft's surface fibers and become zero on its neutral axis, which equates with the central, longitudinal axis of the shaft. Witness that if loaded in flexure a neutral *plane* arises, while for a shaft or bone carrying torque a neutral *line* or axis arises.

(2) *Compression Stress and Strain*: These reach their greatest magnitudes at 90 degrees from the tension stress and strain, and also at 45 degrees from the longitudinal axis of the shaft. Like tension, they become greatest at the shaft's surface fibers, and zero on its neutral axis.

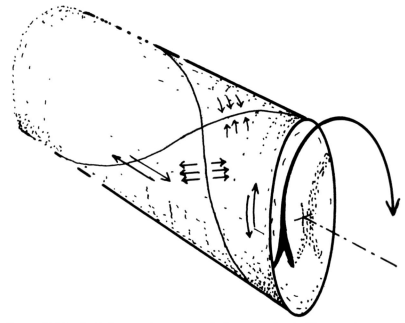

Figure 11.09. A shaft carrying an applied torque load (the curving arrow at the right), develops all of the three principal stresses within its substance. Their maximum values align as shown. Note that both compression and tension stresses now align at 45° to the long axis (but still at 90° to each other), while, as in flexural loading, two planes of shear arise at 90° to each other and at 45° from the tension and compression stresses, and so one parallel to and one perpendicular to the long axis (neutral axis) of the shaft.

(3) *Shear Stress and Strain*: These arise in two planes lying at right angles to each other. A transverse shearing strain in effect tries to twist the ends apart in a plane perpendicular to the longitudinal axis of the shaft. A longitudinal shearing strain in effect tries to displace one side of the shaft north, the other south, as in Figure 11.09, and aligns parallel to the longitudinal axis. Both of these systems of stress and strain become maximal at the surface fibers of the shaft and zero on its neutral axis.

Remember: The surface fibers of structures loaded in torque carry the largest stresses and develop the greatest strains.

(4) *Polar moment of inertia*: This constitutes a figure of merit expressing how well a given cross section can carry torque loads. It performs for structures loaded in torque the same function that I_o does for flexural loading. The formula for computing it for a circular cross section follows:

$$J_o = \frac{d^4}{32} \qquad \text{\textit{Equation 11.03}}$$

Where d signifies the diameter of the section. Observe that as one doubles the shaft diameter he increases 16 fold (i.e., by 2^4 power) its strength in torque. For hollow cylinders (such as bones) one simply computes J_o separately for the cross section of the lumen and subtracts it from J_o for the whole outside diameter (See Special Table 17 in Part III). Given that, then the maximum shearing stress in a shaft carrying torque (only) equals:

$$\sigma = \frac{Tr}{J_o} \qquad \text{\textit{Equation 11.04}}$$

Where r signifies the radius of the shaft, and T the torque in units such as inch-lb. Recall that, as holds generally true for all formulas in this book, whatever units the answer comes out in will depend upon the units in which one expresses the numbers used for its various terms.

Of course when one applies a torque to a shaft it strains in torque, and by an amount that relates to its stiffness. In fact, a twist of θ radians, given torque T, length of shaft L and shear modulus E, can be computed with this equation:

$$\theta = \frac{T\,L}{E_s\,J_o} \qquad \text{\textit{Equation 11.05}}$$

II: COMBINED LOADS

In real structures, both animate and inanimate, loading conditions seldom present pure situations, and usually combine the three primary kinds of loads, that is, uniaxial, flexural and torque. Bending, uniaxial compression and internal hydraulic effects as well often combine in nature. These

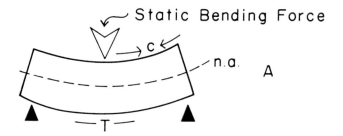

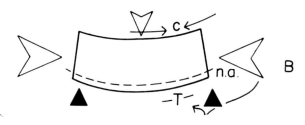

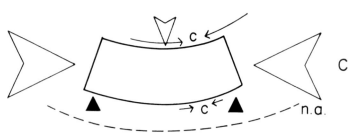

Figure 11.10. *Top:* A beam carrying a *flexural load,* and developing the flexural strain and stress patterns previously described. Note location of the neutral axis (n.a.).

Middle: Now, while maintaining the flexural load, add some end compression load. The unit compression stresses it adds equally over the cross section will augment the flexurally derived one on the top surface fibers but will subtract from the tension stresses in the bottom fibers. Observe that the neutral axis (actually a plane in the case of flexure of a beam) has now moved towards the convex tending surface, downwards here.

combinations can increase stresses in some parts and directions of the structure, and relieve them at others, in ways that may prove difficult to divine by intuition alone. Four such combinations outlined next commonly occur in the musculoskeletal system.

1) Combined Uniaxial Compression and Flexure: One of the commonest loading combinations in nature, it arises in most bones as well as in arthropod exoskeletons, in trees, in building columns and in the earth's crust. See Figure 11.10. Here, a flexureal load of the static bending arrangement causes tension stress at the bottom surface fibers, compression at the top (216). When a uniaxial compression load (and here a horizontally acting one) adds to the flexural one, the stresses it adds will act to cancel out some of the original tension stress (one considers compression stresses as positive values, tension as negative ones), and to boost the original compression ones. Given the proper ratio between the two loads and both surfaces can end up carrying net compression stress and strain, although in unequal amounts. Consequently one can have a bone developing a dynamic flexural strain without any tension stress developing anywhere along its surface fibers. This situation or one very near to it arises quite commonly if not usually in the healthy, active skeleton.

Bottom: Increase the uniaxial end or compression load even further, so that the stress it creates now exceeds the magnitude of the flexural tension stress on the lower fibers. By this means one adds enough compression to the bottom fibers that it now contains a net compression stress. Thus we now have a flexural loading situation in which no tension stress exists in the structure; and one in which the neutral plane has now moved outside the structure to become a *virtual* n.a. (that is what mathematicians call something when it "disappears" but yet in principle still should exist somewhere). Recall that the n.a. signifies that plane of zero compression and tension stress (*not* the plane of zero shear stress).

Witness: The bottom situation exemplifies the actual and typical loading situation in the long bones of all vertebrate mammalian endoskeletons, and also in exoskeletons of all insects, arthropods and the like. Furthermore, exactly that combination makes the flexural neutralization principle described in Part II work.

2) PRESSURE WITHIN CLOSED CONTAINERS: From the standpoint of its cortical walls, a bone forms a closed container, somewhat like a soup can, but into which (unlike a soup can) blood enters under varying arterial pressure some eighty times a minute. At each systolic pulse pressure wave (which equals about 140mm of mercury, or .185 atmosphere) the walls of the container bulge minutely, thereby stretching its circumference. And each time one stands up on his lower extremities, his body weight in effect tries to drive the wedge shaped piston of metaphyseal spongiosa in the proximal tibial metaphysis down into the enveloping cortical enclosure. As a result of such loads tension stress and strain develop parallel to and circumferentially around these walls, and compression stress and strain develop perpendicular to their surfaces. The thicker the walls of such containers, the less the unit stresses and strains in them, while the larger the volume inside the container, the greater the total tension load, stress and strain in the walls.

In the example illustrated in Figure 11.11 a hollow sphere contains an internal medium under pressure. The pressure tends to burst or explode the sphere while the tensile strength of its walls resist that tendency (210). The total load acting to burst it equals the area of the circle exposed by hemisect-

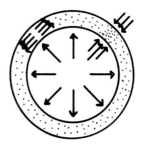

Figure 11.11. A hollow spherical vessel containing a fluid under pressure within it, and then cut in half, illustrates the manner in which the shell of such a vessel strains, and the stresses developed in it. Analogous situations arise in the skull in response to the systolic pressure wave, and in metaphyseal and vertebral central regions of the skeleton under dynamic loading.

ing or cutting the sphere in half, i.e., $\frac{1}{4}$ π D^2, multiplied by the unit pressure, σ, or:

$$P = \sigma \; \frac{1}{4} \; \pi \; D^2 \qquad\qquad Equation \; 11.06$$

Now, P, the total bursting load acting on the area of the sphere's wall exposed by the hemisection, reduces to the unit load by dividing by the area of that wall. Verbally: unit tension load on wall of hollow sphere = (cross section area of outer diameter) — (cross section area of inner diameter) divided into total pressure, P.

3) FLEXURE AND TORQUE: As already noted, both of these forms of loading generate maximal stresses at the surface fibers of the structure. Consequently the tension stress due to the flexural load can add (vectorially speaking) to that

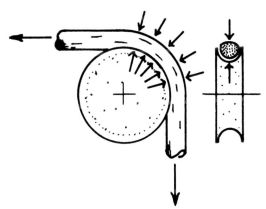

Figure 11.12. A tendon running around an anatomical pulley develops many of the strain and stress patterns found in a rope running around a man-made pulley. Thus a compression strain shortens its vertical diameter parallel to a radius from the pulley as shown, while a tension strain expands its transverse diameter. These produce the intuitively obvious shearing strains. In addition, longitudinal shearing strains arise which attain their maximal values in the middle of the tendon and which may account for some of the fibroma-like reactions that lead to trigger fingers and one type of De Quervain's disease.

Note: In anatomical pulleys the tendon *slides* on the underlying bone and a hydrodynamic-style lubrication mechanism minimizes the ensuing wear. The self-repair mechanisms described in later chapters correct what wear does arise so that normally net wear equals zero.

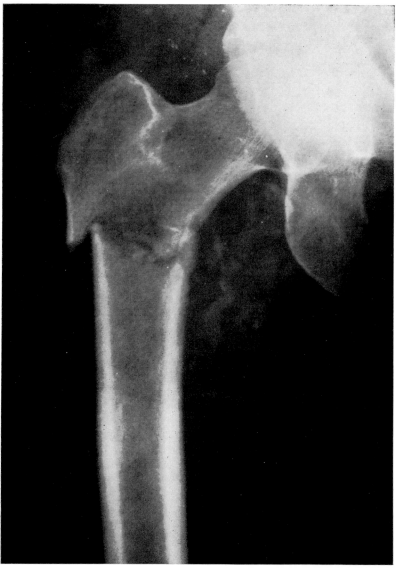

Figure 11.13. This gentleman fell on and "hurt" his hip. He hurt it so much in fact that after several weeks (during which he worked every day as a salesclerk) he came to our E.R. for advice, whereupon this x-ray was taken. Given then that his body weight represented a superimposed compression load on the femoral head and one considerably eccentric to the shaft, why did the fracture not angulate and go into varus?

arising from the torque, causing the direction of greatest tension stress, or its resultant, to lie somewhere intermediate between the vectors representing either stress alone. The compression and shearing stresses add in the same manner. For a given sized load, *much larger surface stresses arise by combining bending and torque than by any other two load combination.* And, of some interest, it seems that many bone fractures caused by accidents of various kinds probably follow such load combinations which, in effect, apply load combinations and kinds the bones were not designed to carry.

4) TENSION PLUS FLEXURE: When a rope running around a pulley, or a tendon curving over the anatomical equivalent (peroneals at the lateral malleolus; finger flexors through the pulleys in the hand) also carries a tension load, a complex of strains and stresses arises which helps to understand some of the clinical pathology arising in such tendons.

As the drawing in Figure 11.12 illustrates, longitudinal tension strains arise which attain their maximal degree on the convex surface. A transverse compression strain arises which decreases the diameter in that direction running towards the pulley's axis. This causes the horizontal diameter to increase, so that the rope or tendon develops an oval cross section where it lies against the pulley. Note that while this increased transverse diameter represents a tension strain, it arises because of an internal compression load acting at right angles to it, and accompanies an internal compression stress. This situation illustrates a point that becomes important when we consider certain biodynamic responses of skeletal

---

Clearly we see a condition of static equilibrium. And so, even though the x-rays do not show them, the contractural forces of the proximally inserted adductor muscles must have generated an opposite static-bending-arrangement set of moments which neutralized the cantilever-arrangement ones the x-ray and his body weight confront us with.

Not the usual consequence of such a chain of events, nevertheless this one proves instructive and should you feel uncomfortable or unsafe about this way of deducing cause from effect, you better practice some, because it works and you can use it (!).

tissues to mechanical loads, and represents one reason for preferring to discuss things in terms of strain rather than of stress as the basic operative parameter.

Finally, the rope traveling around the pulley develops transverse and longitudinal shearing strains. The longitudinal shear, maximal in the middle of the tendon, lies where small fibromatous hyperplasias can arise (called xanthomata and/or fibromata) in the flexor tendons of the hand, causing binding of the tendon within its sheath. This condition has become known as trigger finger.

Now see Figure 11.13.

QUESTIONS: CHAPTER 11

1) Name the primary classes of mechanical loads.
2) What constitutes a mechanical moment?
3) a) What does the rectangular moment of inertia, I_o, define? b) and the polar moment of inertia, J_o?
4) a) As defined in the text, cantilever bending relates the change in load with time to the flexural strain. True or false? b) Static bending as defined herein means a constant, unchanging load. True or false?
5) What manner of loading a structure most effectively threatens to break it?
6) List some of the special bulk properties one can obtain with fiber-reenforced structural materials.
7) In obtaining an optimum match strength-wise between matrix and fiber in uniaxial loading, what ratio constitutes the fundamental one?
8) Do dislocations emerge as important in the bulk properties of fiber-reenforced materials, given fibers of minute diameter?
9) The subject: your right elbow, flexed to a 90° angle, while you push hard towards the left on the handle of a wrench attached to a rusted tight nut on your car wheel (a flat tire on a night out with your darlin'). Clearly the muscles attached to the upper end of your humerus must

apply a very considerable torque to it, and that torque must transfer across your elbow joint. Now:

a) The torque must tend to open up the elbow on its medial side. Given your freshman anatomy, how would you prevent it from opening up?

b) The torque transmitted through the humerus tends to cause a spiral fracture of that bone, and our bones do not demonstrate any great strength in torque, tending to fracture along the perpendicular to the tension resultant which lies at 45° to the long axis. But of course the humerus does not fracture (although the bolt may) so your date will not end with you in a hospital. Why?

c) The torque transmitted to the lever arm of the fore-arm bones tends to strain them in flexure, convexly towards your left. But they don't so strain. Why?

d) Obviously you don't think about these matters as you lean on that wrench; rather you probably think about the persnicketyness of a malicious fate in making your tire flat on that of all nights. Yet these things occur automatically, with unerring consistency and with dazzling effectiveness. Any inferences to draw?

Chapter 12

Bearings

Let us now consider what actually represents a machine (for man-made bearings fall into that category). We will do so for several reasons, all related to the basic purpose of this book. A brief discussion of bearings will serve us thus:

It will make clear their basic and primal purpose, separate from all properties subsidiary to that purpose.

It will introduce some material on friction (265), which we need to understand joints.

It can convey at least the basic ideas underlying joint design, so that one can more easily grasp the nuances nature found in solving problems common to both joints and machine bearings.

Let us begin with a bearing's usual function.

Bearing Function: All bearings, whether artificially made or natural, have as one basic overriding function *allowing one rigid part to move on another*. A major subobjective that such a mechanism should satisfy to constitute a practical and economical one: it must endure a long time in the face of much use. And to achieve that two subproperties must appear and, in order of decreasing importance, consist of: (*a*) *Achieving minimal net wear* of the bearing surfaces; (*b*) and achieving *minimal friction*, i.e., mechanical resistance to motion (248). Here again lay experience tends to get us in trouble, for that experience has led most people to consider reduction of friction as the prime purpose of bearings, when in fact it simply constitutes a third order function underlying the true and overriding one as just stated. Table 12.01 lists some of the design priorities found in bearing construction and, equally if in analogy, in our own joints.

TABLE 12.01
DESIGN PRIORITIES OF MECHANICAL JOURNALS

First order function (1°f) :		To allow one solid object to move on another;		
2nd ° f:		To last a long time,		
3rd ° f:		And minimize wear,		
4th ° f:		And minimize friction		
5th ° f:	Smooth bearing surface	Rigid alignment of bearing surface	Lubricant	
6th ° f:	Physical properties of bearing material	backing under-neath bearing surface	Physical properties	Chemical properties	Pumping mechanism

1) THE JOURNAL: Many different kinds of bearings appear in engineering practice* but here we will consider only one, for it best analogizes the bearing mechanisms found in the human musculoskeletal system and so most aptly serves as a jumping off point in clarifying a few major design features of those living mechanisms. Engineers call such a bearing a journal. A journal uses a thin film of lubricating liquid, pumped in between its moving surfaces under pressure, to float and thus keep the moving metal bearing surfaces from touching each other. When those surfaces do touch, rapid and destructive wear ensues due to tiny upwards projecting regions from each surface where abrasion goes on, and others where seizure occurs as welding of the contacting regions actually plucks material out of one or both of the bearing surfaces (37). And while we can replace worn out machine bearings, that practice in human joints still meets with little favor on the part of its recipients, and furthermore still fails to provide a replacement possessing the most valuable attributes of our own joints: reliable, durable, painless, normal function. Remember then that bearings have the major purposes of allowing one part to move on another. In order to last a useful period of time, this must occur with as little net wear as possible, and subsidiary to that objective one should reduce friction because most of the things that increase friction also increase wear. But to review some material com-

---

* For example, ball and roller bearings; keyways; magnetic, pneumatic, and dry.

ing up later, decreasing friction formed only one of several devices nature has used to decrease *net* wear.

(*a*) *Journal Construction*: A mechanical journal has five parts (see Figure 12.01) : a rotating shaft (S) of some strong material; (B) a fixed, curved backing also made of strong material which fits around the shaft, partially or wholly; (BA) a thin layer of soft metal called Babbitt and soundly bonded to the backing, to provide the physical surface on which the shaft actually rests; a lubricant which flows between the moving shaft and the stationary Babbitt to separate or float their moving surfaces; and some sort of pumping mechanism which assures a continuous flow of lubricant between the moving bearing surfaces. In order for the lubricant to perform its major task of keeping the metal surfaces apart, the geometry of a journal's surfaces must satisfy two underlying conditions; accurate concentricity of those surfaces somehow must exist and persist under all operating conditions, and they must have sufficiently large areas to reduce the unit compression loads carried by the fluid film between them below the point at which the shaft can penetrate that film to touch the Babbitt, given the operating loads and shaft surface speeds expected, and given the known limitations of the lubricant's physical and chemical properties.

(*b*) *The Lubricant*: In order to help preserve the fluid film under slow speed or start-and-stop conditions, it helps

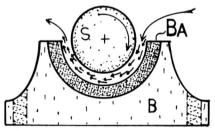

Figure 12.01. The elements of a mechanical journal seen in cross section. It consists of a shaft (S) turning on a Babbitt bearing surface (BA), supported by a rigid (usually steel) backing (B). Lubricant continuously supplied in fresh quantities at the trailing edge on the right "floats" the shaft on the Babbitt.

if the lubricant bonds chemically to the surfaces of the bearing, for that makes it resist being scrubbed or wiped off. One can achieve this by suitable choices of bearing and lubricant chemistry. If possible the lubricant should actually permeate the surface layers of the bearing material. This bonding and permeation make it hard to rub off all of the lubricant molecules as the starting shaft turns, and it greatly reduces starting friction. Bearing surfaces usually do touch and rub on each other to some extent when the shaft starts to turn (due to starting friction), and this causes wear. For that reason some expensive cars have a starting-timing sequence in which the engine's oil pump begins functioning before the starter motor engages, and only after oil pressure in the channels feeding lubricant to the bearings has risen to operating levels does the starter then turn the crankshaft.

(c) *The Babbitt*: When two bare and dry metal surfaces touch, no matter how smooth they may seem to the eye they contact each other only at microscopic surface irregularities or high spots or asperities. These projections have such small area in comparison to the whole area of the bearing (typically 0.1% of it) that the bearing load concentrates heavily on them, leading to microscopic unit loading values that can actually pressure weld them together. Thus a bearing surface carrying say 150 lb/in^2 of load may rest on only .002 part of each in^2, raising the unit loads on those asperities to some 75,000 psi. Motion beginning across such welds will then literally pluck small bits of material out of one or both of the surfaces, and that represents wear. It also makes starting friction depend upon (the mathematician says: "a function of") the mechanical strength of the bearing materials, particularly to shearing and tensile loading. Once the shaft begins moving, then if one of the bearing surface materials has a lower melting point than the other, the heat of their frictional motion upon physical contact simply temporarily melts the lower melting point asperities. The resulting wear first decreases compared to that of a dry bearing with two surfaces of equal melting point materials, and second, it concentrates upon the softer material. This makes the moving friction of a dry bearing a function of the melting points and specific and latent heats of the bearing materials. For this reason metal sliding on plastic—such as nylon—bearings see increasing use in the manufacture of machines; the relatively low melting point of the plastic protects the metal surface. Car designers solved that one by making the softer bearing materials replaceable.

When two identical metal surfaces slide on each other a combination occurs of pressure welding-plucking out of asperities, of abrasion or grinding of one surface by asperities on the other, and by shearing displacement of one asperity under the hammer of a larger one. These processes produce a very finely powdered debris of metal particles, the result of wear due to sliding friction. We shall hear more of this in Part II, although briefly.

(*d*) *The Lubricant Pumping Mechanism*: A fluid lubricated turning shaft pressed towards the Babbitt enveloping it tends to squeeze the lubricant out from between the bearing surfaces so they can touch. Consequently, something must constantly pump fresh supplies of lubricant between the surfaces, a requirement met in a number of ways in machines. For example, a separate pump may do the job; or oil soaked porous material may lie in contact with part of its surface to constantly wipe on a layer of new lubricant; or the moving parts may lie submerged in oil in a liquid tight system as in modern automobile gear boxes.

(*e*) *Surface Concentricity*: The problem of maintaining the bearing surfaces essentially parallel and evenly spaced over wide areas, one encountered in making man-made journals last, nature has solved in an unusual way in our own joints. But as for journals, the axes of the shaft on one side and the backing on the other must remain precisely parallel to each other under all operating conditions. Otherwise at one edge or corner of the journal the shaft would rub so hard against the Babbitt that it would break the lubricant film, leading to rapid and destructive wear (see Figure 12.02), and less good remaining bearing surface to carry on after-

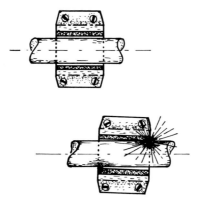

Figure 12.02. Looking down on top of a journal, one can see that when the bearing surfaces of shaft and Babbitt remain accurately concentric the full area of lubricant film between them can act to prevent contact and excessive wear. But even a relatively small malalignment as in the bottom drawing can cause metal to metal contact at one edge, drastically increasing the wear rate and decreasing the useful life of the bearing. This wear also generates heat and particulate debris, representing particles of the bearing surface abraded or plucked out of the body of the bearing metals.

wards. Accordingly, we make bearings in machines large, massive and rigid to maintain alignment of its parts under all load conditions. The requirement of maintaining concentricity derives from the fact that a thin film of a given lubricant can take only so much squeeze per cm² or in² without disrupting, and anything in excess of that can lead to bearing surface contact and accelerated wear. We will describe nature's solutions to some of these problems later; engineers might find food for thought in them.

2) FRICTION: In general friction signifies the resistance of one material body to moving on another lying in physical contact with it. We recognize a variety of types of friction but the present remarks will focus primarily on only a few of them.

Pushing a chair across a smooth floor takes more push to start it than to keep it moving once it has been started. This high resistance to maintaining motion thereafter represents moving friction. A major cause of starting friction arises from the fact that at rest, the two surfaces (floor and chair leg) stick together chemically or even weld together at many microscopic places. Any motion between them breaks these bonds, implying (correctly) that starting friction should depend on the mechanical strengths of the two bearing materials. In moving friction, the microscopic high spots or asperities either grind each other down, or if the melting points of the materials of the two bearing surfaces differ, the high spots of the one with the lower melting point will simply melt, implying (correctly) that moving friction of dry bearings depends on the shearing strengths or the melting points of the bearing surface materials.

The coefficient of friction signifies that fraction of the total load transferred perpendicularly across the bearing surfaces that proves required to keep its surfaces moving at a uniform rate. It usually forms a constant fraction of a total load in the face of a considerable range of variations in the total loads, but in human joints it does not because of the nonNewtonian property of our joint lubricant. Table 12.02 shows some coefficients of friction.

Engineers recognize still other kinds of friction. We mentioned starting and moving friction; in addition, dry friction exists when no fluid lubricant is used, while rolling friction applies to roller and ball bearings, sliding friction applies to boundary layer situations (see below), and fluid friction applies to hydrodynamic ones (see below).

3) PROPERTIES OF FRICTION: Some rather general properties of friction apply primarily to unlubricated, dry bearing surfaces and to most (but not all) ordinary situations.

TABLE 12.02
COEFFICIENTS OF FRICTION*

Gold on Gold	.2	Nylon on Nylon	.3
Aluminum on Aluminum	.8	Teflon	.1
Iron on Iron	1.0	Methacrylate	.5
Chromium on Chromium	.4	Teflon in sintered copper	
Steel on Ice	.03	on same material	.05
Steel on Copper	2.5	Sapphire on Sapphire	.2
Graphite on Graphite	.1	Sapphire on Steel	.15
Hydrodynamic lubrication	.01–.001	Ball Bearing	.01–.001
Bone on steel (dry) 162	.1 –.2	Boundary layer	.1

* The number forms the decimal fraction of the load transferred across the bearing, and needed to keep the bearing moving at constant speed.

(*a*) The force we name friction acts parallel to the contacting surfaces, and thus perpendicularly to any loading force transmitted perpendicularly across those surfaces. In machines and in the moving surfaces of the human skeletal surfaces those perpendicular forces (engineers like to call them normal forces, for in geometry the word normal often means perpendicular to) constitute compression loads.

(*b*) The magnitude of the frictional force represents some decimal fraction of the perpendicular or normal forces and that remains true independently of the total area of the bearing surface. Thus given that the coefficient of friction for a given bearing equals 0.2, and that a load of 100 kg compresses its two surfaces against each other, it would require $0.2 \times 100 = 20$kg force parallel to those surfaces to overcome their friction and make them move on each other. And that would remain true whether the bearing area equalled 10 cm^2 (for a unit loading of 10 kg/cm^2), 1 cm^2 or 100 cm^2.

(*c*) Moving friction remains independent of the speed of bearing motion (up to the point where sufficient heat arises to cause bulk melting of the bearing material). Thus, given a coefficient of friction of say 0.3 for a given bearing, thirty per cent of the load normal to its surface will overcome its moving friction, whether its surfaces move on each other at 0.2 mm/second or at 200 mm/second.

(*d*) The coefficient of friction depends heavily upon the chemical and physical nature of the bearing materials and upon their perfection of surface finish.

In algebraic terms then we may write, using Greek lower case mu to signify the coefficient of friction:

$$\mu = F/P \qquad\qquad \textit{Equation 12.01}$$

where F signifies the force required to overcome friction, and P the compression load acting perpendicularly across the bearing surface. Fig. 12.03 diagrams this situation. Given mu, then solving this relation for F we have:

$$F = \mu P \qquad\qquad \textit{Equation 12.02}$$

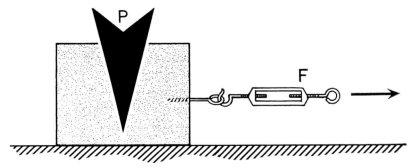

Figure 12.03. Given a weight (P) dragged across a horizontal surface at a uniform speed of motion, and the force (F) required to maintain that motion will represent some constant fraction of the weight. That fraction constitutes the *coefficient of moving friction* for those two materials.

4) HYDRODYNAMIC AND BOUNDARY LAYER LUBRICATION: We recognize two major kinds of liquid lubrication, whose separation upon close examination has come to seem somewhat arbitrary but which remain as quite useful analytical distinctions.

(a) *Hydrodynamic lubrication.* Here a fluid pumped under pressure between two moving bearing surfaces keeps them from touching. In other words, they float on that fluid. This kind of lubrication serves in the crank shaft bearings and cylinder walls of modern automobile engines as well as in other rapidly moving machinery where sliding friction and wear must be overcome. Hydrodynamic lubrication excels at moderately high bearing speeds, but it becomes somewhat inefficient (i.e., unable to eliminate wear) at very low speeds unless the whole bearing including the oil pumping system is designed only for low speeds (a qualification that does not seem to apply to human joints, which know good lubrication in any state). For example, the bearings that support (actually float) the massive yoke of the 200 inch telescope at Mount Palomar actually float it on two bearing pads into which a pump constantly injects oil. Because its many tons thus float wholly on two thin layers of oil one can rotate the many-tonned yoke by hand pressure alone. Hydrodynamic lubrication, if effectively achieved and maintained throughout the service life of the bearing, can provide very low rates of wear, as well as very low coefficients of friction.

(*b*) *Boundary layer lubrication*: This exists in the coarse adjustment slides of older microscopes, in lathe bed slides, in gear teeth, or in a comedian skating wildly and precariously on a cake of soap. It usually depends upon a grease or grease-like substance to minimize metal to metal contact. In doing so its chemical adhesiveness to the bearing substance becomes quite important (far more so than in hydrodynamic situations), and equally one depends upon its great viscosity to retain the necessary amounts of it between the moving surfaces in the face of pressure acting to squeeze it out from between them.

Some bearing wear always occurs under boundary layer conditions and in modern machines one finds it confined to those areas where the total amount of use such a bearing receives does not lead to any serious bearing wear. More critical and constantly moving parts receive different kinds of bearings of greater durability.

QUESTIONS: CHAPTER 12

1) Define the primary function of most bearings.
2) Define the primary function of most lubricating systems.
3) Characterize a journal as to its basic structural features.
4) True or false: a) Starting friction forms a function of the mechanical strength of dry bearing surface materials. b) Moving friction depends upon the melting point of dry bearing surface materials. c) The coefficient of friction varies with the normal load on a bearing. d) Bearing durability depends upon maintaining accurate alignment of the bearing surfaces. e) In effect, hydrodynamic lubrication floats one of the two bearing surfaces on the other.

CONCLUSION, PART I: With those words (reenforced and supplemented by the nine appendices and the nineteen special tables in Part III) let us put aside our conventional consideration of inanimate things as man has conceived them, and see if we can at least obtain a glimpse of how a far better Engineer conceived them through the eyes of our own musculoskeletal system.

PART II

BIOLOGY

Some of the Biological Side
of Biomechanics

THE BASIC GAME plan of Part II consists of the following: the tissue units or structural building stuffs which form the adult skeletal system. Then it will raise its sights to some static and behavioral properties general to the organ level, and then even higher to others, to see how the elementary factors assemble and cooperate (215). Finally it will describe a few pertinent properties of selected orthopaedic implants and procedures. Throughout, the text will provide specific examples *in the sense that they illustrate generalities,* ones which apply to whole classes of problems.

It may clarify several aspects of the upcoming text, before we actually dive into it, to note the following:

The overriding preoccupation of the text constitutes *function,* as Volume II defined this often ambiguously used term.

Function in that special sense implies *cause-effect relationships,* which this text concerns itself with far more than, and sometimes to the exclusion of, descriptions of uninterpreted and possibly even meaningless facts.

Cause-effect relationships imply some sort of game rules in a system that make a cause lead necessarily to a predictable effect. The text devotes much of its verbiage in one or another way towards such rules which, in previous volumes and articles, were sometimes termed *principles of action.*

Some of the game-rule stuff herein turned up in my own research activities since 1953.

But my own main work constitutes clinical orthopaedic surgery and teaching (not research and *not* writing books) and that experience afforded valuable and special insight into orthopaedic research matters. For one's problem patients, particularly when trapped in situations where we really cannot help them even in today's supposedly advanced state of medical expertise, tend to keep one's research eye on the compass and the heading, the hand to the helm and the trim of the sheets, the ear attuned to the pitch of the weather shrouds and any luffing of the canvas. . . Given that, and one must lack intelligence or courage or both to overlook an error in course and/or fail to try to correct it, regardless of any resistance in the fo'c'sle by ones possibly less well equipped to determine such matters.

All right. *This book aims at clinicians,* those who want to understand biomechanical aspects of our bodies better than any of my vintage or before did at graduation from medical school. Those clinicians may know this: the material herein does serve clinical needs, has that reliability assured by time, consistency and repetition, and will handily survive any noises from the fo'c'sle. A good friend of mine, Dr. R. H. Ramsey, once observed that when a stone drops into a penful of animals, the one that squeals (or grunts or moos or brays) probably was the one it struck.

So, not really wishing or intending to heave any kinds of stones into any kinds of pens, let us clinicians who actually care for the patients look at selected biological aspects of biomechanics.

Chapter 13

Some Basic Properties of Bone

THE BASIC BIOMECHANICAL building materials of man and other higher animals include *bone, tendon, ligament, fascia* and *cartilage,* with *muscles* providing the motive force and power, and the *nervous system* providing the control and computing faculties. Before tackling some of the design principles underlying the tissue and organ level functions of these things, the text will state a few of their pertinent properties insofar as we know them at this writing, including their physical and compositional properties, and some of their biological characteristics that seem pertinent. For the benefit of engineers and allied nonbiological people trying to tread water in this area, the text includes some material which physicians may find quite elementary. The latter will perhaps forgive this, as engineers probably forgave us the elementary nature of Part I on this book. Figure 13.00 describes some of the upcoming nomenclature (114).

I: THE SKELETAL ALPHABET

Let us begin with an intriguing and useful (and original) generalizing concept concerning the composition of the skeletal system. We can express its tissue composition readily in an alphabet context, outlined originally in more detail in Volume II of this series. Simply abstracted here, we define the skeleton's tissues as *all of its bony, cartilaginous and fibrous tissue parts.* The immediate discussion will ignore the contribution of the striated muscles, nervous system and teeth. This forms an arbitrary choice tailored to our clinical level and systems oriented main concerns. Prof. W. S. S. Jee (141-144) for example, in instructing some of his N.I.D.R. dental trainees in work which has given him international recognition, need not so generalize their studies and could legitimately restrict the focus of their concern to a mandible,

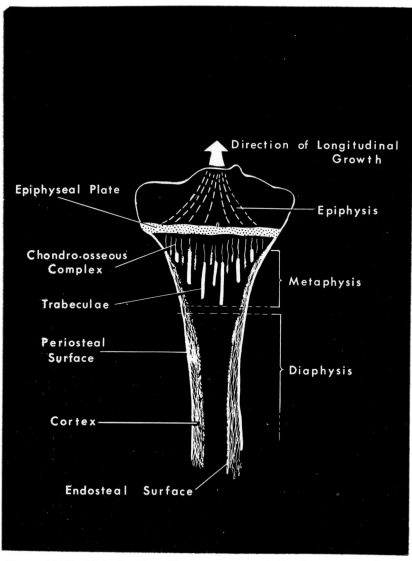

Figure 13.00. This drawing illustrates some of the bone nomenclature, primarily for nonmedical readers. It represents a vertical section cut through a child's tibia. The *chondroosseous complex* forms a synonym for primary spongiosa, while *trabeculae* designate the secondary spongiosa. In adults only the latter exists. The periosteal and endosteal surfaces are also becoming known as the respective *envelopes*. Articular cartilage lies on top of the epiphysis. As to the specifics of the modeling patterns on these elements during growth, the interested reader might consult Prof. Donald Enlow's excellent monograph (66), Dr. P. Rubin's textbook (225), or Volume II and IV of this series, or most modern textbooks of medical histology.

or even one tooth, while Profs. G. Armelagos (9) or J. Dewey might focus their arthropology students' minds on the length-breadth ratio of a single bone.

1) SIMPLE TISSUES: Then we can say this: *Nature used an alphabet of only five letters to construct the whole human skeleton.* Each of these letters constitutes what we will name a simple tissue. All skeletal development, growth, aging and disease phenomena turn out to represent simple combinations, sequences and temporal transitions (i.e., replacements of one by another) of these five biological letters.

To understand in first approximation state* the biomechanics of the adult skeletal system we will need to describe particularly the properties of three of the above five letters: lamellar bone, hyaline cartilage, and fibrous tissue.

Mechanically and rather generally speaking, simple tissues tend to exhibit little overall mechanical order or structural grain at eye level and grosser resolutions. Consequently, they tend to display strain isotropic mechanical properties when studied in bulk. They have readily defineable and usually quite simple chemical compositions, histological structural features, biodynamic responses to a variety of environmental challenges, and mechanical properties.

For future reference, let us list the simple skeletal tissues that will concern us most here.

Fibrous bone	*Lamellar bone*
Fibrocartilage	*Hyaline cartilage*
Fibrous tissue	*others* (teeth, elastic cartilage, etc.)

A more comprehensive list would have to include elastic cartilage and elastic tissue, dentine, enamel, chondroosseoid, and cementum, and one could make a good case for adding the tissues also normally found inside the bone marrow.

2) COMPLEX TISSUES: These represent simple tissues *to which some additional structural property has been added.* This addition may come about in any one of four ways:

---

* The limited objective of this book.

(a) by increasing the long range internal order and uniformity of orientation of the basic fibrillar phase (collagen) common to all of these simple tissues;

(b) or by using the simple tissue to produce gross structures with grossly visible net—and new—architectural external order;

(c) or by combining two or more tissues, simple or complex, in particular temporally and architecturally ordered ways to create a new construct;

(d) or by some combination of the above.

As an example of imposed external order, the cortex of a long bone (a complex tissue) possesses the highly space-oriented mechanical properties endowed by a hollow cylindrical columnar geometry; those properties exist in addition to or superimposed upon the basic materials properties of the lamellar bone (a simple tissue) which composes that cortex. In similar fashion a smokestack has overall and useful mechanical properties which exist superimposed upon (or built with) the basic mechanical properties of the bricks and mortar composing it. And an automobile wheel has properties which exist in addition to the raw steel composing it.

As an example of imposed internal order, the complex tissues named articular cartilage and epiphyseal plate cartilage possess ordered orientation of their internal collagen fibers and ordered spatial segregation of some of their internal cellular activities (demonstrated in some beautiful experiments and microchemical studies by Dr. R. Schenk, and separately by Dr. David Howell) which one finds lacking in the simple tissue form of hyaline cartilage. That superimposed structural order, without involving any alterations of the chemical composition or of the kinds of cellular activities going on, nevertheless endows the newer constructs or complex tissues with useful mechanical and growth properties which do not appear in the simple tissue form. To repeat: simple chemical analyses of these simple and complex tissues reveal identical compositions, because their essential differences seem to lie, not in any changes in their composition but rather in their supracellular and supramolecular level physical organizations (61). Just so, chemical analyses of sawdust and oak beams will never reveal why a good chandler would choose to build a ship only with the latter.

As an example of combining simple tissues, one would include the primary spongiosa beneath the growth plate, a combination of mineralized hyaline cartilage and fibrous bone.

Accordingly I have termed all more highly evolved, and architecturally speaking, more meaningful tissues, still lacking enough structural order and integration to justify naming them as organs, as complex tissues. Figure 13.01 names and diagrams the ones most important to our biomechanical interests.

The complex tissues of an entire bone as an organ would include its cortical bone, its spongy bone, (both made of the

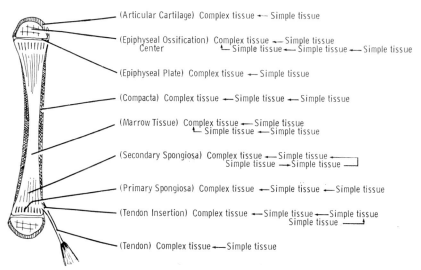

Figure 13.01. This diagram names the major parts of our bones (the terms within the parentheses on the left), and diagrams briefly how they came into being in the skeletal alphabet context. Note that the assemblage of all these complex tissues in the particular architectural relationships shown here constitutes an organ: a "typical" bone. The arrows indicate either a conversion of a simple to a complex tissue by added internal or external order, or as a replacement of one by another, matters gone into in far more detail in Volume II of this series.

simple tissue, lamellar bone), its articular cartilage and epiphyseal plates (made of the simple tissue, hyaline cartilage) plus that cartilage which attaches all tendons, ligaments, and fascial attachments to the osseous skeleton, and its fibrous tissue structures (made solely of the simple tissue, fibrous tissue) which include its tendons, ligaments, and fascia. Table 13.01 lists some complex tissues of biomechanical concern. Understand this, throughout the following chapters: *The biomechanics of the adult human skeleton deals almost exclusively with the properties of its complex tissues.* Most of our predecessors understood this quite well, as you will find reflected in the unstated but quite obvious

TABLE 13.01

SOME COMPLEX SKELETAL TISSUES

Name	Simple Tissues Forming it	Sequence in its Formation
Cortical bone	Lamellar bone	Fibrous bone → replacement by lamellar bone → intermittent deposition of further layers of lamellar bone.
Secondary spongiosa	Lamellar bone	Hyaline cartilage production → replacement by fibrous bone → replacement by lamellar bone.
Articular cartilage	Hyaline cartilage	Hyaline cartilage produced with added internal architecture already established.
Epiphysis	Hyaline cartilage, lamellar bone, fibrous bone.	Chondral growth, partial fibrous bone replacement, complete lamellar bone replacement.
Epiphyseal cartilage	Hyaline cartilage	Same as for articular cartilage.
Tendon attachment to bone	Tendon, cartilage plus cortical bone	Same as for cortical bone; see Volume II.
Tendon	Fibrous tissue	Collagen fibers deposited with internal order already established around one axis or line of action.
Ligament	Fibrous tissue	Same as for tendon.
Fascia	Fibrous tissue	Same as for tendon but order established on two intersecting axes, i.e., in a plane.
Muscle	Fibrous tissue plus muscle cells	Both arise from primitive mesenchym in the embryo.

This table lists in the left column the major complex tissues on the skeleton, in the middle their simple tissue components, and on the right some of the basic cell behavioral sequences that produce them. Compare with Figure 13.01. Our biomechanical eyes focus upon the complex tissues; that is where most of the action lies.

assumptions underlying their work (17,20,21,30,48,56,158, 164,213). Simple tissue phenomena play minor roles here, and become of greater importance only when we consider skeletal histogenesis, development, growth and disease.

Now, with respect to bone we must make one more preliminary categorization.

3) KINDS OF BONE: At least two different kinds of bone exist, a matter causing some confusion among students because our older literature called them by the same name bone, and because only recently have we realized that they represent quite different stuffs mechanically, biologically, and in their physiological responses and evolutionary functions and roles (223). These two kinds of bone (both simple tissues) constitute lamellar bone (our primary concern here), and fibrous bone. Table 13.02 lists some of the behavioral differences of these two types of bone, differences which, while quite unequivocal, still remain little recognized or used by scientists working with skeletal physiology. That is unfortunate, for trying to do skeletal research in ignorance of such facts resembles trying to do thoracic surgery without bothering to learn the anatomy and function of the chest cage contents. And this ignorance shows, sometimes flagrantly, in the strategy, design and interpretation of some skeletal research reports (but some modern authors including Arnold (14,15); Epker (68,69); Z. F. Jaworski, Duncan (59,60); Jee (141,143); Shifrin (240–243); Takahashi (260–263); D. Baylink; P. Meunier (188–190); and K. Wu are gradually changing that).

Lamellar bone: As to their distributions in the skeleton, the osseous complex tissues of the *adult skeleton* (i.e., its compact and spongy bone parts) comprise almost exclusively lamellar bone (1,122,283). In its various complex tissue forms, its collagen fibers exhibit uniform average orientation which parallels the resultants of the time-averaged compression and/or tension strains developed in bones in normal usage. The needle-like apatite crystals in its mineral salts align similarly simply because they adopt the alignment of the collagen

TABLE 13.02

PHYSIOLOGICAL PROPERTIES OF LAMELLAR AND FIBROUS BONE

Agent	*Effect on Lamellar Bone Producton*	*Effect on Fibrous Bone Production*	*Sources*
Hypercorticoid state	Inhibits profoundly	Little or no effect	Follis, R.H.; Proc. Soc.
Estrogen therapy	Inhibits profoundly	Little or no effect	Explt. Biol. and Med., 76: 722, 1951.
Thyrotoxic state	Accelerates profoundly	Little effect	Endocrinol. 28:83, 1941
Hyperparathyroid state	Variable	Variable	
Initial reaction to trauma	0	+	
Initial reaction to infection	0	+	
Initial reaction to nonosteogenic neoplasm	0	+	
Tissue culture can produce this kind	0	+	
Lamellae present	+	0	Ascenzi, A.; in *L'Osteoporose*, Masson and Co., Paris, p. 42, 1964.
Regular geometric overall organization of collagen	+	0	
Regular overall orientation of hydroxyapatite crystals	+	0	
Structure oriented parallel to physical forces on the bone	+	0	"Wolff's law"
Can deposit directly on calcified cartilage	0	+	
Fate in body	Stable for decades	Always replaced by other kinds of tissue	
Mechanical durability	Strong, fatigue resistant	Weak, fatigue prone	

This table simply compares some of the physiological properties of lamellar and fibrous bone. While we have known of their structural and distributional differences for generations, the further concept that at least two *behaviorally* different kinds of bone exist in the skeleton, which the author began pushing *ca* 1960[55], has now become widely accepted and along with it the parallel acknowledgement that you cannot really understand skeletal disease, neoplasia, or even its normal physiology, until you understand many of these differences.

fibers.* The average direction of the collagen fibers and apatite crystals in lamellar bone represents the direction of its grain (71,72) (See Fig. 13.02).

---

* While the bone mineral (largely apatite) exists in dynamic equilibrium with the blood and constantly turns over in response to processes not directly related to bone formation, it maintains a stable average set of physical properties (see Volume IV).

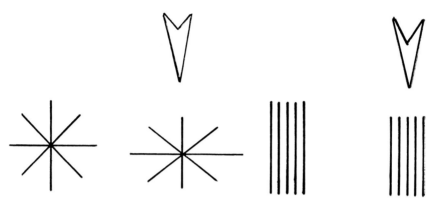

Figure 13.02. This diagrams a mechanically important aspect of the spatial distribution of both the collagen fibers and the trabeculae of fibrous (i.e., woven) bone. The mineral phase which provides the bulk of its strength and stiffness in shear has been omitted for clarity. Observe that only a portion of the total fiber mass lies oriented in space in such a way as to carry directly and with optimal efficiency a compression load. The remainder of its fibers contribute inefficiently to the support of that load because of their variably oblique inclinations to the line of action of the load.

Right: In lamellar bone long range order of the fibrillar phase exists. Thus the material has a grain at the macro level of resolution, and along one particular direction it possesses its maximal tension and compression strengths and stiffness, while along directions perpendicular to that it has its greatest strength in shear. Accordingly lamellar bone potentially forms a superior structural material, provided some ways exist first to stereotype the orientations of the load resultants, and then second to align the grain of the bone so it conforms to those resultants. Significantly, nature has actually evolved mechanisms which do both, and deposit lamellar bone exactly in that way which aligns its maximum strengths with the time-averaged and stereotyped (spatially speaking) maximum load resultants it carries.

As to its basic functions as a simple tissue, lamellar bone provides a material whose microscopic level grain permits aligning its directions of maximum strength parallel to the maximum time-averaged load resultants it carries (92) ; it contains a signalling or communication system of some type capable of making the living cells that can alter its shape do so in just that way that makes most effective use of its strength (26,27,29,99) ; it provides a building material rigid to all three principal strains, strong in each of them, and of

Hookean behavior over most of its useful strength range. It also possesses respectable mechanical toughness.

Fibrous bone: (synonyms: fiber bone, woven bone, reactive bone, primitive bone). This stuff participates intimately in bone creation and development in the embryo, and in the longitudinal bone growth process in childhood; otherwise one sees it primarily in the defensive processes of walling off infections, and certain tumors in bone, during normal *bone healing* processes and in some rare developmental disorders of bone (1,139). We will describe shortly its role in fracture healing, a description which also applies to some extent to bone grafting problems. Fibrous bone lacks any overall of bulk mechanical grain (see Fig. 13.03) and so in the purely structural and mechanical sense makes somewhat inefficient use of its component fibers (85).

With those matters expressed now let us take a look at some of the physical aspects of lamellar bone.

II: STATIC PROPERTIES OF BONE

1) RELATION BETWEEN STRUCTURE AND LOADS: Both microscopically and grossly, the architecture and grain of structures made of lamellar bone intimately relate to and derive from the mechanical loads they typically carry. We will describe this, as the operationally useful flexure-drift law, representing the *bone modeling/force-response characteristic* or principle of action, in a later chapter. For the moment let us settle for a few rather general remarks.

During its deposition, the microscopic grain of lamellar bone becomes parallel to the time-averaged direction or resultant of the greatest tension and/or compression loads it carries. Furthermore the overall external and internal gross or macrostructure, and the lie in tissue space of a bony shaft or cortex demonstrate the same correspondence. This grain-alignment property so disposes the organic fibers and mineral crystals in a given mass of bone as to make maximum use of their inherently oriented mechanical properties, as Figure 13.03 illustrates. Such obeisance of structure to the needs

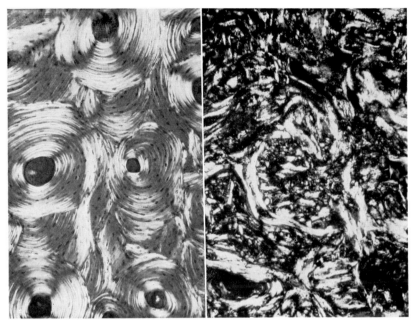

Figure 13.03. *Left:* An undecalcified thin cross section of human compact lamellar bone seen at medium magnification (about 300×) between crossed polars. The alternating bright and dark lamellae show clearly, and the bright ones exhibit birefringence due primarily to the molecular-level long-range order of its fibrillar and apatite phases or components. This stuff comprises most of the bony parts of the adult skeleton.

Right: A similarly prepared and viewed section of fibrous bone, showing the lack of long range order in arrangement of its two birefringent phases. This stuff represents the growth facilitating, healing and defense type of bone which, when present, by some means always self-stimulates its own replacement by lamellar bone.

of physical usage derives from a special negative feedback system, in which the strain patterns on bone surfaces somehow generate signals that guide its special kinds of cells. Due to this guidance the cells alter the size and shape of a bone in just that way which minimizes future strains by the same loading patterns.

2) MECHANICAL STRENGTH: Tables 13.03 and 13.04 list the basic strength properties of adult human wet bone. They reveal for compact bone typical breaking strengths of 11

TABLE 13.03

MECHANICAL PROPERTIES OF SOME HUMAN BONES

Bone	Ultimate tensile strength		Modulus of elasticity	
	Wet (kg/mm²)	Dry	Wet (kg/mm²)	Dry
Femur	12.4	15.4	1760	2060
Tibia	14.3	17.4	1840	2100
Fibula	14.9	17.9	1890	2150
Humerus	12.5	15.8	1750	2040
Radius	15.2	18.3	1890	2180
Ulna	15.1	18.1	1880	2160
Mean	14.0	17.2	1830	2120

To convert the moduli in the two right hand columns to the perhaps more familiar English units of psi $\times$ 10^6, multiply by 1.5 and move the decimal three places towards the left. Thus the mean E, wet, of 1830 kg/mm² becomes 2.6 $\times$ 10^6 psi. The data reveal only minor differences in strength and stiffness, in different bones, when expressed as unit materials properties. Obviously the total strength in compression of the large femur will exceed greatly that of the much smaller ulna.

To convert the unit stress values in the two left hand columns to English units of psi in thousands, multiply by 1.1 and leave the decimal where you find it. Thus the mean wet tensile strength of 14.0 kg/mm² becomes 15.5 thousands of psi, or 15,500 psi.

Quantitative tetracycline-based histological studies of bone turnover reveal that in human adults, annual turnover in the femur and humerus exceeds that in the more distal bones, the tibia, fibula, radius and ulna. The increased MSA this causes may account for the increased E that associates with it.

(Data in this and subsequent tables taken largely from the book by Yamada, and several publications by F. G. Evans).

TABLE 13.04

MECHANICAL PROPERTIES OF WET HUMAN FEMORAL COMPACTA*

Test	Age			
	25	45	65	Mean
Ultimate tensile strength, kg/mm²	12.5	11.4	8.8	10.9
Per cent elongation at failure	1.4	1.3	1.2	1.3
Ultimate compression strength, kg/mm²	17.0	16.4	14.8	16.2
Per cent shortening at failure	1.9	1.8	1.8	1.8
Shear strength across grain, kg/mm²	9.0	8.6	8.2	8.6
Ultimate flextural tension stress at failure, kg/mm²	17.7	16.5	14.2	16.0
Ultimate torque stress at failure, kg/mm²	5.8	5.4	4.9	5.4

* From H. Yamada.[293] Hookean up to 70% of failure point in tension, nearly to the failure point in compression, and elastic up to the failure point in both.

Taking wet femoral compacta as fairly generally representative of human bone, this table provides basic data on its unit properties. You can see that its strength declines somewhat with age. While the table does not show it directly, its stiffness too decreases mildly with age.

kg/mm² in tension, 16 kg/mm² in compression (both parallel to the grain) and 8.5 kg/mm² in shear across the grain. These strengths decline modestly with aging ($\approx$10%–20% from age 25 to 65), and associate with small increases in E, Young's modulus (10,12). The material behaves elastically nearly up to its breaking point, and in the Hookean manner up to about seventy per cent of its breaking stress.

We lack good data on the unit properties of trabecular bone; that available suggests it remains similar to compact bone but has about fifteen per cent less stiffness and lower breaking stresses. Its bulk properties depend upon how densely trabeculae pack in it and upon their individual sizes. Thus in Table 13.06 a cm^3 from the greater trochanter fails at only 97 psi, while that in the femoral neck can sustain some 630 psi, differences reflecting the amount of bony tissue in that cm^3, rather than any alterations in its basic unit materials properties. Note that where the modulus of elasticity of compact bone runs around 2.6×10^6 psi/in^2, that for spongy bone in bulk can run as low as $.04 \times 10^6$ psi/in^2, or about 65 times less stiff. And while compact bone has an E value of 2.6 in tension parallel to the grain, it has only half that tension stiffness or 1.1- 1.3 $\times$ 10^6 psi, when tested perpendicular to the grain, according to S. B. Lang.

Also, Table 13.04 records the fact that while a mean unit tension stress in uniaxial loading of only 12.5 kg/-mm^2 causes fracture of compact bone at age twenty-five, it does not fail in flexure until the surface tension stress, *computed on the assumption that the material has uniform stiffness across the diameter* of the bone's cross section, becomes 17.7 kg/mm^2; or if you will it seems some forty per cent stronger in flexure than in uniaxial tension. This comes about for an intriguing reason with several roots. First, that represents the assumed surface stress, computed on the assumption that the bone has uniform stiffness across the diameter of its cross section. But second, as we have shown (100,103), turnover or re-modeling of cortical bone usually proceeds more rapidly near the periosteal surface than deeper with the cortex. That causes periosteal bone to have a younger mean skeletal age or MSA, and so to have more mechanical compliance and tensile toughness than bone lying deeper in the cortex (89). And P. Blaimont (32) has shown by direct microhardness testing that this subperiosteal layer of bone is softer than the deeper bone, probably as a direct result of its lesser MSA. As a result the tension loaded surface bone can yield enough more than the deeper bone during flexure to stress—relieve the extreme surface fibers, and that spreads the surface flexural strain energy over a deeper layer, some 100–500 microns thick. Consequently, the computed surface stresses exceed nearly twofold the true ones. This mechanism makes living bones tougher to flexural impact.

Recall in our earlier discussions of impact that a stiff material, because it causes momentum transfer to occur more quickly, develops larger stresses during impact. In that regard, Kimura (156) and Kuroma (165) in Kyoto found wet bone (less stiff) to require some 0.14 kg-cm/mm^2 of energy to fail in flexure but dry bone failed at only .09 kg-cm/mm^2, or at only some sixty per cent of the energy absorption when wet. Since children's bones have less stiffness than adult's, one can see at least one reason why their bones break less easily than those of grownups.

The above property relates to a kind of viscoelastic deformation which fresh bone can demonstrate when loaded close to its upper limit. Dr. H. Roth and the writer first demonstrated this phenomenon in 1961 (104,224) and it was recently rediscovered by Burstein *et al** who proposed that it accounted for the tension stress-relieving phenomenon just described.

3) STRUCTURE: Grossly, bones form hollow, closed containers whose walls, made of the simple tissue lamellar bone, we call the cortex. The resulting construct, by virtue of added external order, becomes a complex tissue. Many tiny, usually tortuous channels perforate the cortex (Volkmann's canals) to allow blood vessels to enter and leave the bone. The large hollow cavity within, named the marrow cavity or medullary cavity, contains bars and plates also made of lamellar bone and called trabeculae or spongy bone, another complex tissue made of the same simple lamellar bone one. Trabeculae lie mostly at either end of the bone. They also

---

* Burstein, Currey, Frankel, Reilly; J. Biomech., 1972.

align parallel to the major *time-averaged compression load resultants* carried by the local part of the bone in which they lie. Between the trabecular bars lie the marrow soft tissues consisting of a combination of blood forming elements, blood vessels, nerves and supporting fatty tissues. See Figure 13.04.

To repeat, the building material for both of these bony parts constitutes the simple tissue, lamellar bone. Cortex and trabecula relate to lamellar bone as building and fence do to boards and nails; the same materials, assembled in layers in the same basic way, can serve to make grossly different structural forms with quite different aggregate mechanical (and even physiological) properties.

We call the external surface of a bone its periosteal surface because a membrane called the periosteum often covers it. The inner surface, which also forms the outer wall of the

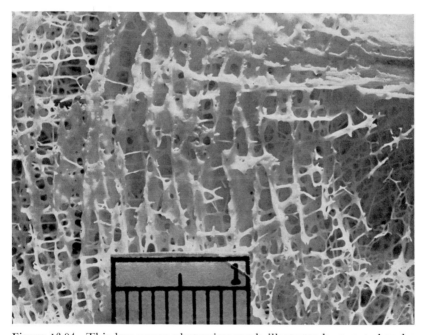

Figure 13.04. This low power photomicrograph illustrates human trabecular bone from the upper end of a bivalved femur, as you might see it under a magnifying glass after removal of all soft tissue elements from the marrow spaces lying between these trabecular bars and plates. The scale represents one centimeter divided into millimeter intervals.

marrow cavity, we name the endosteal surface. Table 13.05 lists and illustrates two ways of classifying bone types, one according to classical descriptive morphological properties, and a newer one according to mechanical function. At the microscopic structural level, the orientation of the collagen fibers in an intact bone parallels its gross anatomical length *only in terms of the average*. When one looks into this matter with a polarizing microscope, two significant features emerge. One, both in the form of its secondary osteons or haversian systems, and in the form of the sub-periosteal layers of bone, alternating lamellae (i.e., layers of optically distinguishable fiber directions) exist, as shown in Figure 13.03, left side. Two, the fibers in a given lamella tend to spiral around the long axis of the whole structure, whether osteon or intact bone, and if it has a right hand twist

TABLE 13.05
CLASSIFICATION OF BONES

Anatomical Basis	Examples
Long bones	Femur, tibia, fibula, radius, ulna, humerus, clavicle, rib
Short bones	Phalanges, metacarpals, metatarsals
Flat bones	Bones of the skull; scapula; ilium of the pelvis
Irregular bones	Vertebrae, carpals, tarsals, sesamoids
Biomechanical Basis	
a) Bone Modeling dependent	
Flexure-compression loaded bones (column-beams)	Femur, tibia, humerus, rib, radius, metacarpal, posterior vertebral elements, pelvic bones
Compression loaded bones (pure columns)	Vertebral bodies; navicular; cuboid
Tension loaded bones	Cranial vault
b) Bone modeling independent	
Bone-modeling- inactivated bones	All sesamoids; dental surfaces of mandible and maxilla

The top classification abstracts the venerable and purely morphological way of categorizing the different bones in the skeleton.

The bottom or biomechanical basis provides a more modern (and original) classification into two basic groups: those in which bone modeling operates as we define the term herein, and those in which only chondral modeling operates. Of the former, some serve as combined column-beams and this includes all of our long bones and parts of others such as the laminae of the vertebrae. Other of our bones serve only as pure columns, for example the vertebral centra, while a very few others carry only trivial compression and flexural loads at best, as in the cranial vault.

The chondral modeling dependent bones include all sesamoids, and most of the small bones of the carpus and tarsus.

then the lamellae on either side of it will have left hand twists, and the ones beyond them right twists, and so on. This situation resembles (strikingly to my mind) the alternating right and left twist helices described in Chapter X under the discussion of fiber-reenforced composite structural materials. One may reasonably suspect that from the engineering aspect it serves the same function in bone: to boost the tangential or circumferential tension strength of cylinders made of a grained material which otherwise would remain inherently very weak in tension perpendicular to the grain. Thus bone's actual tension strength in this tangential direction of some 5000 psi probably arises by virtue of this helically based reenforcement. Should one isolate one of these lamellae and then test its tension strength perpendicular to the fiber direction, it might well fail below 1000 psi.

4) GROWING BONE: The bones of children differ from those of adults in an important way: they usually have growth centers at the ends.

We call the growth center itself the epiphysis, and a layer of hyaline cartilage called the epiphyseal plate separates it from the main metaphyseal part of the bone. At this plate arises most of the growth in any bone's length, as well as in the overall body height of an intact man. A complex series or sequence of cellular events and simple tissue replacements converts this cartilage to (literally, replaces it by) new lamellar bone (160); we signify that series, which one can legitimately think of as one process, by a term that cropped up before: endochondral ossification. This process stops for practical purposes at the time of skeletal maturity (i.e., 18 years±), and it leaves behind as one of its specific final residues the trabecular or spongy bone already referred to.* While several ways occur in nature of producing trabecular bone, over ninety-five per cent of that in the healthy adult human skeleton derives from the endochondral ossification process. Professor Pierre LaCroix, now departed from us,

---

* Another residue: the size, shape and alignment of the neighboring joint.

described these matters quite well in a pioneering synthesis more than twenty years ago (166).

5) BLOOD AND NERVE SUPPLY: The three general routes of entry of blood into bone include the metaphyseal vessels, the periosteal vessels and the nutrient artery (114). The numerous small metaphyseal vessels enter the bone through special holes (Volkmann's canals) in the thin metaphyseal cortex, to connect with each other, with vessels lying within and nourishing the cells in the cortex, and with vessels from the nutrient artery inside the medullary cavity (268,269). The periosteal vessels supply blood (via more Volmmann's canals) to approximately the outer third of the thickness of the cortex in the diaphysis of the bone. The nutrient artery, usually a good sized vessel, perforates the cortex at midshaft and nourishes the medullary contents and the inner two-thirds of the diaphyseal cortex (229,237). At least in some laboratory animals various investigators have shown a definite trend for the arterial blood entering the medullary cavity to flow via the numerous intracortical channels *centrifugally towards the periosteum* on its way out of the bone and back to the heart. Veins usually accompany the above arteries. In fracture healing the periosteal blood supply usually constitutes the most important in the repair process, primarily for biomechanical reasons. In a few special places however, such as the femoral neck, this does not hold true.

Bone contains nerve fibers, both in the medullary cavity and in the cortex, as Miller and Kashara found (194), and others in New Orleans and Rochester subsequently confirmed. Bones also go through a series of age-related changes which affect in a minor way their overall structural strength, stiffness and toughness (107,234,249,250).

6) PHYSICAL PROPERTIES: Most of what follows applies to lamellar bone; biochemical and engineering studies have not yet attempted to compare specifically the compositional and mechanical properties of the two basic types of bone (259).

Density 2.3 (degreased, and dried in air at 100 C to constant weight) ; 2.4 (wet) (3,12,125) . Proportional limit, rupture strength and ultimate strength of lamellar bone approximately equal, i.e., it represents a brittle material which, however, displays significantly greater toughness in its natural hydrated state than it does after drying. It provides the intriguing situation of increased breaking strength (by some 20%) but decreased toughness (by some 40%) following drying. It also demonstrates nearly twice as much toughness at high speed loading rates as at slow ones (156,165) . It has a Rockwell hardness (H scale) of 32–48, Brinell of some 24–27, and Vickers of 25. Tensile strength (wet) about 11,000 psi, compression strength about 15,000 psi, shear strength 4,000 psi parallel to and 8,000 psi perpendicular to its grain (See Tables 13.03, 13.04, 13.06, 13.07) . Young's compression modulus ≈ 2.8 × 10⁶ psi parallel to the grain. All tests of these properties† have demonstrated the usual noise or scatter in the values of different samples. Because in the absence of disease bone mineral deposits and quantity of organic matrix remain interdependent, one finds total strength

† Which are listed for wet bone.

TABLE 13.06
MECHANICAL PROPERTIES OF HUMAN SPONGY BONE

Sample	Ultimate Compression Stress psi	% contraction	Modulus of Elasticity psi	Density gm/cc
Head of femur	545	3.3	.041 × 10⁶	.75
Lateral femoral condyle	362	2.7	.04 × 10⁶	.66
Medial femoral condyle	333	2.2	.030 × 10⁶	.66
Greater trochanter	97	2.6	.005 × 10⁶	.59
Femoral neck	627	2.0	0.50 × 10⁶	.82

This table lists unit loads to failure in compression of trabecular bone from a variety of sampling sites. Do not overlook the much lower Young's modulus, compared to that of compact bone listed in earlier tables. Observe, too, the good correlation between density and ultimate strength. For one thing, this means that trabecular bone which cuts easily under the osteotome will prove weaker in normal use than that which cuts with greater difficulty. This table does not illustrate effects of disease or aging on these properties. Dr. Claude Gendreau[108], in a pioneering study of trabecular bone dynamics while at Guelph, Ontario, showed that its volume-based turnover considerably exceeds that of compact bone, leading one to infer a significantly lower mean skeletal age (MSA) for the former. Thus its materials properties as well as its geometry must enter somewhat into its increased static compliance. R. Hattner, B. N. Epker, L. Ilnicki and the author defined MSA (mean skeletal age) some years ago (See Bone Remodeling Dynamics) .

TABLE 13.07

ULTIMATE COMPRESSION LOADS OF INTACT WET HUMAN MALE BONES (Age 50)

Bone	Ultimate Compression Strength			Ultimate Tension Strength			Cross section
	Total (kg)	Unit (kg/mm²)	ΔL %	Total (kg)	Unit (kg/mm²)	ΔL %	Area mm²
Cervical vertebra	337	1.08	6.7	90	.31	.70	305
Thoracic vertebra	373	.73	5.3	270	.34	.73	540
Lumbar vertebra	477	.45	4.2	380	.37	.75	1000
Femur	4780	15.4	1.7	3,800	12.4	1.4	310
Tibia	3660	13.3	1.8	3,920	14.3	1.5	275
Fibula	860	13.5	1.8	950	14.9	1.6	64
Humerus	2580	13.0	1.8	2,500	12.5	1.4	200
Radius	950	11.0	1.9	1,310	15.2	1.5	86

Total loads to failure of intact bones. A later chapter will make the point that the relative total strengths of bones probably reflect reasonably well the relative differences in the time-averaged mechanical loads they carried, mostly during their growth, and to a much lesser degree after skeletal maturity. In comparing spongy to compact bone, keep in mind that their unit properties probably do not differ greatly. The whole spongy bones prove weaker than the compact ones because more than half of their volume is filled with marrow tissue, not bone. One excellent series of studies on this trabecular-compact comparison has been published by Gong, Arnold and Cohn[112,113].

to prove a function of total ash (11,73,267,276). The values obtained also depend on the rate of application of the test loads, most biological structural materials appearing significantly tougher as well as stronger upon impact than under static testing.‡ Tables 13.06, 13.07 provide additional materials—properties testing data, the first for spongy bone from several anatomical locations, the second as total loads at failure for eight different bones.

Ash weight about 65 per cent, and oxidizable organic fraction about 30 per cent by weight; water 5 per cent (219, 220,291) (see Fig. 13.05). Water forms about 11–12 per cent of the mass of fresh wet bone, and some 2.7 per cent of that

---

‡ Fortunately for those who would like to do some work in this field, a tremendous amount of basic study still needs doing before we can state the static and dynamic properties of the biological structural substances with as much confidence and completeness as we can for nonliving structural materials.

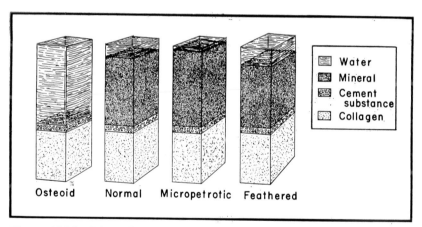

Osteoid   Normal   Micropetrotic   Feathered

Water
Mineral
Cement substance
Collagen

Figure 13.05. These bar graphs illustrate diagrammatically the absolute and relative changes in the amounts of organic bone matrix (composed of collagen and cement substances), and the water and inorganic mineral phases, which one finds typically in unmineralized new bone matrix on the left, usually termed osteoid or osteoid seam, in normally mineralized bone second from the left, in micropetrotic bone and in any other type of dead bone as well, and at the far right in so-called feathered bone (i.e., incompletely mineralized). As the mineral fraction increases, the mechanical compliance and the toughness both decrease while the rigidity or Young's modulus increases. The organic matrix remains constant while the volumes of the mineral and water phases vary reciprocally to each other. (Reprinted by permission, author and publisher, ref. no. 89.)

of air dried bone (10). Grain (of lamellar bone); pronounced. Endurance limit: unknown, although F. G. Evans studied this property some years ago. Hardness: variable, see above.[§] A *Hookean and three phase fiber-reenforced composite material* which generates weak (millivolt range) voltages of opposite polarity on the concave tending and convex tending surfaces when loaded in flexure, very likely by some type of piezoelectric effect (183,238). Normal bone also probably exhibits some mechanical creep, and osteomalacic bone certainly does.

As to its microscopic structure and to repeat, lamellar bone comprises a three phase composite solid material, the phases constituting collagen (95% of the organic content by weight), mucopolysaccharide (5% of the organic) and the inorganic mineral salts (67% by weight of the whole after drying and degreasing) (89). *Note:* the collagen orientation determines the grain of the whole (6,18,218), and possibly we should consider the water in bone a fourth phase.

Fibrous Bone. This material serves to initiate one of the only two mechanisms known in all of nature for creating new bony tissue where none existed before (87). It possesses rigidity to all three principal strains, medium strength and compliance to each, and the poorly understood but consistent and physiologically important property of self-initiating its own replacement by lamellar bone. Figure 13.03 illustrates examples of fibrous and lamellar bone. Up to this writing most of the studies of mechanical properties of bone have dealt with lamellar bone, not fibrous bone. Consequently, we have a fair amount of information only about the materials properties of lamellar bone.

With these physical matters disposed of, let us now describe some of the dynamic properties of bone and bones.

III: BIODYNAMIC PROPERTIES

1) THE FIVE MAJOR FACES OF BONE PHYSIOLOGY: For biomechanical needs we must characterize briefly five bio-

---

§ See Sedlin, E.: Suppl. 83 Acta Orthop. Scand. Vol. 36, 1965.

dynamic properties of living bone: its growth, modeling, remodeling, repair, and blood-bone exchange faculties. Understand that we now discuss bone tissue in a rather broad sense, and primarily as a building material, but do not yet consider specific osseous structures, or articulations, or the attachments to bone of ligament and fascia. These latter will receive some separate attention in later chapters. Thus:

(*a*) *Growth: Definition. Enlarging skeletal parts from fetal to adult size.* In this series of texts, growth exists as a behavioral entity separated from another (termed modeling, coming up next) which determines many of the architectural features and details of the finished product.* Consequently the relatively tiny bones present in the fetus by the 4th month after conception, ultimately enlarge to adult size by summing up the contributions of two different classes of cellular activity, one of which drives or conducts the duet, the other of which follows.

The driving process, named simply the growth process, itself sums up the contributions of two cellularly based and separate subprocesses, the longitudinally acting chondral growth process which establishes the overall lengths of bones (119) (and a few other features we will describe later), and the appositional bone growth process which acts transversely to the long axis of a bone to establish its outside diameter.

It seems that systemic endocrine (i.e., hormone based) factors actually drive the chondral growth process, in particular growth hormone and thyroxine. The sex and adrenal cortical hormones play major roles in stopping it after puberty, producing what clinicians call skeletal maturity. Thus sharks, mice and trees lack the property of skeletal maturation and so continue to grow as long as they live, but man's skeleton matures around age eighteen or so, as a consequence of which his body ceases to grow for practical purposes but

---

* This separation does not represent conventional thinking as yet so you will not likely find it in other contemporary literature except that from this laboratory. However the unambiguous basis for the distinction indicates it will become conventional concept within a decade or so.

he continues to live (and, one hopes, continues growing in other more abstract but equally essential ways). And in fact some gradual increase in skeletal size postmaturity appears the rule in man and other mammals (107,150,151, 154,262).

When allowed to proceed together in the absence of all applied external mechanical loads, we infer that these two growth processes, the chondral and the osseous, should tend to produce perfectly straight sided, cylindrical bones with circular cross sections. A clinical situation in which one may observe some (note: only some, not all) of these effects: lower limb paralysis of congenital origin, such as in severe myelomeningocele producing paralysis above the T-12 level. Another one, a rather rare disease: hyperphosphatasia.

Function: Growth has a simple prime purpose: to enlarge the tiny fetal skeleton to adult size.

(b) *Modeling*: *Definition. Establishing and maintaining the architectural features of the skeleton as it grows from fetal to adult size.* In other words, the term signifies a kind of sculpting. It exists as a separate entity from the growth processes' effects on overall skeletal size. We deal here with bone modeling or shaping, and will say a few brief words in the next chapter about an analogus cartilage activity, chondral modeling.

When a growing bone also carries the externally applied mechanical loads arising from muscle pulls, body weight and inertia, plus the varying arterial pulse pressure within its enclosed marrow cavity, the mechanical strains (including particularly the flexural ones) its cortex develops as a consequence thereof cause its periosteal and endosteal surfaces to move or drift through tissue space in predictable ways and in conformance to stereotyped overall patterns (teeth do likewise, a phenomenon used by orthodontists to control tooth movement and facial development) (172,195,200,202). And, systematic deposition of layer after layer of new bone by batches of osteoblasts on a given region of a bone's grossly visible surface will build that region up (252), while a similar pattern of erosion in another region by batches of osteoclasts

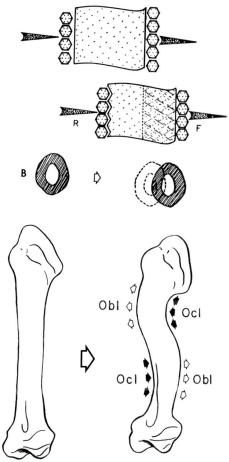

Figure 13.06. *Top:* Modeling activity in the skeleton begins as separate motions of individual bone surfaces through tissue space, called *drifts*. An *osteoblastic drift* on the right, and an *osteoclastic drift* on the left, appear on opposite sides of a single bone cortex. Each hexagon analogizes a separate drift BMU.

Middle: Any long bone seen in cross section. By properly patterning its surface drifts as to kind and location, as actually occurs in life, the whole middle half of the bone can move towards the right from its original location, and relative to its fixed ends, as diagrammed here.

Bottom: In addition to patterning drifts around a cross section, when one also patterns them further along the length of the bone, rather complex shapes can result—or undergo correction—via the drift mechanism. This drawing illustrates how a bone, originally straight in the fetus, could develop an S-shaped curve by bone modeling activity, or patterned drifts, on its surfaces. All of the bone surface drift activities combined constitute the entity we term *bone modeling*. Somewhat analogous modeling phenomena affect cartilage growth.

will cause it to melt away. When properly coordinated (as forms the usual case) a local region of a whole bone can move sideways through tissue space to create a longitudinal curve, such as one finds in ribs, clavicles, femurs and radii. See Figure 13.06. When one bone surface moves through tissue space in this manner we call it a drift. The sum and patterns of all drifts going on in a bone constitutes modeling.

As described in Volume IV, the modeling system functions in response to mechanical factors in such a way that all the internal and external surfaces (i.e., the periosteal and endosteal envelopes, but not the haversian envelope) of a bone drift towards the concavity that arises during a series of stereotyped dynamic flexures.* Because of particular general features of the anatomy of muscles, this causes a bone to become, and then to remain, primarily a column (perhaps we should really call it a column-beam) of that size and shape and location in tissue space most suitable for carrying the loads applied to it by the geographic sources of those loads. In addition, the cellular and physicochemical mechanisms underlying this behavior average all of the flexural strains a bone develops, and over some period of time which we will term sigma for lamellar bone modeling. The duration of the sigma value for that averaging process approximates one-half year in a year old infant, and increases to well in excess of one hundred years by the time of skeletal maturation around age eighteen years.

Thus as Becker *et al.* inferred (29) in part, we can state this: *With respect to dynamic flexure a negative feedback control system governs the architecture of lamellar bone.* Figure 13.07 diagrams part of it. The error it specifically

---

Note: That operational description constitutes a consistent, reliable and clinically highly useful phenomenon, and the author discovered and reported it solely from clinical observations (92). Consequently its validity and clinical usefulness stand on its own feet, and very solidly so and in that respect will neither gain nor lose from whatever may develop in the very active—and intriguing—studies of bioelectrical phenomena currently in progress around the world. The students of bioelectric phenomena *ca* 1964 recognized that they probably studied one element in a feedback system (29) but they were tuned in, analytically speaking, to principal stress, not flexure (a complex strain), as a brief review of relevant publications prior to 1965 will make clear.

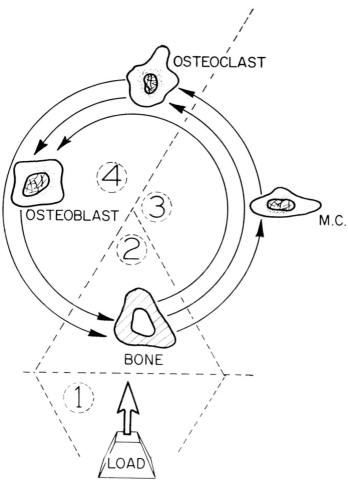

Figure 13.07. A diagram of the essential cause-effect interactions which relate mechanical factors to lamellar bone architecture (a later chapter will present specific morphological properties of this system in action). Thus: (1) Mechanical loads arising from muscle forces act upon the bones and strain them. (2) The bones then develop appropriate signals on their surfaces which mesenchymal cells (3) receive and react to, as well probably too the osteoclasts and the osteoblasts. (4) Those cells then modify the structure of the bones, and in exactly that way which reduces subsequent strains provided the loads remain stereotyped as to their timing and spatial orientations (and they do). The cellular sequences involved in this negative feedback system combine with some mechanical factors the text discusses in a later chapter. (Reprinted by permission of author and publisher, ref. no. 92.)

detects and corrects constitutes excessive osseous dynamic mechanical flexure.

Probably an underlying requirement for an effective and/ or rapidly acting modeling process represents active skeletal growth. Paraphrased, bone modeling probably represents a tune played upon a kind of bone growth keyboard. Accordingly, given rapid growth, and rapid and highly effective modeling activity can occur, but without any active growth little effective modeling apparently can develop. Of this, we remain somewhat uncertain at present because of a lack of relevant experimental data. However, in normal people most of the modeling activity that sculpts or shapes the skeleton occurs during the rapid growth period (birth to age 10 years) and ceases at skeletal maturity (age 18 years) for practical purposes.

Function of modeling: The bone modeling process appears to have two major purposes. It makes bones function primarily and in the overall sense as columns rather than as beams, as just noted, another way of saying it adapts bone architecture to the dictates of muscle forces according to a particular set of some rules (11,29,54,213,231,279); and it maintains the overall architecture and the proportions of a given bone while it enlarges far more than one hundred-fold in volume in the period of life lying between the 4th intrauterine mouth to the age of skeletal maturity (67,76,207).

(c) Remodeling: Definition. A special kind of lifelong turnover or renewal of lamellar bone tissue.

Remodeling of bone appears in discrete packets, arranged in such a way that no great or rapid changes in its total net amount, nor in its gross architecture, need occur during the remodeling process. A multicellular unit I have named the BMU causes it; each such BMU turns over approximately .05mm^3 of bone, a practically constant property defined by O. Landeros in 1964 (169) which has some rather profound effects upon the functional organization of this system (98). The remodeling activity proceeds throughout our whole life (185), i.e., it does not stop at skeletal maturity, and so in this respect differs from the modeling process (287). It has other differences too, and Drs. Charles Hansen (124), L. C. Johnson (146–149), and A. F. Jaworski: (three among the North American continent's really competent bone physiological systems experts) sometimes have felt that they had to spend more time transmitting these ideas to their own fellows and students than they could trying to learn more new things about bone for themselves. As to its spatial orientation, the BMU-based remodeling process parallels the major compression stress resultants arising within bony tissue in response to the gravitic and muscular loads imposed upon it. Volume III of this series described the very important BMU-based remodeling activity in some detail, and in spite of the fact that we have known of its existence and behavior for ten years, at this writing that volume represents the only written source in any language where one can find an adequate description of these matters. Fig. 13.08 illustrates some of them.

Functions: We believe (at present) that the BMU-based turnover process serves two prime needs: First, it eradicates mechanical fatigue-like damage of bone while it remains trivial and microscopic in extent; paraphrased, it constitutes a lamellar bone tissue self-repair mechanism which can make the whole organ immune in the operational sense to gross fatigue failures, even though the organs's building material lacks any such immunity (65).

Second, it replenishes continuously the skeleton's supply of osteocytes (at a rate varying from $>$ 100%/year in infants to $\approx$ 10%/year in adults) *, cells which seem intimately involved in triggering the self repair process as well as in managing blood-bone exchange of buffer and electrolyte, thereby maintaining the effectiveness of the skeleton as a sink reservoir system for use by the blood (34,36,125,131). A chapter

---

* We have obtained reasonably good data on this activity only within the past 15 years, as a result of new methods developed and put into use since then (40,41, 45,63,75,134,171,179,188,263).

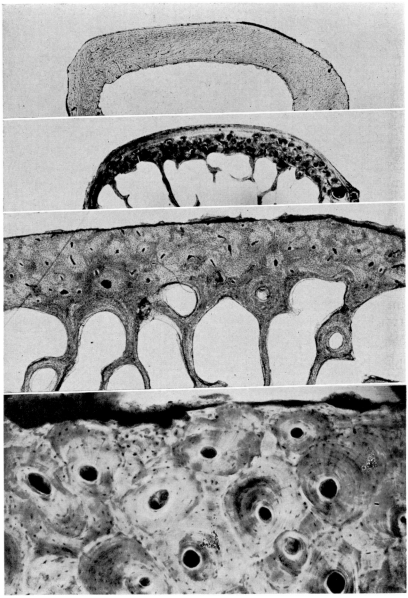

Figure 13.08. All photomicrographs represent undecalcified cross sections of long bones taken in ordinary transmitted light.

Top: Rabbit femur, post pubertal. While this animal and bone may provide a good model of the modeling and growth processes, it lacks significant amounts of the remodeling activity as defined in these volumes.

in Volume IV and an article by J. S. Arnold (13) deals with this quite important but sometime misunderstood—and misconceived—activity. The older concept that osteoclasts and osteoblasts themselves served that homeostatic function directly and primarily (and which one finds embodied in a wide range of articles and symposium proceedings over the 1950–1972 period), now falls into increasing disfavor (190,191), a circumstance that pleases Roy Talmage (264) and your author (94), who both felt compelled to challenge that conclusion *ca* 1960–1962 when such challenge proved generally unpopular. While those cells can and probably do have such actions, equally probably they account for less than twenty per cent of the skeleton's total homeostatic and buffering activities.

(d) *Repair*: *Definition*: This word serves in two contexts: (1) *restoring mechanical competence to a mechanically damaged bone;* (2) *defending bone from some damaging process, whether of intrinsic or extrinsic origin.*

Repair forms a naked eye level phenomenon where the BMU-based remodeling process forms a purely microscopic one.

Practically *all* of the cortical bone shown here deposited under the aegis of the growth and modeling processes defined in the text.

Second: Rib of a young woman, compacta above and marrow cavity and trabeculae below. This bone exhibits considerable remodeling or turnover activity, which occurs in temporally and spatially discrete packets called BMU.

Third: Also a rib but another and younger subject at greater magnification to zero in on the morphological tell-tales of discrete BMU. See lowest cut.

Bottom: Rib from still another subject, now one much older. Here we see at higher power (200×) various secondary osteons or haversian systems, each the end product of a remodeling BMU. Each has a small round canal containing blood vessels (and looking black because of overstaining), and lies surrounded by a thick, tubular cylindrical wall of lamellar bone. Most of the circumferential lamellae originally deposited during her growth by the modeling and growth processes have now become *replaced* by such secondary osteonal bone.

As to its cellular basis, the tissues lying adjacent to all of the surfaces of a living bone contain special pluripotent populations of cells we term mesenchymal cells. When gross injury occurs to a bone, such as a fracture, these mesenchymal cells receive some kind of message from the damaged tissue (292) which makes them begin to divide, producing thereby newly and locally generated populations of specialized cells of various types (211,266). Those specialized or differentiated cells then proceed to heal or repair the damage. The bone repair process proceeds through a number of identifiable stages which we will discuss later.

In addition to gross fractures, other phenomena can also trigger off repair type bone reactions, and they include burns, some types of chemical injury, the injury of a surgical procedure, the physical, chemical and biological irritation of some implant materials and designs, plus contusions, many kinds of infection and certain neoplasms. The repair process forms a physiological entity which follows its own rules or principles of action, ones separate from those affecting remodeling, modeling and growth. Curiously while competent and astute clinicians (such as R. Menke; L. Van Herpe; C. L. Klasinski; G. Hoover; E. Thompson; B. Mayo; D. Carlson; H. Schoene, or D. B. Auchard) have little difficulty in grasping—and making intelligent use of—that fact, the bone research community lags far behind in doing so.

Function: Clearly, the repair mechanism exists to restore mechanical integrity of broken or otherwise physically damaged bone. But it can also serve to wall off or defend the organ—and thus the man—from a variety of noxious and irritative processes, such as infections and some neoplasms.

(e) Homeostasis: Definition: This signifies maintaining constant pH, composition and ion concentrations of the body's extracellular fluids (including the blood plasma). This represents an important function because changes of relatively small magnitude in the concentration of many of the ions in those fluids can incapacitate or even kill a man. In subserving that function, by some means the skeleton can

and does make available to the blood, and rather promptly so, some of its very large reservoirs of, or its ability to serve as a sink for large amounts of, acid, base, calcium, magnesium, phosphate, sodium, and other ions (235). It can also store and/or release many trace elements, some helpful, some innocuous and some harmful. We currently believe that the osteocytes in bone play a major role in regulating and making possible these activities (13). Volume IV discussed one aspect of this function (245).

Having characterized briefly some of the skeleton's basic physiological activities or faces, let us next say a bit more about the repair process, for we will need that background

TABLE 13.08
SOME PHYSIOLOGICAL DIFFERENCES IN REMODELING AND REPAIR

Agent	*Effect on Bone Remodeling*	*Effect on Bone repair*
Adrenalcortical steroids	Profoundly inhibits	None
Thyroxine	Greatly accelerates	Delays
Growth hormone	Accelerates	??
Ageing	Associates with declining speed	Little
Zero remodeling activity	—	Does not imply repaired healing
Zero repair activity	Need not imply zero remodeling	—
Primary hyperparathyroidism	Variable	May impair
Mechanical compression loads	Undetermined	Usually potentiate
Mechanical stress trajectories	Grain conforms to	Does not conform to
Space defect	Cannot fill it directly	Can fill it directly

This categorizes several differences between bone remodeling and bone repair. One must take them into appropriate account in clinical work or in trying to interpret research results which supposedly relate directly to clinical problems. In going over this table keep in mind one purely operational but quite rigid definition of bone repair: *It acts to restore normal mechanical strength to the part.* Consequently the only direct measure of its efficacy constitutes a direct measure of its mechanical strength, not its histologic or radiographic appearance, not the various enzymes one can measure in it, not its chemical composition, not its uptake of various isotopes.

Clinicians need not fall into the common trap of believing that what some laboratory finds a hormone or chemical compound does to bone remodeling will of necessity apply to your patients with healing fractures. For example, systemically administered steroids can totally turn off human bone remodeling but they do not seem to impair human bone repair (regardless of what they may do to rabbits or guinea pigs or rats). In fact steroids to some degree seem actually necessary for a biologically competent repair faculty.

material in later chapters which discuss some biomechanical problems found in fracture healing, joint arthrodesis, and joint arthroplasty.

2) THE BONE REPAIR PROCESS: Understand that *bone remodeling and bone repair differ rather fundamentally in their effects, responses, and reactions to a variety of challenges.* Table 13.08 lists some of these differences. In the past, the semantic fact that both involve stuffs we call by the same name, bone, as well as cells to which we assign the same names, osteoclasts and osteoblasts, has tended (mistakenly) to equate these things in our minds (see Volumes II and III).

When bone becomes injured, a special sequence of events follows, diagrammed in Figure 13.09. The injury may constitute a fracture, or a surgical operation, or the effects of some infection or of a malignant tumor (177,182,228,244,256,269, 270).

(*a*) *The Callus:* The sequence begins with the production by mesenchymal cell proliferation of new populations of several kinds of cells, and of new tiny blood vessels called capillaries. Then some of these new cells differentiate or specialize into special ones which we may name fibrous osteoblasts; they lay down bars or trabeculae of new fibrous bone organic matrix which, when it subsequently mineralizes (i.e., calcifies) soon afterwards, becomes a kind of biological solder known as fracture callus. Soundly and permanently adherent to the underlying bone at special adhesive lines termed (aptly) cementing lines or reversal lines, this biological solder repairs the fracture sufficiently well in the mechanical sense to allow function of the part to resume.* The callus producing mechanism can also fill in small holes and other structural defects in bone. The whole repair process

---

* Those who seek a strong and durable cement or adhesive suitable for use in the body's aqueous and ionic environment should turn their attention to that already functioning as such in our own bones, and leave the study of the adhesive which attaches barnacles to rocks and ship hulls to marine biologists. After all the adhesive mechanism evolved in our own bones and, acting at the cementing lines, already exists there perfectly adapted to our needs in the chemical, mechanical and biological respects.

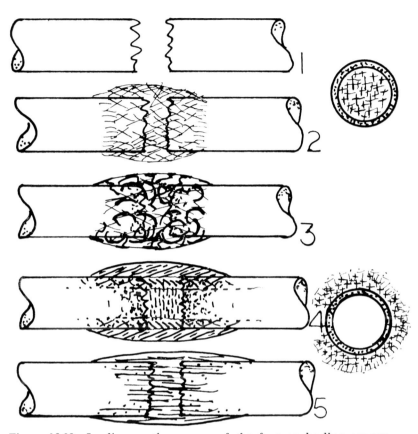

Figure 13.09. In diagram the essence of the fracture healing process.

(1) An *acute fracture* usually leads to the production of a hematoma and a

(2) *fibrin clot* which then undergoes organization, or invasion by blood vessels and supporting tissues. Within this granulation tissue

(3) there then appear new *osteoblasts,* and often chondroblasts, which deposit the various tissue components of the

(4) fracture *callus.* This then undergoes replacement by

(5) *lamellar bone* with its mechanical grain properly aligned paralleled to the major, time-averaged, stereotyped local stress trajectories. (Reprinted by permission of author and publisher, ref. no. 94.)

typically takes from three to twenty weeks in man (less in animals) to evolve. It happens sooner in children than adults, and sooner in trabecular than in cortical bone injuries, provided the local blood supply stays intact. Often considerable hyaline cartilage formation accompanies it, especially when undue motion of the fragments exists in the early stages of healing. Fracture callus does not deposit according to the lines of mechanical stress in the part; rather, it follows the lines of growth of the new capillaries.

(*b*) *Remodeling of the Callus*: Next, and after normal function has resumed, the callus tissue becomes gradually replaced by newly generated populations of typical lamellar bone remodeling BMU, in each of which a batch of osteoclasts first removes a moiety of the preexisting callus and then deposits in its place a newly made moiety of lamellar bone, one made by a batch of *lamellar osteoblasts*. This replacement process, named as such in Volumes II and IV, has elsewhere been termed the remodeling of the callus, a source of potential semantic confusion.* Note that lamellar bone always lays down according to the lines of the mechanical stress and strain resultants within the part, and in that respect its conformance to the local stress trajectories spans the resolution range extending from $1000\times$ optical magnification up to the gross, naked eye level. A variety of different biological, biochemical and physicochemical phenomena contribute to establishing that conformance at various levels of organization but this does not form an appropriate podium for discussing or speculating on them. Another good subject for more research.

In man it usually takes one to five years for the remodeling process to replace the fracture callus essentially completely with lamellar bone; a process that investigators such as Schmidt, D. Wilde and R. Schenk in Europe have described beautifully. Fortunately, the fracture repair usually attains sufficient mechanical strength to allow function to resume within some five to twenty weeks, depending on the injury, its location, the age of the person and some other factors.

(*c*) *The Chain of Events in Repair*: Effective fracture

---

* The text asks no debate with others who may use some of its terms in different contexts and meanings; it merely acquaints you with its own usages so we may communicate effectively.

repair depends upon and requires each of the following, which occur in temporal sequence in the order given:

1) a good local blood supply to the fragments;
2) good reduction and immobilization of the fragments;
3) the ability of special progenitor or mesenchymal cells to detect and react to the injury by dividing repeatedly;
4) thereby producing as new daughters the new differentiated cells called osteoclasts and osteoblasts,*
5) whose specialized intracellular biochemical machinery then actually makes and mineralizes the new organic matrix of the callus, which in the mechanical sense actually and directly repairs the damage.

Regard: *A break at any link of this five link chain will render the whole repair process ineffective.* A sixth link consists of modeling the fracture, and we will discuss it in a later chapter. While numerically speaking, in past times breaks of links (1) and (2) provided far and away the commonest sources of improper bone healing (i.e., 98%), now and in this country it seems that failings of links (3), (4) and (5) become increasingly common (i.e., $\approx$ 30–50%) (97,98,274), and as you might guess, we do not yet understand them very well.† With this material behind us, and after a brief quiz let us turn our attention to the stuff which usually caps the ends of bones and follows its own behavioral conductor: cartilage.

---

* Plus capillaries and other cells of the supporting tissues.

† As a rule, things that you really understand are not problems, only the things we do not understand are problems. This includes love, hate, war, the common cold, healing, and man.

QUESTIONS: CHAPTER 13

1) List the simple tissues of the skeletal alphabet.
2) Name the basic ways of creating a complex tissue.
3) True or False:
   a) Fibrous and lamellar bone differ in their chemical composition.

 b) Fibrocartilage and hyaline cartilage differ in their internal structural organization.

 c) Genetic factors directly determine the architecture of any given bone.

 d) Cortical bone has a different chemical composition than trabecular bone.

4) Name some of the physiological compositions nature "plays" upon the simple tissue keyboard.

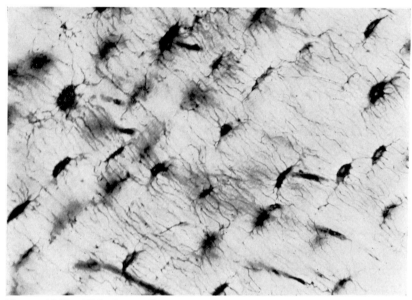

Figure 13.10. This figure illustrates the osteocyte lacunae and canaliculae of lamellar bone, as seen with appropriate contrast-enhancing filters in the light microscope at about 800×, in an undecalcified cross section of bone stained with the simple Frost basic fuchsin technique. In essence this provides a negative shadow of the physical holes in bone, rather than any information on its chemical composition.

 Record these numerical properties of the osteocyte lacunae (within which the cells called osteocytes reside): Lamellar bone contains about 18,000/mm³; each contains about 70–100 canaliculae, the very fine hollow tubes interconnecting the lacunae; the mean canalicular diameter equals 0.45 micron (different values characterize rodents and canines). A generation or more ago, Wassermann, J. Albert Key and M. Heller-Steinberg believed these cells might play a role in homeostasis and as the evidence now shapes up from laboratories such as those of P. Meunier, D. Baylink, J. Marshall, L. Belanger, R. Talmage, W. S. S. Jee, Dr. Hoshino, and J. S. Arnold (to name a few) that projection appears correct.

5) Name three cellular activities basic to all bone bio-dynamics.
6) Name the higher activities created by "playing" on three basic ones.
7) How many separate mechanical phases does bone combine?
8) a) Can lamellar bone signal pain to the brain? b) or its orientation in space? c) or mechanical strain? d) or injury?
9) Refer to Figure 13.10. Given the numerical data therein, find the following:
    a) The mean separation of individual osteocytes along three orthogonal axes, assuming regular cubic stacking.
    b) The mean canalicular length.
    c) The total canalicular surface per mm³ of bone; per liter ABV.
    d) The surface/volume ratio of the canaliculae.

Chapter 14

The Properties of Hyaline Cartilage

U NDERSTAND THAT THE cartilaginous tissues serve different roles in skeletal biology than bone, and those roles relate to specific properties of cartilage in the multiple senses of structure, composition, and most important of all, behavior. The exposition then will begin by summarizing some of the properties of hyaline cartilage, and then cope with its behavioral aspects.

1) PHYSICAL PROPERTIES

Density 1.3; water content: 75 per cent. Organic content 20 per cent of wet, 90 per cent of dry cartilage. Collagen: 39 per cent of organic content. Ash: 5 per cent. The above properties vary moderately according to the anatomical site under study (35,47). It behaves like a gel which, although elastic, has poor resilience, lacks brittleness and, especially over long periods of time, behaves in a non-Hookean manner. Elastic limit: unknown. Yield point: unknown. Ultimate strength: unknown. Approximate tensile strength: 1,000 psi. Shear strength: unknown. Grain: none as a simple tissue but pronounced in its complex tissue forms; it varies depending upon the sampling site one chooses. Thus, articular and epiphyseal cartilage (termed complex tissues in Volume II) have a pronounced grain but cartilage in a healing fracture (a simple tissue in this instance) does not (58). Cartilage has a mechanical compliance more than fifty times larger than that of bone.

Cartilage exhibits creep under shear. The amount remains relatively small in normal cartilage but can attain pathological amounts if the layer of cartilage becomes abnormally thick, or if some disease alters its mechanical properties in a way that increases its shear susceptibility, or if a combination of both occur. And such phenomena do occur, for examples in the varied kinds of rickets (77,78) , Morquio's disease, Hurler's disease, in slipped capital femoral epiphysis of adolescence and possibly in idiopathic scoliosis.

2) COMPOSITION AND STRUCTURE:

A relatively easily deformed, largely organic and gel-like material, hyaline cartilage contains large amounts of water loosely bound to its organic part. The organic part forms about a third collagen and two-thirds cementing substances which differ chemically and characteristically from the cementing substances of bone and teeth. Thus, cartilage (of all types) constitutes a fiber reenforced composite structural material, and since it does not mineralize to any significant extent except under special circumstances, it usually retains its rather large mechanical compliance. This endows it with the stress-relieving property when it interposes between two stiffer materials carrying loads across some incongruity at their mechanical interface. When mechanically squeezed for a long time, cartilage can lose much of its water and so decrease in volume. After removing the squeeze, it imbibes the water again. Because this takes time, cartilage does not behave very resiliently or in a Hookean manner, although it remains essentially elastic in its behavior and various authors now report studies of this phenomenon under the heading of its viscoelastic properties. While I once inferred and proposed the immediately challenged idea that cartilage might exhibit some creep with time (83) ; to repeat, we now know for a fact that it does. That creep plays some interesting and even essential roles in normal joint physiology, as well as in diseases such as scoliosis and slipped capital femoral epiphysis, roles we cannot discuss in detail because of space limitations. To continue now:

We recognize three kinds of cartilage as simple tissues: hyaline cartilage, elastic cartilage and fibrocartilage. Hyaline cartilage forms the one of major interest in biomechanics, since it serves as the Babbitt or bearing surface material in our joints and as a barrier to bone surface modeling activity in other locations which we will mention briefly later on.

TABLE 14.01
MECHANICAL PROPERTIES OF HYALINE CARTILAGE

Property	(*Wet Costal Cartilage*) Age			Fibro-cartilage
	15	35	55	
Ultimate compression strength (kg/mm²)	1.16	0.96	0.72	—
% contraction	17.0	14.0	13.0	—
Ultimate tension strength (kg/mm²)	0.46	0.42	0.25	5.3 (8%)
% elongation	28.0	25.0	17.0	
Shearing strength (kg/mm²)	.50	.45	.31	

Consider these values for cartilage strength (largely from Yamada's tables) only as ball-park or order-of-magnitude estimates for human articular and epiphyseal cartilage. We not only lack detailed studies of the mechanical properties of hyaline and fibrocartilage in their simple and complex tissue forms; determining them provides a sticky technical challenge.

Table 14.01 lists probable approximations of a few of its mechanical properties.

3) BIODYNAMICS:

(*a*) *Occurrence and Function*: New hyaline cartilage arises during the longitudinally acting growth processes, as well as at tendon and ligament attachments to bone, and in certain kinds of repair. In the evolutionary sense, it probably represents the most primitive of the hard skeletal tissues (223). It certainly represents the most primitive in the embryologic sense, for the initial models (anlages) of many bones formed in embryonic life derive from hyaline cartilage, and without them we simply would not be. Hyaline cartilage also serves as a special kind of glue which aids as a tension bonding agent to anchor to bone a variety of structures made of collagen and called tendon, ligament and fascia, and others called interosseous membranes. We will discuss these tension transfer mechanisms separately in a later chapter. Of major concern here, cartilage also forms the surfaces of all sliding or diarthrodial joints, and so represents a kind of special, biological Babbitt.

(*b*) *Growth*: Special differentiated cells called chondroblasts make cartilage. They reside in holes called lacunae inside the cartilage and they make the components of the organic intercellular matrix. And, while bone grows like a brick wall or a tree, that is by progressive additions of new layers to its outside surfaces, cartilage grows like a puff of smoke, by essentially uniform internal expansion. The progenitor cells that make new chondroblasts usually come to lie in a plane in the tissue which we will name the germinal layer. And *division of those cells represents the essential first step in chondral growth or enlargement, upon which depends one's body height and the lengths of all long bones.* Destruction of these progenitor cells (meaning of the germinal layer) will interfere with the subsequent growth, nutrition and function of growing cartilage (see Fig. 14.01) (251). Hence surgeons operating upon children's skeletons need to exercise care not to damage germinal planes inadvertently.

Cartilage does not turn over in the same packet-like fashion that lamellar bone does; a turnover of its molecular constituents does take place however, and fairly actively so for H. Mankin estimates the fifty per cent turnover time in rabbit articular cartilage as some eight days. It usually can undergo resorption (by special cells called chondroclasts) *only after it has become mineralized* (i.e., calcified), by which time most of its cells are either dead or dying. The overall frequency of the division of its progenitor cells falls in large part under the aegis of growth hormone and thyroxine, so those two hormones regulate overall cartilage growth (271,288) .*

A failure of cartilage growth due to subnormal cell division causes various forms of dwarfism (22). The spatial direction of growth of cartilage in tissue space responds to biomechanical factors (64,202), outlined shortly and well described for clinical needs in Volume II. In essence, under physiologic loads that direction of growth parallels the time averaged direction of the compression and/or tension load resultants acting across the cartilage, and its speed responds predictably to the magnitudes of those resultants. That explains why epiphyses and joint surfaces in children grow in

---

* Physiologists just begin to think about the natural question raised by this reasonably well established fact: what then turns off that response to produce maturity, i.e., a cessation of growth, when modern studies reveal it does not occur because we stop making either hormone?

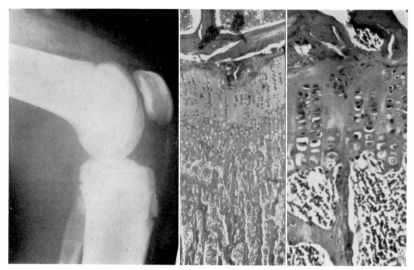

Figure 14.01. *Left:* Lateral x-ray of an adolescent child's knee. The thin, transverse radiolucent lines represent the *epiphyseal plates* of the distal femur and proximal tibia.

Middle: Photomicrograph of a longitudinal, hematoxylin and eosin stained section through the proximal tibial epiphyseal plate of a normal rat. The unmineralized cartilage lies opposite the patella on the left, and demonstrates vertical columns of chondrocytes residing within lacunae.

Right: High powered view of the epiphyseal plate of a rat, demonstrating the lacunae within which the chondrocytes reside. This rat was not normal; we treated him with toxic doses of an adrenal corticosteroid.

Growth at these plates determines overall body height and bone length (200,201,209). Any failure of it leads to dwarfism. And such growth depends primarily upon chondroblast cell division in the cell layer at the top of the plate. Local modifications in the rate of that growth can control limb alignment and a later chapter will describe some examples of such control.

the proper directions: The outside forces or loads acting on the part actually determine both the direction and speed.

(*c*) *Blood Supply and Innervation:* Hyaline cartilage has no direct blood supply. In order to maintain their viability its cells depend upon diffusion through the gel-like chondral substance of the nutrients, gasses and wastes they use and excrete (8). Repeated mechanical straining or working of the cartilage during normal function probably aids these diffusion processes. This arrangement makes cartilage able to take very large compression loads without harming the viability of its cells, and only bone and tooth of all of the body's other tissues have this same property.

In joints the synovial fluid nourishes the cells of the joint cartilage tissue, allowing it to live independently of the viability of the underlying bone. Mechanical circulation of that synovial fluid between the articular cartilage and the joint lining or synovia (richly supplied with nerves and blood vessels) must occur to maintain optimum chondral nutrition, and the usual daily motions of the joint ordinarily achieve that circulation. Cartilage contains no nerves whatsoever and so totally lacks any sensation.

(d) *Repair*: Hyaline cartilage heals mechanical injuries slowly and very poorly, particularly in adults. But it does try to heal and on about the same time scale as bone healing, although definitely longer. The healing involves initial proliferation of some of the chondral cells, their differentiation into cells capable of synthesizing the organic matrix of new cartilage, and then that synthesis. Such healing can respond to mechanical factors in the immediate environment, endowing even mature (but injured) cartilage with a limited ability to adapt to such factors. An important area for future biomechanical research represents learning to identify, understand and become able to manipulate or control this adaptive faculty, for it would enhance measureably our clinical diagnostic and therapeutic expertise.

4) BASIC FUNCTIONS:

The five we have identified so far for hyaline cartilage include:

It initiates one of the only two routes known in all of nature for producing or creating new hard skeletal tissue in mammalian life;

In that capacity it plays essential roles in the creation, development and growth of bones *in utero* and during childhood (42,58,66,67).

Its biomechanical force/growth-response characteristic (the principle of action which describes how it responds to mechanical factors) plays an essential role in aligning limb joints and in determining articular architecture;

It inactivates the flexure-drift law on any bone surface it covers;

And makes an excellent bearing surface material.* Keep in mind that each of the above functions or roles of cartilage depends for its effective realization upon selected properties of cartilage.

5) CHONDRAL GROWTH/RESPONSE CHARACTERISTIC:

Volume II quite recently defined for the first time if in a general way the characteristic responses of growing cartilage to mechanical forces. With respect to tension and compression loads applied parallel to the direction of overall growth, the accompanying figure provides a curve which in the operational (i.e., clinically useable) sense defines these responses. In essence, *cartilage grows more slowly under tension than under compression, but a point exists on the ascending compression-loading portion of the curve at which growth begins to retard.* And with further increases in compression load growth ultimately arrests (184). The physiologic range of tension compression forces, that is, the range of load magnitudes experienced in a normal skeleton during a typical year, covers only a portion of the total curve. Volume II outlined these matters at greater length.

In action in the growing skeleton, this growth/force-response characteristic determines and then maintains normal alignment of limbs about joints according to the negative feedback situation described in figures 14, 15, Chapter XIX. It does so by regulating the speed of cartilage growth on each side of a joint in the appropriate way. As a result of the behavioral properties of this characteristic, minor abnormalities in limb alignment act in the mechanical sense to change the cartilage growth rates in exactly that way which tends to restore the normal alignment. Only when the malalignment

---

* To wit: it can carry large loads continuously without loss of its viability, because that viability does not depend upon fragile, pressure sensitive capillary blood vessels.

exceeds some limit (as yet undefined in absolute number) so that one side of the joint becomes loaded over onto the descending compression limb or pathological range of forces of Figure 14.02, does such a deformity become a self perpetuating, positive feedback (i.e., self aggravating or vicious cycle) type of thing.

Like the analogous bone and fibrous tissue phenomena, this chondral response characteristic exhibits the very important time-averaging property, in that its actual response conforms to the dictates of all the loads taken by the region and averaged over some period of time, one named sigma but not exactly defined as yet, and ranging from a few weeks in a newborn to far longer than man's whole life span by skeletal maturity. To use a concept delineated in Volume III, that time period represents sigma for the chondral modeling process. And where intermittent and dynamic changes in loads appear to provide the most effective stimulus of biomechanical origin that controls the biomechanical force-response characteristics of lamellar bone and fibrous tissue, cartilage growth may also respond to steady or constant loads in its appropriate fashion. Relatively recently recognized, we have no good studies of such matters at this writing which would permit us to replace our uncertainties and our verbally phrased recognition of important principles of action with hard, numerically expressed knowledge.

Epiphyseal plates receive effective mechanical shielding from unequal unit loadings over their areas, shielding provided by the ossification center within the epiphysis itself, which acts as a thick, somewhat stiff pad protecting plate from joint surface. As you can see in Figure 14.01 left, that protects the plates from any unusual local load concentrations that might arise at and act directly on the growing articular cartilage surfaces. Thus *these plates tend to determine the overall alignment of our joints.* On the other hand, lying in direct, unprotected contact with the opposing joint surface, *the articular growing cartilage tends to respond in that manner which will determine the external joint shape.* While some controversy should exist over the propriety of these

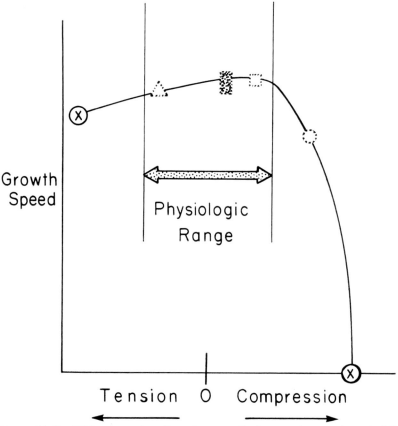

Growth
Speed

Physiologic
Range

Tension　0　Compression

Figure 14.02. This curve describes the *growth force-response characteristic* of healthy cartilage growing under normal (i.e., perpendicular) forces. The vertical axis plots growth rate, the horizontal axis plots stress ranging from tension on the left down towards zero and over into compression on the right. The curve has an *ascending limb* and a *descending limb,* and the peak dividing them lies towards the limit of the physiological compression range of forces. The horizontal rectangle simply indicates the *physiologic range*; forces outside of that range are abnormal ones or we say they lie in the *pathological range*. Over the physiologic range, growth proceeds slightly faster in compression than in tension (a readily and repeatedly demonstrable fact, not an hypothesis, as Volume II described). As loading enters into the pathological range of compression, growth retards reversibly for most of the span, but with excessive loading complete arrest can occur. This characteristic accounts for the bulk of normal limb alignment and normal articular architecture, given only as a basis for it to begin working on, the fetal cartilaginous skeletal anlages, normal muscle anatomy, and neural integration. This mode of behavior appears consistently during growth and one finds it hidden or concealed by "noise" only in special circumstances such as during local repair processes or in the presence of some intrinsic chondral disease such as occurs in rickets or slipped epiphysis. (Reprinted by permission of author and publishers, ref. no. 94.)

laconically stated rules of thumb in the coming ten years, in the clinical action they function with apparently flawless consistency and consequently the interested reader may speculate less over the accuracy of the behavioral predictions they generate, and more upon the cellular and biochemical mechanisms which underly these responses.

As far as skeletal architecture goes and taking these matters one analytical step further, these aspects of the chondral growth/force-response characteristic imply that the *overall alignment of limbs must derive basically from the patterns of muscular contraction that affect them,* beginning from the time such contractions first arise in the fetus. Those patterns must derive just as much from the neural integration mechanisms which determine those contractural patterns as from the anatomical dispositions of individual muscles. The chondral growth/force-response characteristic also implies this: *the gross articular surface shape represents a predictable adaptation of growing articular cartilage to the dynamic muscle forces carried by the joint during its development,* particularly during its phase of most explosive relative growth, which lies between the third month of intrauterine life and age one year of postuterine life.

Let us now write all of that as a verbal equation:

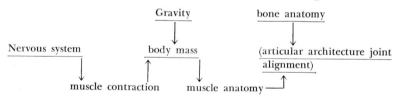

As we near skeletal maturation, the ability of cartilage to grow becomes actively suppressed by some means* so that only trivial amounts of chondrocyte division and true cartilage growth occurs throughout that part of man's normal life span following his skeletal maturation (132). However,

---

* The clue that this represents active suppression rather than some kind of exhaustion: when taken out of the adult body and placed in cell culture media *ex vivo,* these cartilage cells recommence the active cellular division which forms the inescapable initial requirement for chondral growth.

various injuries and joint diseases, including particularly the so-called degenerative or traumatic forms of arthritis, can somehow reactivate the cartilage growth potential, usually at the periphery of the affected joints, leading initially to the production of large, unmineralized cartilage spurs which one can feel but cannot see on x-rays (196). These then become replaced (inevitably) by bone from their base, to produce ultimately the bony spurs that do become visible upon x-ray. Also injury can reactivate both cartilage production and growth, a fact we make use of each time we perform a mould arthroplasty, or drill into the bony bed that shed a free floating osteochondritis dissecans.

6) FIBROCARTILAGE:

We will discuss this tissue only briefly. Like hyaline cartilage, it represents a mixture of the same collagen and hydrophilic cementing substances, but unlike hyaline cartilage it has a great deal more collagen in it in terms of gm/cc, and correspondingly less water. Its sparsely distributed cells lying in lacunae, receive their nutrition by diffusion through its substance, for it contains no blood vessels, nor any lymphatics or nerves. Thus it, too, remains totally insensate (any pain generated by a torn meniscus such as may occur in football players, arises from severe mechanical distortion of adjacent, well innervated tissues by the meniscus, and not in the meniscus itself).

In its simple tissue form its fiber phase lacks uniform architectural organization. But in its complex tissue form (examples: medial and lateral menisci of the knee), the collagen bundles always exhibit an overall preferential spatial orientation, one which parallels the time averaged tension load resultant acting on it. That resultant usually also parallels the gross anatomical length of the meniscus. Accordingly a meniscus in bulk possesses great tension strength and rigidity but equally respectable flexural and shearing compliance. We will propose one role of menisci, and thus of the complex tissue form generally, in a succeeding chapter.

QUESTIONS: CHAPTER 14

1) Name three basic functions of hyaline cartilage.
2) How many mechanically separate phases does cartilage contain?
3) a) Can cartilage signal pain to the brain? b) or orientation in space? c) or strain? d) or stress? e) or injury?
4) Name the major features of the chondral growth/force-response curve.

Chapter 15

The Properties of Fibrous Tissues

1) Composition and Structure:

Ligaments, joint capsules, fascia, tendons and interosseous membranes, all form important structures of the skeletal system in a biomechanical sense, even if one must classify them as soft tissues. A common basic fiber building stuff serves in all of them to endow them all with similar basic functions and mechanical and biological properties. Of this group we will consider tendon primarily, as fairly typical and illustrative of this whole group of structures.

The major organic constituent of all fibrous tissues and fibrous tissue organs consists of the fibrous, crystalline protein named collagen. Existing as bundles of parallel fibers, *collagen supplies one simple basic mechanical function: strength and rigidity in tension, and in tension only.* It thus permits great flexural and shearing compliance or flexibility, where bone supplies strength plus rigidity in all three principal modes: compression, shear and tension. Table 15.01 lists some mechanical moduli for collagen, and also for some of the other constituents of skeletal building materials. Note that per unit cross section area, plain collagen has less than ten per cent of the stiffness in tension of bone. This bonus of compliance in tendons and ligaments has one predictable effect: it provides real protection to their bony attachments from impact in tension. That is a sudden muscle contraction or ligament pull produces lower impact stresses on the anchoring bone than it would if it had the same E, or tension stiffness, as bone itself. The magnitude of this effect conforms approximately to this relation:

$$\text{Impact reduction factor} = \frac{\text{E bone} \times \text{Cross section area bone}}{\text{E tendon} \times \text{Cross section area tendon}}$$

or, in symbols:

$$f\ (D) = \frac{E_b\ A_b}{E_t\ A_t} \qquad Equation\ 15.01$$

Fibrous tissues actually constitute composite, fiber-reenforced materials with two phases. The first constitutes the collagen fibers, and the second an embedding gel-like, water-soaked matrix of the mucopolysaccharide named hyaluronic acid. The cell (the fibroblast) manufactures tropocollagen fibers as helical molecules wound of individual, and also helical substrands, each with a defined and constant number and sequence of amino acids. Outside the cell that manufactures them (whether fibroblast, osteoblast or chondroblast), these tropocollagen units serve as mers to construct long chain collagen polymers (75,110). Some cross linking of these fibers exists and it usually increases with age. And some form of bonding must also occur with the embedding, compliant gel of MPS. The gel allows shearing displacements between adjacent collagen bundles to occur readily parallel

TABLE 15.01
MODULI OF STRUCTURAL TISSUE COMPONENTS

Material	Moduli, 10^{11} dynes/cm^4			Tension, 10^6 psi	Poisson's ratio
	Bulk	Shear	Tension		
Collagen	0.14	.046	0.12	.18	.35*
Bone	1.5	.71	1.9	2.7	.30
Dentin (bovine)	1.8	.80	2.1	3.1	.30
Enamel (bovine)	4.6	3.0	7.4	11.0	.23
Fluorapatite	9.4	4.6	12.0	17.6	.28
Hydroxyapatite	8.9	4.4	11.4	16.7	.27

* Poisson's ratio estimated.

This lists the mechanical moduli for collagen, a basic organic constitutent of all of the skeletal structural simple tissues except tooth enamel. Enamel has a special but non-fibrillar organic matrix. Keep in mind that these moduli define *stiffness*, not strength. Witness the more than 10-fold increases in stiffness over plain collagen that arises when hydroxyapatite crystals deposit on and among them to form bone and tooth dentin (from reports by J. L. Katz and K. Ukrainik; and R. S. Gilmore and J. L. Katz, *J Biomech*, 4, 1971).

Note too that to convert 10^{11} dynes/cm^2 c.g.s. moduli to English 10^6 psi units, multiply the former by 1.5 and leave the decimal alone; to convert from English to c.g.s., multiply the former by 0.66. Finally, observe that the isolated apatite crystal has six times greater stiffness than the bulk bone of which it forms a part, and in the region of 100 times greater stiffness than the collagen in that bone.

to their grain, which explains the high gross flexural compliance of fibrous tissue structures.

In its simple tissue form, no uniform order appears in the overall orientation of the fiber bundles in fibrous tissue, and it looks like felt under a magnifying glass. We call such a mass a scar. By simply producing uniform fiber alignment in space, the same chemical constituents transform to the complex tissue form which one finds composing ligaments, fascia and tendons. An occasional blood vessel and tendon cell (fibrocyte) lies within these tissues, and their special cementing substance or hyaluronic acid molecules appear in the EM very like bristles on a test tube brush, attached to a protein core or backbone.

As for the function of the complex tissue forms, by definition a tendon attaches a muscle at one end to something else on the other, which may consist of a bone, another tendon, a ligament or a sheet of fascia, and it does so to transfer a tension load from one to the other. Ligaments bridge joints in part to prevent laxity or excess mobility in certain directions not well stabilized by muscle forces, while fascia forms a kind of biological fabric which wraps up or flexibly encases some organs, such as muscles. Fascia may also serve as part of a load transmitting attachment to other structures. Fascia envelops other structures as its skin does an orange; it serves as a source of flexible structural support to some organs (as a burlap bag gives shape to 80 pounds of sand) , and it isolates some parts of the body from others.

Table 15.02 lists some approximate mechanical properties of living, intact fibrous tissue structures, all examples of complex tissues.

2) BIODYNAMICS:

(a) *Function and Growth*: As for function and as just noted, the basic role of a tendon constitutes transfer of a tension load from a muscle to another structure (usually a bone) . As for its manufacture, special cells called fibroblasts or tenoblasts make the extracellular constituents of tendons. Like bone and trees, nature provides separate means for the

TABLE 15.02
MECHANICAL PROPERTIES OF FIBROUS TISSUES (WET)

Tissue	Ultimate tensile strength kg/mm²	% Elongation
Fascia, thigh (human)	1.14	16.7
Fascia, leg (human)	1.04	15.6
Tendon, Achillis, age 25 (man)	5.6	9.9
Tendon, Achillis, age 75 (man)	4.4	9.1
Extensor Pollicis longus, age 35 (man)	6.7	9.9
Tendo Achillis (horse)	8.4	8.0
Tail tendon, (rat aged 12 mos.)	4.7	

Again these values for the tension strength of the complex tissues fascia and tendon must be considered approximate. The seemingly great differences between tendon and fascia reflect two things; one constitutes the nonuniform fiber orientation in fascia which, remember, has two coplanar axes of fiber orientation. The second factor represents the technical difficulties in measuring accurately what fraction of a mm² of tendon or fascial cross section forms its collagen, and what forms the interfibrillar water and MPS. Clearly a one mm² cross section containing 50 per cent collagen will prove twice as strong as another one containing only 25 per cent collagen.

It follows that the differences in various tendons probably reflect more some differences in collagen packing density than in its inherent nature.

longitudinal growth, and for transverse or sideways growth. Longitudinal growth responds to the growth control mechanisms of the body generally, which appear largely hormonal in nature. Like bone, a tendon's transverse growth responds to the mechanical tension forces applied to it according to a simple negative feedback system that reacts to excessive stretch by causing the cells residing in it to add new tendon substance laterally.

(b) *Turnover*: Healthy, uninjured tendon turns over fairly slowly in normal adults, and its rate of turnover (in the region of 1 to 5 per cent per year) probably compares with that found in human adult bone compacta in some parts of the skeleton (157,221). While such turnover was once disputed (based upon studies in lower animals using not-too-sensitive methods) it has now become clear that it does occur. Presumably this turnover represents at least in part a way to repair mechanical microdamage due to fatigue or injury.

(c) *Blood Supply and Innervation*: Tendon receives nourishment from arteries which enter its substance from the surrounding loose connective tissue. Where tendons go through confining tunnels, a structure called the mesotenon carries the nourishing vessels and nerves. Tendons also contain strain sensitive, specialized nerve endings and pain fibers. One must infer from a considerable variety of clinical facts that these strain and pain sensitive endings serve at least this role: via their connections with the central nervous system they provide a fail-safe mechanism which, by detecting and warning of impending failure in tension (in terms of excessive tension strain) and thereby evoking protective reaction from appropriate muscles, do in fact serve to protect the system from destruction by the contractural forces of its own muscles.

3) REPAIR:

A tendon injury, like that of bone, heals in two stages. In the first stage, progenitor cells (ubiquitous in all tissues of mesodermal origin) that in some way the injury stimulated begin proliferating to make new fibroblasts. Those latter cells then produce a tangled mass of new collagen fibers embedded in newly elaborated cementing gel, a mass called a scar when it occurs in other soft tissues and named tendon callus when it develops in an injured tendon. It may take about five weeks to finish producing the tendon callus. The fibers of this callus or scar lie randomly oriented in space, and so provide suboptimal bulk mechanical tension strength. Figure 15.01 diagrams the basis for this. After deposition of this callus function of the part can resume. And during that function and while the living subject remains unaware of any subsequent events, a remodeling process arises, quite analogous in several ways to that developing in fracture callus, one which gradually replaces the tendon callus by new tendon, i.e., new collagen fibers embedded in mucopolysaccharide, and with the new fibers aligned reasonably uniformly parallel to the pull or tension load carried by the tendon (or ligament, capsule or fascia). This replacement stage, which probably occurs in quantized packets analogous to the fracture callus replacement process, may take some three years

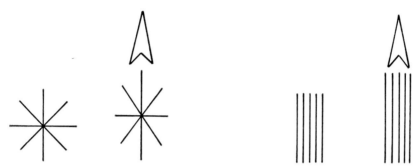

Figure 15.01. *Left:* The random orientation of the collagen fibers in a fresh scar (a simple tissue) of any type provides relatively poor bulk strength in tension in any direction.

Right: But when uniform alignment of these fibers arises, as one finds it does in normal tendon, ligament and fascia (now complex tissues because of this added structural order), the identical mass of collagen can have more than five times greater bulk strength and rigidity in tension.

or so to reach completion, a time period that depends in part upon the subject's age, the replacement process finishing sooner in children than in adults.

For those delving more deeply into the biology of this and related problems than most pure clinicians may care to, we must note here a fact held in common by bone, cartilage and fibrous tissue organs: The physiology of the mechanisms that normally turn them over or remodel them in the rather specific context of that term in these five volumes, differs in many fundamental ways from that of the mechanism of the initial repair process appropriate to each. Much research gets off on the wrong foot, or leads to silly and embarassing errors in interpretation, because of a certain lack of awareness of that fact.

4) FUNCTIONS:

Collagen has one simple basic mechanical function, while living fibrous tissue has that plus one further biological function. The first (already named twice) held in common by both constitutes the purely passive one of providing *rigidity and strength in mechanical tension alone,* and those all in one direction or axis. While neither collagen nor fibrous

tissue lack rigidity in compression and shear according to our
fairly rigorous definition of rigidity in an earlier chapter
in Part I, at the levels of resolution that concern us here they
lack any great stiffness in compression and shear, and so provide fairly high compliance to them, as well as to flexural and
torque loads. Thus *collagen provides a basic biological fiber
or thread*. With it, nature weaves ropes of tendons and ligaments providing mechanical rigidity in only one axis and
principal strain—tension—as well as fabrics called fascia
which provide tensile rigidity along two coplanar axes but
in only one principal strain—still tension. And as noted in
preceding chapters, it participates in bony tissue (and dentine and cementum) in combination with mineral salts to
provide rigidity and strength to all three principal strains,
and in all three spatial planes, simultaneously.*

The second function of fibrous tissue represents a dynamic
and biological one which we will define as the stretch hypertrophy rule, signifying the capacity of living fibrous tissue
structures to adapt their total strength to the mechanical demands made of them, given time to do so and provided that
living populations of mechanically competent cells reside
within them. We describe it next.

The Stretch Hypertrophy Rule: Living fibrous tissue
structures respond in a particular fashion to mechanical
loads. Under most shearing and compression loads, they
appear to exhibit no detectable response that can change the
architecture of any organ made of fibrous tissue. But when
a series of intermittent tension loads elongate it repeatedly
beyond some minimum degree (termed elsewhere the minimum effective strain) (97), this appears to generate and deliver some type of signal to the cells within and around the
tendon which in sum, and ignoring here the details, stimulates them to produce additional collagen. This additional
collagen of course adds to the total preexisting cross section
area of the structure, whether it constitutes a tendon, a liga-

---

* These statements suggest some intriguing possibilities ré making composite
materials with unusual bulk mechanical properties. Perhaps we shall see some
of them materialize in the coming years in industry.

ment or a sheet of fascia. Increasing its cross section area also increases its net total tension strength and its total tensile rigidity, and in direct and probably equal proportion (153). Increasing its rigidity of course then decreases the amount of elongation it will develop under subsequent tension loads

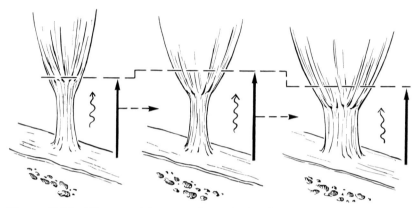

Figure 15.02. The stretch-hypertrophy rule in diagram.

Left: A tendon attaching the muscle above to the bone below for purpose of transferring tension loads. The curly vertical arrow immediately alongside it represents the tendon's length with the muscle at rest, while the bold and slightly longer one represents the tension strain or stretch developed in the tendon each time the muscle contracts. Clearly the amount of that stretch will depend on the strength of the muscle and the cross section area of the tendon.

Middle: Assume the muscle increases in strength, perhaps due to growth, or to a weight lifting program attendant to a sudden interest in a particular member of the opposite sex. Consequently the increased force of its contractions increases the time-averaged, intermittent tension strains of the tendon.

Right: Somehow that phenomenon leads to the production of additional tendon substance which increases its cross section area, and thus its size and total strength *and stiffness,* until its time-averaged tension strains again reduce to the normal or limiting amount. Of some interest analytically, tendons also produce electrical surface phenomena when strained and as for the case of bone those phenomena may play a role in controlling the collagen-making cells in this set-up. But whether yea or nay the operational rule epitomized here exists and proves consistently applicable, and exists on its own merits quite independently of the electrical problem. One finds it "drowned," and so hidden, by other phenomena only in special circumstances, for example during active fibrous tissue repair processes, or in the presence of pathological-range loads, or in the presence of devitalization of the tissue.

of similar magnitudes. The system continues to act in this manner until enough augmentation of tensile stiffness has arisen to reduce its typical tension strains again below the minimum effective strain level (which probably lies somewhere in the region of 1–3% elongation). Figure 15.02 diagrams this mechanism, which we may also write as a verbal equation, as follows:

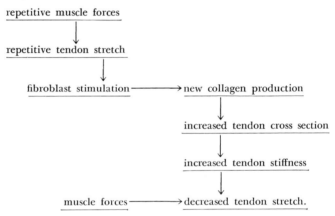

This hypertrophy in cross section area following excessive intermittent stretch represents the stretch hypertrophy rule. In action in our bodies, this stretch-hypertrophy rule demonstrates the following three additional significant properties. We emphasize "intermittent" because a single tension strain, and most likely a constant one, do not appear to actuate this system or principle of action. In fact a constant strain leads to a definite stress relaxation phenomenon analogous to that reported in Part I under the consideration of viscoelastic behavior of polymeric plastics.

The tissue has some means of time averaging the loads it carries and thus the strains it develops, and the total cross section area ultimately attained represents that most suited to the time averaged conditions. We do not know the exact length of this time averaging period (i.e., its sigma value as we call it elsewhere) but it probably constitutes a few months.

The creep property: In addition, when observed in some clinical stituations (particularly when placed under a constant tension load by some form of traction) structures made of fibrous tissue appear to demonstrate a significant amount of mechanical creep, and will elongate significantly under relatively small tension loads maintained constantly over long periods of time, even though they may demonstrate enormously greater strength and rigidity under large tension loads applied for only brief periods of time. If fibrous tissue does possess the creep property, then the fact that tendons, ligaments, and fascia do not progressively stretch out during the fifty or so years of a man's adult life span under the influence of normal resting muscle tonus suggests further that a creep compensatory mechanism must exist within the tissue. We do not yet know whether this represents a cellularly driven process, or a purely physical chemical one, or a combination of both.

The curvature effect: On the convex-tending side of a fibrous tissue structure carrying a tension load around a curved trajectory, the stretch-hypertrophy rule consistently becomes somehow inactivated. We have only recently recognized this effect (although some of its clinical manifestations have been long known) and we have no adequate physical chemical and/or biological explanation for it.

5) LIGAMENT FUNCTION:

In one important aspect, ligament function appears to enlarge in scope over that of tendon function. Both have the common role of transfer of mechanical tension loads, most ligaments of course transferring them from bone to bone* where tendon transfers them from muscle to bone. And the purpose of that transfer in ligaments differs from that in tendon for the former provides a mechanical restraint to certain undesired motions of a joint, usually motions not directly controlled by the muscles serving as its prime movers.

However, ligaments seem to play another special active

---

* The annulus fibrosus of the intercentral vertebral joints seems to function as a circumferential pressure container which prevents hydrostatic pressure within the nucleus pulposus from extruding it transversely. The longitudinal spinal ligaments more likely serve the role for the spine that we discuss here for the extremity joints.

role in addition to the purely passive one just categorized. The relevant facts and inferences in this regard include the following.

Ligaments contain abundant nerves, including special end organs responsive to mechanical tension strain, and fired off (i.e., made to send afferent impulses back to the CNS) by mechanical stretch of the intact ligament.

In the living conscious subject one cannot rupture ligaments by deliberately applied forces, for example by forcing a knee into valgus to load the tibial collateral ligament in tension. This remains true because a point comes at which the patient's muscles will contract beyond his power to inhibit them and *in such a way as to relieve the ligament of that load*. And that remains true whether he tries to overload it deliberately himself, or whether another person tries to overload it by manual means. Under an anesthetic, of course one could rupture the ligament by such means.

From those and numerous clinical facts it becomes reasonable, even necessary, to infer that ligaments provide a strain-sensitive monitoring device which, in the presence of dangerously high levels of internal tension stress, fire off warning signals to the CNS which result (via some special reflex arc) in immediate muscle contractural activities which act to stress-relieve the ligament.

Of course, such a behavioral mode would have to have the effect of protecting the joint from disruption by and during normal function.

Now let us look at how this might apply to some clinical matters of biomechanical nature. *Examples in action*:

Shoulder dislocation: Bankhart's original concept of the basis for recurrent dislocation of the shoulder represented a capsular laxity plus a geometric defect of the anterior margin of the shallow glenoid socket, which allowed the humeral head to slide forwards, down and out and to luxate repeatedly under physiologic motions and usage. The corrective operation he devised does permanently snug up the anterior capsule and so permanently restricts external rotation of the shoulder (it also cures the problem of repeated dislocations).

If that pathophysiologic concept correctly epitomized the problem, then it should follow that operations which neither correct glenoid labral defects nor permanently restrict external rotation should not cure the dislocation problem.

Fact: The Magnuson Stack procedure does cure the problem in some ninety-seven per cent of persons accepting it, yet it rarely causes permanent loss of mobility.* The procedure consists simply of elevating the insertion of the subscapularis tendon (combined with its fusion with the anterior joint capsule) from the lesser tuberosity of the humerus, and moving it laterally and distally and anchoring it by some means to the humerus lateral to the biceps groove. The glenoid labral defect (which I find in only about half of these shoulders) remains untouched in this procedure.

My explanation for its success (as well as that of the seemingly equally good Putti—Platt reconstruction) goes something like this:

Normally a mechanically unstable joint because of its shallow socket, the capsular ligaments of the shoulder by virtue of the strain monitoring property referred to above prevent dislocations in normal usage and circumstances, by making the shoulder muscles contract in those ways needed to avert impending sublaxation. But if the capsule heals in a lax state after a traumatic dislocation, the shoulder must at least partly sublux to tauten the ligaments enough to activate this strain—sensitive monitor. Since this usually occurs during some fast moving dynamic function, the few tens of milliseconds delay this causes in the muscular reaction to the warning signals provides enough time for the subluxation to proceed to a full luxation before the muscles can avert it. It follows then that a corrective surgical procedure which eliminated the capsular laxity without damaging the capsular innervation should correct the usual case of recurrent dislocation of the shoulder (and that proves correct). It

---

* And this does not constitute an opinion; it is a fact of the author's own 20+ years of clinical experience with this procedure, and one duplicated and duly reported in our literature by many other orthopaedists.

follows too that if one does not immobilize an initial traumatic dislocation long enough (and in the correct position of internal rotation and adduction) for primary healing of the torn capsular ligaments to occur (this takes some five weeks), recurrent dislocation should ensue much more often than otherwise. Clinical experience certainly supports this concept.

Ligament reconstruction: We know from experience that repair of a torn ligament—as in the knee in athletes for example—usually works out quite well as long as one can use and retain the original ligament, and this seems true whether we do the repair immediately after injury, or do a later procedure which corrects any laxity of the ligament (we will ignore here some special technical problems posed by particular ligaments such as the anterior and posterior cruciates of the knee).

We also know from experience that most ligament reconstructions done with free grafts (whether of tendon or fascia) fail in that they progressively stretch out over several months after resumption of function. Furthermore, such joints prove unusually prone to reinjury later. Clearly a free graft becomes infarcted, and denervated thereby, while one's own ligament should still retain most of its blood supply and innervation, even if torn.

This implies that choosing procedures that retain the strain-monitoring property in surgical ligament reconstruction and/or repair (by preserving its remaining blood supply and innervation) should lead to clearly better long range results than procedures which sacrifice that property, and any free graft must sacrifice it. And it raises the possibility (unanswerable at present) that if one could mechanically protect the latter class of procedures from too large mechanical loads long enough after the operation, that the reconstructed ligament might become reinnervated from its host tissues so as to again become a competent strain monitor.

Note: We discuss elsewhere the probably quite separate problem of mechanical fatigue of a free devitalized ligament graft. If protected long enough postoperatively to become reinvaded from its enveloping living tissues with biomechanically competent lines of mesodermal cells, the stretch-hypertrophy law can again come to operate to increase its cross sectional size to meet demand. This assumes of course that resumption of loading occurs gradually and progressively over a period of some months after the five to six week period of initial healing postop. I have seen examples of this return of competence in my own practice, so its dependability forms the issue, not the possibility.

QUESTIONS: CHAPTER 15

1) Name the separate mechanical phases of all fibrous tissues.
2) Define the stretch-hypertrophy law.
3) a) Define the first order function (s) of fibrous tissue. b) of hyaline cartilage. c) of lamellar bone.
4) Two tendons have identical cross section areas. Must they then have identical strengths?
5) Which should (and does) prove stiffer in tension: young collagen or old? Why?
6) What mechanical test would most effectively measure the degree of cross linking in bulk mature fibrous tissue? Why?
7) A normal conscious person cannot voluntarily make his muscles contract with sufficient force to rupture the tendons, or avulse their bony attachments, or fracture his bones by indirect violence. But in the throes of a convulsion or when an unexpected obstacle suddenly and abruptly halts a forceful motion of a limb, such ruptures and/or fractures can and do occur. a) What does this imply about the functional properties of the nervous system control set-up? b) On that basis, how do you evaluate the practice of injecting painful sprained ligaments of athletes with procaine or xylocain just before a game? c) What does this concept suggest an orthopaedist should favor in choosing ligament reconstruction procedures about major joints?

Chapter 16

Synovial Fluid

1) PROPERTIES: (230) Density: 1.1. Viscosity about 10 to 100 centipoise, and variable. Table 16.01 provides some representative viscosity values. Organic content: 10 per cent. Ash: 2 per cent. Cell: 100/mm³.

2) COMPOSITION. The major constituent in synovial fluid constitutes mucin, which consists of many separate mer molecules of an MPS or cementing substance (hyaluronic acid) joined at one end to a protein backbone to make an elongated composite molecule looking somewhat like a test tube bristle brush, as shown in Figure 16.01. Separate mucin molecules can join or polymerize end-to-end to form polymers of variable length. Normal synovial fluid also contains some dissolved glucose, CO_2, oxygen, amino acids, electrolytes and other cellular nutrient and waste substances in small amounts.

3) BIODYNAMICS.

(a) *Variable Viscosity*: Increasing the amount of mucin, and increasing the number of molecules combined into the average mucin polymer molecule, will both tend to increase the viscosity of the synovial fluid (286). With increased shear rates (i.e., increased speed of joint motion)

TABLE 16.01
VISCOSITY OF SELECTED FLUIDS

	Poises	*Centipoises*	$cm^3/dyne$ *Bulk modulus*
Water	.01005	1.005	50×10^{-12}
Olive oil	.840	84.0	65×10^{-12}
Linseed oil	.331	33.1	
Glycerine	8.30	830.0	22×10^{-12}
Ethyl alcohol	0.12	1.2	80×10^{-12}
Acetone	.0031	.31	
Synovial fluid	.10	10.0	

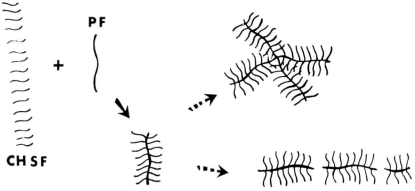

Figure 16.01. The basic mucopolysaccharide molecule (MPS) of the skeletal tissues looks like a test-tube brush under the electron microscope. Its linear core constitutes a long protein molecule and about five per cent of its mass. The bristles represent various chemically closely related polysaccharides, consisting of chondroitin sulfates A and B in bone, A and C in cartilage, and hyaluronic acid (chemically related to heparin) in fibrous tissues and in synovial fluid. Small amounts of another called keratan appear in bone, cartilage and fibrous tissue.

One can readily see that rather complex bulk properties can arise by combining or polymerizing these molecules end-to-end as at the bottom right, or by entangling their bristles as at the top right, or by coiling and folding, as well as by other arrangements.

CHSF: Polysaccharide molecule   PF: Protein filament core.

the rodlike polymers tend to break up into small fragments; this would tend to decrease the viscosity, and thus the drag on the joint surfaces, during high speed joint motion. It might also provide one major factor determining the non-Newtonian behavior of synovial fluid viscosity, which tends to decrease significantly at high shear rates. As to their origin, the mucin molecules come from the synovia, either made by the synovial cells themselves or by the interstitial cells in the tissue just outside of the synovia. They undergo constant turnover as the synovia absorbs and removes old ones and replaces them with new ones. Because as joint motion decreases in speed the viscosity of the lubricant increases (33,286), the variable viscosity acts in that way which makes it harder to squeeze a knee or ankle joint dry by standing still upon it.

Basically two different kinds of stacking of mucin molecules should occur in life in synovial fluid, and it should form no great problem to study them. These two ways constitute what one might term the log jam pattern, and the parallel roller pattern.

1) *The Log Jam Pattern*: When articular surfaces (or a tendon in the tendon sheath) move very slowly or not at all, the mucin molecules should tend to stack quite irregularly, the bristles of one mucin brush entwining at various angles with those of another, and regardless of the mean polymer length. They would thus tend to form a quasi-planar felt-work, somewhat compressed from above by the compression load across the joint. In this form they would add measure-able resistance to shearing displacements of the synovial fluid, for it would require extra force, far above the fluid's normal surface tension, to disentangle the bristles of one brush from those of its neighbor. That implies that the fluid's viscosity should rise at low or zero shearing rates (which it does).

2) *The Parallel Roller Pattern*: When the articular sur-faces begin to move, the elongated mucin molecules should begin to align perpendicular to the direction of motion and to roll between adjacent layers of fluid moving at different rates. This much resembles the way in which one might move a house or garage on rollers made of logs. The mucin polymers, probably as elongated clusters rather than indi-vidual molecules, would thus tend to "log roll" rather than to tumble end over end under high shearing rates, and the longer the polymer and the stronger the bonds joining them end to end, the more striking should this effect become. This should respectably decrease the resistance to shearing dis-placement of the synovial fluid during rapid articular motions (which does actually occur), and it should also produce thixotropic birefringence, mostly of the form variety, which should prove detectable and quantitatively measureable in *in vitro* systems.

(b) *Nutrition and Circulation*: The synovial fluid nour-ishes the chondrocytes buried in the lacunae of the articular

TABLE 16.02
SYNOVIAL FLUID COMPOSITION

Component	Range	Mean
Viscosity (25°C) (centipoise)	10 –1000	235.0
pH	7.2 – 7.4	7.4
Leucocytes/mm^3	13 – 180	60.0
Total solids, gm/100cc	2.4 – 4.8	3.4
Albumin/globulin, gm/100cc	1.02– 2.1	1.7

Fibrinogen, glucose, NPN, electrolytes: same concentration as in the blood plasma.

cartilage.* Circulation of that fluid by joint motion brings its dissolved nutrients close to the articular region overlying a given cell (which they actually reach by diffusion through that cartilage), and takes away from the cellular region its dissolved waste products. Table 16.02 lists some of the constituents of this fluid. That provides a necessary assist to cartilage cell nutrition, for otherwise some of the larger nutrient molecules, such as glucose, the amino acids and hormones, would diffuse so slowly through a fluid as viscous as synovial fluid as to threaten the viability of the cells. Fortunately, frequent joint motions circulate the synovial fluid repeatedly to alternately expose it to both the synovial lining and the cartilaginous surfaces many times a day.

---

* This is as good a place as any to define the meaning of a function in this text, and in musculoskeletal physiology generally. Consider a joint: it allows motion to occur between two or more biological rigid solids, with a minimum of accompanying wear and friction. This motion serves the needs of the rest of the body and constitutes the primary or direct or first order function supplied to the whole man by the joint. This joint also has innumerable other properties, such as size, mass, rigidity, chemical composition, hardness, blood supply, dielectric constant, ohmic resistance, geometry and so on. Some of these properties may prove essential to sustained performance of the joint, but to the rest of the body they have no direct meaning. In other words, function uniquely signifies a relationship, something done by one part for the rest. If this function (such as joint motion) can be substituted satisfactorily by an entirely different kind of inanimate device, the rest of the organism would not care or even know the difference. We get into trouble in biomechanics as often because we do not really know the true functions of biological structures and systems yet, as because of deficiencies in our inanimate structural materials. For example, one function of bone constitutes providing a rigid physical support. But another function consists of generating special surface signals in accordance with the way it strains. These signals control cell activity on its surfaces, and the cell activity then determines the bone's actual size and shape. Our metallic bone replacements do not do this.

When this mechanical circulation effectively stops long enough, the cartilage cells in the region of closest surface contact of the joint surfaces may become embarassed to the point of dying. And when that happens something deleterious also happens to the physical properties of the surrounding cartilage, for as a result it becomes thinner and thinner with subsequent use, leading to joint disease of the bearing failure type.

QUESTIONS: CHAPTER 16

1) a) Define a Newtonian fluid. b) In what sense does synovial fluid form a nonNewtonian one?

2) a) Define log jam pattern of mucin molecule arrangement. b) and the parallel roller pattern.

3) What nourishes articular cartilage? What removes its cellular metabolites? What lubricates our joints? What lubricates our bursae? Our tendon sheaths?

4) a) Does articular cartilage form a simple tissue? b) Does scar? c) Does fracture callus? d) Does synovial fluid? e) Does adult spongy bone? f) Adult cortical bone?

Chapter 17

Voluntary Muscle and Skin

I: MUSCLE

1) COMPOSITION: While the contractile protein in muscle constitutes actomyosin (2), the gross mechanical dynamics of muscle concern us more in this biomechanics text than its compostion or chemistry (135), so we say nothing further here about the latter.

2) BIODYNAMICS:

(*a*) *Kind*s: Of three different kinds of muscle tissue, only one directly concerns us here. Called voluntary or striated muscle, its distinguishing functional property consists of the fact that we can voluntarily control its contractions and relaxations.

(*b*) *Structure*: A typical voluntary muscle contains thousands or millions of long cells, each of which contains the biochemical equipment and internal structures that cause it to shorten when delivered a stimulus to do so. This stimulus comes from a nerve fiber which connects to the muscle cell's outer membrane at a special region called the motor end plate.

(*c*) *The Motor Unit*: One motor nerve fiber (i.e., an axon) leaving the spinal canal divides into many separate fibrils after entering the muscle it supplies, and each of these fibrils then supplies a single muscle cell. Thus, when a single axon delivers a contractile impulse to a muscle, all of the separate muscle cells supplied by its fibrils will develop a contractile twitch, although a latent period of some 0.04 seconds elapses between delivery of the stimulus and the first mechanically observable change in the muscle. The twitch that results takes some .04 seconds to develop, and another .05 seconds to relax. This means that all of these cells form a functional entity, one Sherrington named the

257

motor unit. When given the command to contract, each muscle cell shortens briefly and then relaxes. It can only do this a certain number of times per second, for a brief recovery phase seems required after each contraction for the muscle cell to recover (called the relative refractory period and equalling ≈ .03 seconds) and become ready for its next contraction, and until that recovery has occurred the muscle cell remains only slightly affected by additional strong nerve impulses.

(d) *Control of Gross Contractile Force*: The grossly observed gradation in the contractile force of intact muscles arises primarily and simply by varying the number of its motor units stimulated to contract per second. Because a very large number of motor units exist in most muscles, their gross pulls act as though infinitely adjustable (Table 17.01 provides some numerical data on this). Just so the total fighting strength of large army might vary in an apparently continuous way by varying the number of individual soldiers in it.

(e) *The Force-Length Relation*: The maximum contractile force or pull a muscle can generate depends in part on its length expressed as a fraction of its resting length. Generally as muscles shorten beyond the resting length they can generate only weaker than maximal contractions, and conversely. A curve of the relative contributions to its total contractile force of a muscle's dynamic contractile force, and the purely passive contribution due to its inherent elastic resistance to stretch, appears in Figure 17.01. A typical voluntary muscle cell can contract to about sixty to sixty-five per cent of its resting length, and it retains significant dy-

TABLE 17.01
SOME PROPERTIES OF MUSCLES

Muscle	Mean diameter of muscle cells, microns	Total number of muscle cells	Total number of motor axons	Number of motor units	Muscle cells per motor unit
Platysma	20	27,000	1800	1100	25
Brachioradialis	34	130,000	520	315	410
Tibialis anterior	57	250,000	740	450	657
Gastrocnemious	54	1,100,000	960	580	1900

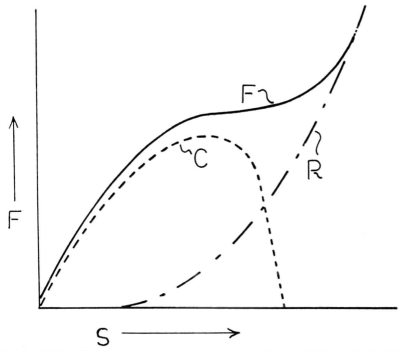

Figure 17.01. The muscle force-length relation. The solid line F, signifies the amount of total tension force a muscle exhibits as one progressively elongates it. It develops that two internal elements cause this. One, the active element, constitutes the contractile force produced following maximal stimulation of the nerve innervating it, and in relation to its degree of shortening or extension it has an ascending limb, a peak and a descending limb which in essence reaches zero at about 30% elongation beyond the resting length.

The second and passive factor constitutes the elastic resistance to tension strain of the muscle cells and interposed fascia and other tissues, which rises sharply on the right towards the rupture point at around 0.5 kg/mm².

namic contractural force out to one hundred thirty per cent or so of its resting length.

When a muscle contracts against some fixed resistance so that no mechanical work is done (i.e., $WL = O$), it still expends chemical kinetic energy which appears as heat carried away by the body's practically universal heat sink, the blood. Physiologists term such as *isometric* contractions. When on the other hand a muscle contracts and shortens against a constant resistance it performs mechanical work, and we name this situation an *isotonic* contraction. Intriguingly, given equal nerve stimulation a given muscle expends more total work during an isotonic than during an isometric contraction.

As to the relationship between cross section and contractile force, a muscle can exert approximately 4–10 kg f/cm² of cross section perpendicular to the muscle cell long axis. The mechanical power it can generate relates proportionally and directly to its mass (or with equal validity, its volume). Note that muscle's passive strength to rupture in tension approximates 50 kg/cm², which represents a considerable safety factor in preventing it from rupturing itself.

(*f*) *Anatomical Types of Muscle*: By differing the mechanical arrangements of muscle cells, and of muscle cell attachments to tendons, a variety of functional types of muscle organs occur in nature. Muscles which have a long distance between their extended and contracted position (i.e., a long range of contraction) tend to consist of strap muscles, in which all the muscle cells lie parallel to the gross anatomical length. Such muscles sacrifice overall contractile force for increased contractile speed and increased absolute linear excursion* of their contractile motion.

Where a very large contractile pull or force seems needed, muscle cells weave in complicated ways which, in essence, provide large pulls (i.e., force multiplication) at the expense of speed of contraction and excursion of motion. We call such muscles pennate muscles, and the strongest among them consist of the multipennate muscles (See Figure 17.02).

(*a*) *Nomenclature of Attachments*: Muscles must attach to something solid at each end in order to do mechanical work. It has become anatomical convention to consider the attachment closest to the center of the body the origin, and that farthest away, or that to which its tendon connects it, the insertion, of a muscle. Functionally and dynamically, of course, these terms simply form different and

---

* Given that any muscle has an active contraction range equal to 60% of its resting length, then the range in cm (i.e., in absolute number) of the sartorious may approximate 20 cm, but that in the palmaris brevis only 0.5 cm.

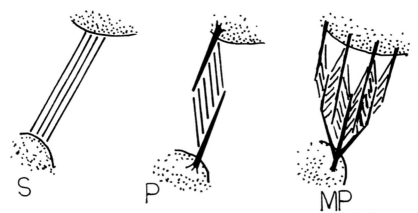

Figure 17.02. A strap muscle in which the uniformly parallel alignment of the muscle fibers provides maximal contractile range and speed of the whole muscle.

Middle and right: By interweaving the muscle cells in the manner shown one obtains increased contractile force at the expense of decreased range and speed or linear velocity of contraction.

arbitrary points of view, like loads and stresses (See Figure 17.03).

(*h*) *Repair*: As far as we now know, muscle cells (like the neurons in the central nervous system) do not turn over significantly in adult man, so we have to do the best we can throughout life with the number of fibers we come endowed with in early childhood. Nor does striated muscle repair itself following injury by generating new striated muscle. Instead it heals, or becomes stitched back together, by scar tissue, which (as reported earlier) forms initially as a felt-like interwoven network of collagen fibers.

(*i*) *Intermuscle Relations*: A muscle that directly causes a motion (of interest at any moment) we call an agonist, and other muscles that may assist it we call synergists. The muscles which oppose those actions then form the antagonists. Clearly this nomenclature also reflects as much a difference in point of view as the differences between democrat and republican.

3) EXERCISE: We may identify two separate behavioral properties of muscles of some importance in every day life, both affected by exercise.

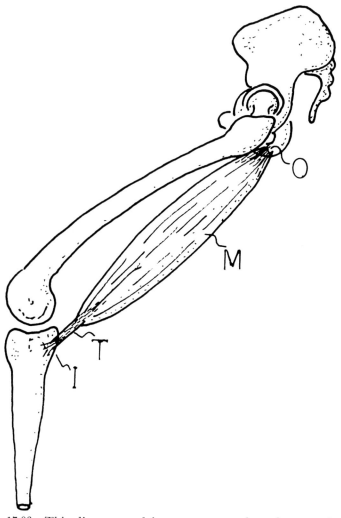

Figure 17.03. This diagram explains some nomenclatural conventions for nonmedical readers. Human thigh from the left side. M: a muscle *belley,* the actively contractile part of the organ, lying below the femur bone. O: its proximal attachment to the ischial tuberosity of the pelvis bone, named the *origin.* T: the *tendon* which transfers its tension load to the posterior surface of the tibia bone. I: the *insertion,* or attachment of the tendon to the tibia.

(a) *Total Strength*: The maximal contractile force a muscle can exert can build up through periodic exercises involving contracting against maximal resistance. One need only do these exercises briefly several times a week (as weight lifters do). They will lead to a visible and measureable hypertrophy in the diameter and cross section area of a muscle, although only up to some limit inherent and predetermined in a given person. The hypertrophy represents a true increase in the cross sectional size of individual muscle cells, not an increase in their number, and without a real change in their length. This behavioral property underlies the use of progressive resistance exercises in clinical orthopaedics. This consists of evoking a series of maximal contractions of a muscle or muscle group (which vary from 10–50 in different parts of the country) against some form of resistance (springs, or weights and pulleys for example), with week-to-week increase in the resistance as the muscle gains strength.

(*b*) *Endurance*: This constitutes a quite separate property of a muscle and signifies its ability to repeat a given amount of mechanical work a great many times. This work lies much lower in magnitude than that produced by a maximum effort exerted through a maximal range. Thus a long distance runner's lower limb muscles may fatigue quickly if asked to exert a maximum effort, but can take him twenty plus miles in a marathon if properly trained. One achieves endurance in a muscle by daily exercise which taxes it to its limit of endurance, and it does not associate with increased muscular cross section, nor any change in the length or cross section of individual muscle cells.

Note: Great strength does not provide great endurance, nor conversely (152).

II: THE SKIN

We will describe some of the properties of this organ very briefly. Thus it consists basically of three layers, each subdividable into others but that concerns dermatologists and internists more than this text. These layers include:

Epithelial layer, including the living epithelial cells and the outer, keratinized layer of harder, tougher dead cells.

Dermis, composed chiefly of collagen fibers which provide the bulk of the tissue's strength in tension parallel to the surface of the skin.

Tela subcutanea, composed of the fatty tissue, blood vessels, nerves, hair follicles and sweat glands. The vessels in this region nourish the whole skin.

Properties: the skin provides a tough, quite elastic but poorly resilient external surface to the body which protects underlying structures from mechanical abrasion, which effectively damps out impacts from external hard objects and surfaces, and which limits body water loss by limiting fluid evaporation. Normal skin can accept very large compression loads if only briefly applied.

Of considerable orthopaedic interest, even normal skin has a low tolerance for continuous pressure, this tolerance lying in the range of 0.5–3 lb/in^2. The harmful effect of this pressure arises by interference with flow of blood in the blood vessels in the underlying tela subcutanea. This becomes quite important in applying casts, braces, elastic circumferential bandages and like devices which the patient will wear continuously for many hours, days or even months. Fortunately in normal conscious persons an impending pressure sore or ulcer signals itself by generating a considerable amount of pain which neither patient nor physician can easily ignore. But this mechanism may fail in infants and young children, in comatose or stuporous patients at any age, and in regions lacking normal sensation because of underlying neurological disease such as post CVA, myelomeningocele, traumatic paraplegia, peripheral nerve injuries, some neuropathies and the like.

Also the absolute tolerance of skin to continuous pressure falls in the presence of anemia below ten grams per cent of hemoglobin as well as in severe nutritional deficiencies, whether due to poor food intake or to chronic, wasting illnesses.

For obvious reasons persons with little fat in their skin prove more prone to pressure sores than fat people, for extra fat acts as a stress relieving pad over various bony prominences. In thin, poorly padded patients a bulky implant on a subcutaneous bony region may create a large enough bump or rise in local contour as to cause local skin necrosis, now not from external pressure but from the elastic stretching of the skin over the underlying device, a stretching which damages the fragile capillaries in the tela subcutanea on which skin viability depends. A fracture fragment jutting up beyond the periosteal level of a major fragment can also lead to a local necrosis by this mechanism, and require its removal.

Precisely this intolerance to continuous pressure has led to the development of some forms and techniques of internal fixation and of skeletal traction, as means of bypassing the limits otherwise imposed upon therapeutic need by the skin.

Repair: When incised (whether therapeutically by a surgeon, or as a means of resolving "social disagreements") and then sutured back together, the skin will heal. A layer of new epithelial cells will grow over the surface, while a feltwork of collagen fibers called the scar will stitch together all of the deeper layers over a period of 1–3 weeks. But the scar requires an additional 3–6 months before it will accept in normal fashion local contusions and undue tangential tension loads. The scar exhibits both the stretch-hypertrophy rule and the curvature rule behavior mentioned in an earlier chapter dealing with fibrous tissues. During that 3–6 months time the scar usually contracts significantly in volume, and undergoes internal replacement and remodeling so its fiber directions conform to the local tension load resultants.

Anything that impairs local perfusion by the blood will retard the wound healing process, and the commonest factor here arises in the surgeon: he tends to tie the sutures in skin and tela subcutanea too tightly, creating a local slough which prolongs healing and adds to the total eventual amount of scar.

We have now established our mechanical and physiological foundations, a basis for comprehending some of the biomechanical properties of the intact musculoskeletal system. Accordingly in the remaining chapters we will consider an illustrative constellation of bodily problems or systems, such as an intact joint, force-structure relations in an intact and real bone, spine function, a limb alignment problem, some biomechanics of fracture healing and some of the tension load transfer mechanisms evolved by nature, as well as some others.

The particular examples serve simply to illustrate general cases. One expects the reader can and will extrapolate from those particulars to the general situation for himself.

After disposing of those matters the text will finally discuss a variety of problems related to the use of implant devices, kinds of problems that every practicing orthopaedic surgeon will meet one or another way, and some many times over. At the conclusion of that material the formal text ends and Part III comes along.

QUESTIONS: CHAPTER 17

1) A muscle's power proves proportional to what property? b) Its contractile force proportional to what? c) Its active range of contractile motion to what?

2) a) Define isotonic contraction. b) Isometric.

3) What is the motor unit?

4) What determines directly the patterns of muscular contractions?

5) What determines the types of loads a muscle can apply to any structure?

Chapter 18

The Structure, Design and Function of Joints

I: BASIC STRUCTURE

IN THIS CHAPTER we will try to take a system-oriented view of a typical sliding human joint, meaning we will try to relate its various anatomical and physiological properties to the purposes that it seems to us they serve at this time (23,24, 222).

Table 18.01 lists a simple anatomical classification of the basic kinds of joints. Figure 18.01 sketches some important features of the mammalian diarthrodial (i.e., sliding) joints. Basically, it possesses two apposing smooth cartilaginous articular surfaces. When no load crosses the joint, their surface curves do not match perfectly, and in such a way that a small wedge-shaped gap arises between them at the joint edges. As a result, the load transferred across the unloaded joint tends to concentrate on a relatively small region of the whole joint surface. But the fall-off in unit loading, as one goes centrifugally from the central region of highest unit loading towards that peripheral one of lowest unit loading, occurs quite gradually. Between these two surfaces lies a

TABLE 18.01
ANATOMICAL CLASSIFICATION OF JOINTS

Synarthroses (immovable)	Synchondrosis (cartilage, hyaline) (ex: epiphyseal plate) Symphysis (fibrocartilage) (ex: symphysis pubis) Suture (fibrous tissue) (ex: skull) Syndesmosis* (ligament) ex: coracoclavicular ligaments)
Diarthroses (movable)	Enarthrosis (ball and socket) (ex: hip, shoulder) Ginglymus (hinge joint) (ex: knee, elbow) Screw joint (ex: atlantoaxial) Trochoidal joint (ex: radioulnar) Saddle joint (ex: carpometacarpal of thumb) Irregular joint (many carpometacarpal joints)

* Motion of the two parts may occur, the coracoclavicular syndesmosis being an example; in others it may not, the coracoacromial syndesmosis being an example.

267

film of the viscous synovial fluid, which adheres chemically to the cartilage, and which to some extent permeates into it. And we may state this literal truth: *Our ability to live, play and work depends on maintaining over our life span a reasonable mechanical integrity of these thin films of fluid.* The need to keep them unbroken throughout all conditions of use dominates many of the details of joint design.

Note bene: One of the reasons nature probably chose cartilage to construct our Babbitt with seems quite simple: joints must take large compression loads, such loads would crush fine blood vessels, and cartilage seams the only living tissue in the body whose viability does not depend upon a patent, functioning internal capillary bed.

Underneath the articular cartilage lies a thin layer of subchondral bone, joined to the cartilage by a basal layer of calcified cartilage of irregular contour. This irregular but interdigitating contour, combined with the fact that all such joints carry sizeable compression loads acting perpendicularly to their surfaces (typical maximum unit loads in compression during active function approximate 50–70 kg/cm^2, and during one's lazy periods less that 10% of that) acts to lock or press the cartilage hills down into the bone valleys, giving rise to a mechanically effective resistance to any relative displacement of bone on cartilage in shear.*

The collagen fibers in articular cartilage do not align randomly within its substance. It forms a complex tissue, not a simple one, and they tend to come perpendicularly out of the subchondral bone, but then curve as they approach the joint surface to become parallel to it, as shown in "A" in Figure 18.01. At the surface, the overall direction of these fibers tends to lie perpendicular to the direction of the usual or time averaged shearing motions of the two surfaces on each other. This probably arises as a consequence of a gradual

---

* This shear, representing the viscous drag of the moving joint surfaces on each other, equals ≈ 1% of the superimposed compression load. By actually measuring the mean angles of the slopes of the hills and valleys referred to one can show that this shear-locking mechanism has approximately 20× greater strength than needed to prevent dislodging the chondral/subchondral joining under this shearing load.

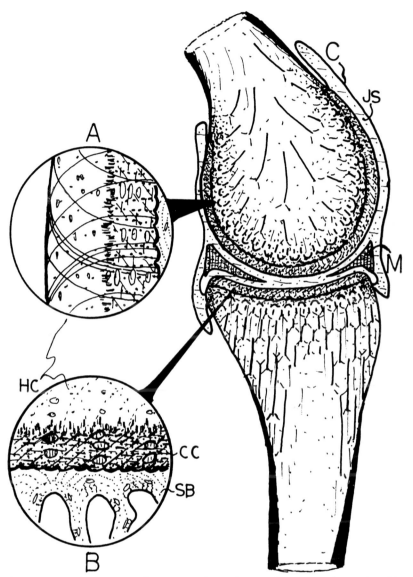

Figure 18.01. A diagram of a typical joint, here a knee seen from the side. C: capsule and synovial membrane lining. JS: the synovial fluid of the joint, normally less than 5cc in volume in a healthy knee. M: the meniscus (only a few joints possess them). HC: Hyaline articular cartilage. CC: The calcified or mineralized layer of cartilage at the base of all articular cartilage in adults, and supported by the underlying SB, or subchondral bone.

Note the "fanout" of the trabecular bone supporting the articular cartilage as one moves from joint towards diaphysis.

mechanical creep or flow in the cartilaginous substance in response to the compression and shearing strains that arise during joint motion under load. It analogizes the orientation of sea weed or marsh grass in an incoming (or outgoing) tide.

The subchondral bone in its turn lies supported by numerous arches of deeper trabecular bone (secondary spongiosa, a complex tissue), which accept the loads crossing the joint, and distribute them gradually and progressively towards and onto the more distant cortex of the bone as the accompanying x-ray illustrates.

Ligaments (complex tissue structures not shown in Fig. 18.01 but discussed briefly in an earlier chapter) stabilize joints in those planes in which dynamic muscle forces do not move or protect them, and a lax, enveloping capsule folds and unfolds in the plane of greatest motion. This capsule (another fabric-like structure made largely of collagen) creates a closed joint cavity or space whose lining tissue (subsynovial fat and synovial membrane) prevents mechanical extrusion and loss of the synovial fluid. Muscles and tendons cross joints but need not actually touch or attach to them; they provide the dynamic forces which move the joint against the resistances of body inertia, gravity and other mechanical reactions.

Table 18.02 summarizes some of the design priorities of human joints, which we consider next.

Functions: The diarthrodial joints all have one basic, primal first order purpose and function: *To allow one rigid skeletal member to move upon another.*

In achieving that function, a second order purpose arose: The capability should last over a man's life span (i.e., it should possess service life durability). That led to a second order function: *minimization of net wear.** And many of the

---

* Why "net"? Because of two things. First, durability of the prime purpose of a joint need not depend at all upon life long protection from disabling wear by making perfect use of perfect inanimate materials. Equally it could depend on a biological and dynamic factor added to it which constantly and effectively repairs imperfect materials and use-caused deterioration thereof, to allow a joint as a functional entity to remain normally functional throughout our life span. Second, nature actually chose the latter route.

TABLE 18.02

DESIGN PRIORITIES OF HUMAN JOINTS

JOINT

First order function: Allow motion of one solid body on another

1° f: Allow motion of one solid body on another

2° f: to last a long time

3° f: to minimize wear

4° f: minimize friction

5° f: lubricant smooth surfaces

6° f: Pumps   Phys   supply
                chem
                props

7° f, *etc.*

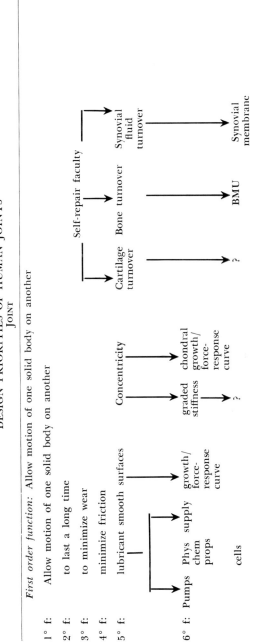

Table 18.02

For human joints and from a systems behavioral viewpoint rather than a morphological one, this lists the purposes existing at varying levels of organization, and their priorities as the author finds them. "One degree f" signifies first order function, i.e., its immediate and direct purpose in the whole system.

third and higher order design features and functions of joints focus upon that single, second order one. The reduction of friction in joints thus becomes, not the major purpose of a joint but rather one means nature used in joint design simply to minimize net wear. As we begin to implant artificial joints in people with increasing frequency, we increasingly face the hard proof that wear, not friction, constitutes one of the major and direct design challenges they pose us, and its solution deserves the higher priority.

II: BASIC DESIGN FEATURES

1) INTEGRITY OF THE LUBRICANT FILM: Inadvertently compromising or destroying one of the properties of joints essential to lasting and reliable function, for example by operation or injury or improper use of a cast or a brace (the author still calls them that, and leaves to others the use of terms such as orthosis and sanitary engineers), can lead to what one could call a bearing failure, and which in clinical practice we term degenerative joint disease (See Figure 18.02), or if a known injury caused the problem, a traumatic arthritis. Many specific design features of joints serve (directly or indirectly) to help to maintain the continuity of the very thin film of synovial fluid between the moving joint surfaces, thereby minimizing wear by minimizing their actual contact (57,80,83,94,146,195,196).

2) GRADUATED STIFFNESS AND COMPLIANCE: As one goes from the articular cartilage towards the midshaft of the bone, one goes from a region of minimum stiffness* (or max-

---

* While quite true that measured in inches these structures have a very small amount of give, so the trachea has a small diameter if measured in miles; small, but important.

Note bene concerning these two paragraphs: A recent discussion with Dr. Eric Raden exposed a region of possible confusion here which we can resolve by recording two sets of facts.

First, in terms of materials properties, articular cartilage does have much higher unit compliance than the underlying spongy bone, and the latter's unit compliance exceeds that of the diaphyseal compacta. But that's not the whole story, for:

Second, the total thickness of the articular cartilage may equal some 4 mm.

imum compliance) to one of maximum stiffness or rigidity. A solid glass rod represents a quite rigid and brittle structure, which will break easily if bent only slightly, yet the same cross sectional amount of glass in the form of a rope woven of fine glass threads will retain the total tensile strength and tensile rigidity of the original solid glass rod, but now it has great flexural compliance, so that one can tie a knot in it without breaking it. Just so, the systems of thin bony trabeculae under the cartilage provide effective mechanical support but now combined with a considerable increase in overall and particularly flexural, compliance. Table 13.04 and 13.06 make this quite clear in revealing that E, or Young's modulus in compression for compact bone, can exceed that of spongy bone more than sixty-fold. Or if you prefer, spongy bone can have sixty times more compliance than compact bone. This compliance gradually decreases from the articular surface towards the most rigid part, the middle of the bony shaft, as shown in Figure 18.01. Note that per square cm of support cross section, the diaphysis of the bone (its compacta) consists about ninty-five per cent of bone and only five per cent of internal porosities, while trabecular bone

---

but that of the underlying spongiosa in the metaphysis may equal 50 to 70 mm. Since each unit of trabecular thickness adds its own compliance to that of all of the others above and below it, the *total* compliance of the metaphyseal spongiosa may exceed by 3x–30x that of the intact articular cartilage. And here another factor enters in: while a one mm. cube of cartilage may squash to $\frac{1}{3}$ or less its original height under a compression load, it does so by bulging laterally. But in place in a joint, surrounded on all sides by similar unit amounts of cartilage, each securely fastened to the underlying bone, the intact articular cartilage becomes hardly able to bulge laterally at all. Thus *as an intact structure* the compression compliance of an articular cartilage surface loaded uniformly in compression becomes markedly less than that of an isolated, small cube of the stuff, and so markedly less than that of the whole metaphyseal spongiosa.

Similarly, the even lesser unit compliance of the diaphyseal compacta nevertheless adds up over the total length of the diaphysis, and so it contributes significantly to the total compliance in axial compression of the intact bone.

This situation illustrates in one microcosm, the nature and value of a system's approach to skeletal function, and one reason why studying atomistic properties alone cannot ever (and alone) provide an adequate understanding of the neuro-moto-skeletal system.

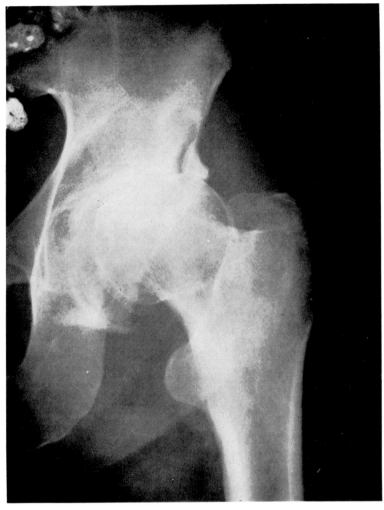

Figure 18.02. This adult's hip undergoes a "bearing failure," having lost first the integrity of its subchondral mechanical support, and that led to high load concentrations on the still properly supported articular cartilage which then wore away. Note, too, the evidence of a lax joint capsule. Underlying cause: tertiary lues, causing an early Charcot joint. As the articular cartilage wore down the bony parts came closer together, and the increased whiteness on either side of the joint indicates bony reaction to the disturbed local loading and other biomechanical properties. This example of an early arthritis of the hip did not arise from any known trauma (i.e., injury).

typically consists of about eighty to eighty-five per cent of the soft, nearly totally compliant marrow tissues in between individual cross section area, and only some 15 to 20 per cent actually represents supporting bone of the trabecular type.

This graduated stiffness appears crucial to durable joint function, although few seem to have appreciated its role in the past Figure 18.03 illustrates several situations in which this compliance become impaired, or never existed.

3) VARIABLE DIRECT BEARING AREA: Let us first discuss those sliding joints which do not have menisci present.

As noted earlier, when at rest without any superimposed large compression loads acting across them, such joints usually exhibit close contact in their center regions, and a slight, wedge-shape gap at their peripheral edges. Because of this and because the backing of the articular surface (i.e., cal-

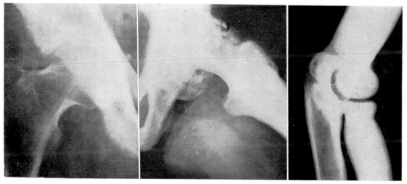

Figure 18.03. *Left:* Paget's disease of the socket in this adult's hip changed the compliance of the bony backing beneath the cartilage, which over a period of years led to breakdown of that articular cartilage and a bearing failure.

Middle: Another patient with the same disease—and result—of the hip joint.

Right: An adult patient, born with a congenital disorder which retarded removal of the mineralized tissue residues of growth from the metaphyseal parts of the marrow cavity of the bones (osteopetrosis). Thus the subchondral bone in this joint has had subnormal compliance since childhood, and clinically it, too, has begun to develop signs and symptoms of a bearing failure (x-rays courtesy of Dr. M. E. Castle of Detroit).

cified cartilage, subchondral bone beneath it and the immediately underlying supporting trabeculae) can yield slightly under superimposed compression loads, the area which effectively transfers the majority of the load across a joint increases as the total load it carries increases. In our hip joint for example the close contact region varies from about fifty per cent of the opposing surfaces at zero load to one hundred per cent at total loads on the order to fifty to seventy-five pounds (116). Thus, unit loads on the synovial fluid film between joint surfaces should not increase in direct proportion to the total loads (See Fig. 18.04). Doubling the total load should increase by less than two-fold the unit loads. We lack any numerical measure of the magnitude of this effect at present.

The Role of Menisci: First a few background facts. Anatomically speaking, a meniscus represents a fibrocartilaginous structure interposed between two sliding joint surfaces which have a larger than average wedge-shaped gap at their outer regions. The meniscus lies in and so fills that gap. In addition, the meniscus either represents a complete (if distorted in outline) circle as in the acromioclavicular and sternoclavicular joints, or if only part of a circle then each of its ends has a very strong attachment to one of the bones participating in the articulation, as in the knee.

Now, the joints which possess menisci all seem to have an unusually large amount of incongruity of their mating cartilaginous surfaces, and one finds the menisci interposed exactly between the regions of greatest incongruity. Furthermore the orientation of the greatest tension strength in such a meniscus exactly matches that which one would deliberately establish if he intended the meniscus to accept a large fraction of the total compression load transmitted across the joint surfaces. The meniscus in other words partially floats one joint surface on the other, relieving in a substantial way the central region of closest contact (the variable bearing area). See Figure 18.05. To achieve such a function, the hoop tension strength parallel to their perimeter and possessed in common by all menisci becomes essential.

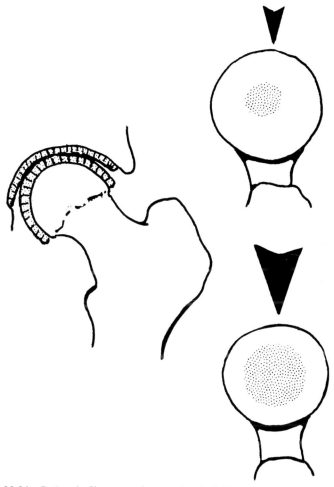

Figure 18.04. *Left:* A diagram of an unloaded hip as seen from the front, illustrating the articular cartilage on the ball and socket, and the slight wedge shaped gap at the periphery.

Right: The closest contact area in the lightly loaded state at the top enlarges significantly as the joint accepts loads, as implied in the bottom diagram. This occurs because of the graduated compliance mentioned in the text, and it serves as a mechanism for reducing unit normal loads on the synovial fluid film between the articular surfaces.

Note: This remains a diagrammatic visualization, for the geometry of the bearing area of the socket of real hip joints actually has a horseshoe shape.

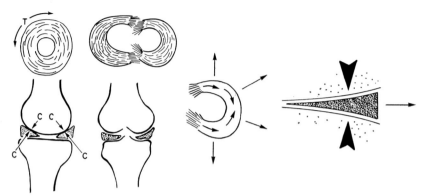

Figure 18.05. *Left:* Given a meniscus forming a complete circle as seen from the top in the top view, and given great "hoop" strength, or tension strength parallel to its circumference, then a bearing surface pressing down on it as shown below *could actually float free of the exposed articular cartilage region lying within the central hole in the meniscus.* Clearly, by adjusting the meniscus form and its tensile properties appropriately, the entire region could be made to bear equal unit loads.

Second: In our knees an analogous situation happens, the modification consisting of the division of this hoop into two halves, the two ends of each half attaching very strongly to the tibial surfaces in the intercondylar regions. Thus these meniscal pads could still carry much of the normal loads across the joint, relieving at least somewhat the central exposed regions of tibial articular cartilage. The author conceives exactly that as one major function of an articular meniscus.

Right: Further cuts which illustrate the above effects. Note that the upwards supporting force on the femur by the meniscus equals the tension load or restraining force (directed to the right) divided by the tangent of the angle of the wedge. If you look up the tangent of 15° in the table of trigonometric functions in Part III you may become impressed.

If true, then one must ask: Why enlarge the total load carrying bearing surface of a joint by such a seemingly awkward means? In this regard all joints containing menisci demonstrate a probably meaningful property which we can illustrate by the knee. While the human knee has only one primary function as far as its motion goes (that of moving the femur on the tibia like a hinge) , in doing so it also develops or carries considerable torque, lateral bending moments and anteroposterior sliding (i.e., shearing) motions of its tibial and femoral components, one upon the other. Because of its obvious incongruities such motions by leading to concentrations of large loads on small, incongruent contact regions, would soon batter those direct bearing regions to death (and almost literally so) during strenuous physical activities, in the absence of any compensating mechanism. But a meniscus provides exactly such a compensating mechanism.

Observe: Longitudinal tension (i.e., hoop) loads develop in it when one stands on the knee. The vertical load across the knee tries to squeeze the meniscus out from between the articular surfaces. But its hoop tension stiffness and stress act against that squeeze, to pull the meniscal wedge in between the apposing joint surfaces in exactly that way which maintains close contact and evenly distributed pressure in the wedge, and which tends to float the femoral condyles above the tibial condyles. Thus the meniscus *must* carry a significant fraction of the compression loads on the joint. During this process, the high compliance in flexure and shear allows the meniscus to deform and adapt readily even to rapidly changing alignments of the articular incongruities, so that unit loading over the whole meniscal surface in contact with cartilage tends to remain uniform.

If this concept has any substance, it should then follow that transecting a meniscus perpendicular to (i.e., in cross section to) its greatest tension strength, thereby interrupting completely its hoop rigidity, should overload the central direct bearing area of that femoral and tibial condyle. Because of the time-averaging process, that should lead that compartment to break down in time, i.e., to develop a degenerative arthritis. Of some interest, it does, and I opened the knee of a woman yesterday in which exactly that cause-effect relationship was found. Note that this concept of meniscal function requires that such a breakdown should occur in time, even though the actual cut (or a transverse tear due to injury) affects only a trivial portion of the total meniscal surface in contact with the articular cartilage.

Numerous clinical observations by my predecessors and contemporaries reveal that exactly this result follows an untreated transverse tear of either the medial or lateral meniscus of the knee. This fairly consistent relation directly suggests that one of our older concepts of meniscal function—to maintain continuous synovial fluid flow—represented a possibly permissible but nevertheless incorrect guess.

One may then wonder whether or not subnormal meniscal hoop strength in tension due to some other cause, perhaps a change in collagen metabolism, might not have analogous consequences. Could tensile weakening of such an origin, leading to overload of the central regions of the joint, cause osteochondritis dissecans in the direct bearing area in growing children? Certainly most of those lesions appear in exactly those parts of joints one would expect to find overloaded in compression if tensionally substandard menisci existed. And equally certainly those lesions separate from the parent body of bone along exactly those lines of greatest shearing strain that photoelastic analyses have shown (in some engineering problems) arise in mechanically analogous situations. I suspect this forms the case, and offer the idea for evaluation by my successors in this field.

4) CONCENTRICITY: The means by which the overall structure maintains two bearing surfaces* aligned accurately parallel (i.e., truly concentric) differs drastically in human joints and man-made machine bearings. One would measure the laxity of a human knee or ankle joint (i.e., movements of one bone on another in planes other than the hinge motions they exist to supply primarily) in whole degrees, typical values ranging from three degrees to fifteen degrees of external-internal rotation of the tibia relative to either the femur at the knee, or to the talus at the ankle (as examples). In a machine on the other hand, the maximum allowable bearing laxity or play of a journal would constitute a very few hundredths of one degree; larger malalignments will lead to burning a corner of the journal, a serious form of thermomechanical damage which can rapidly propagate to involve—and ruin—the whole journal. In our machines, the inherent rigidity of the bearing surface materials (i.e., their

---

* Do not mistake the meaning here: we discuss the true surfaces of the articular cartilage, not the cartilage itself and not its bony backing.

low compliance in compression) makes it mandatory to control the fit or concentricity of the bearing surfaces by maintaining very rigid and strong alignment of the backing and remoter parts they attach to. Those parts of course include the shaft, and the remainder of the machine to which they attach.

In human joints, nature took a fundamentally different approach to maintaining surface concentricity. The bearing material and its backing possess good mechanical compliance, greatest at the joint surface and decreasing to its minimum value at midshaft of the bone. And in joints in which unusually large malalignments occur during normal function, flexible menisci arise which simply extend further the above graduated compliance feature. That compliance permits enough local deformation in response to malalignments under load to preserve continuity of the synovial fluid film under all natural and normal conditions of joint loading and malalignment. Thus when a joint takes a sudden side-load or torque, its tissues can yield enough locally to distribute those loads over a large enough total area of synovial fluid film—and joint bearing area—to hold the unit loads down, and below the point that would rupture the film and allow surface-to-surface contact, and its attendant destructive wear. When this compliance becomes impaired, for example by the production of too much new subchondral bone in healing a local fracture, or because a large metallic (and thus very stiff) implant lies placed too close to the joint surface, the part can become rigid enough locally to cause a bearing failure.

5) SMOOTHNESS: Joint surfaces seem to require two kinds of smoothness to provide durable function: smoothness of *surface contour,* and smoothly distributed *sub-surface compliance.*

(*a*) *Contour*: The joint surfaces require overall mechanical or geometric smoothness because otherwise any local irregularities or asperities could cause local breaks through the lubricant film, allowing contact of the solid surface material of one side with the other, a contact which must accelerate local wear. That region of local mechanical wear or defect, once worn down and thus load relieved, then gives rise to another edge or high spot at its margins which repeats the process but now around a larger perimeter, and so on. Thus such regions show a definite tendency to propagate themselves with use. Note however: At the level of resolution of the scanning electron microscope (we speak particularly of about $500\times-4000\times$), the cartilage surface proves wavy and rather rough, and the tiny hollows and valleys created thereby may serve to trap local tiny pools of lubricant. Thus bearing smoothness proves a relative matter, and this holds for man-made bearings too.

(b) *Compliance or Stiffness*: A smooth and regular distribution of articular cartilage's subsurface compliance proves just as essential to durable joint function as a smooth contour (155). To understand why, consider this analogy: Given: a silver dollar laying flat under a rug. The eye sees no bump nor will any trouble arise in trying to drag a baby's small (and in terms of weight, light) toys across the place on the rug above where the dollar lies. Those toys won't even "see" the dollar. But now attempt to drag a heavy trunk across the same spot. It may slide readily enough until it hits that spot, and there it will stop. Increasing the pushing force on the trunk eventually will move it over that hidden obstruction but at the expense of damage to the rug. A heavy weight squashed or deformed the rug enough to encounter or "see" the effect of the local subsurface bump or region of abnormally low compliance caused by the dollar.

Equally so, a local stiffening under a joint's cartilage surface creates a local hump seen by the opposite joint surface and the intervening synovial fluid rug, whenever the joint carries a heavy load (See Fig. 18.06). The increased unit loads that occur over that hump can then break the lubricant film and lead to accelerated joint wear and disease. As already noted, this can occur when bulky metallic implants lie too close to subchondral bone, or when healing of some irritative disease close to a joint surface causes a lot of new bone to deposit.

6) MALALIGNMENT: The way in which an otherwise

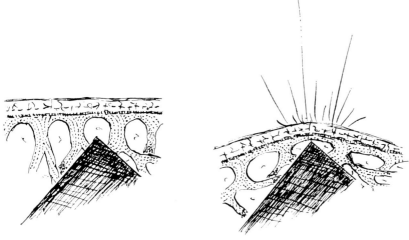

Figure 18.06. Diagramatically, a Smith-Peterson nail lying close to the subchondral bone of this hip joint causes no problems under conditions of light loading. But under heavy loads the nail's stiffness, far greater than that of the surrounding bone and superimposed articular tissue, could lead to a local bearing failure due to excessive unit normal loads on the synovial fluid film above it.

Nature can protect the patient from this by removing enough bone from the immediate neighborhood of the nail to allow its upper end to "float" in fluid and soft tissue. And about 80% of the time when a mechanical situation like this arises, she does just that. This phenomenon—readily visible on x-rays as a thin clear space between nail and bone—forms a kind of biodynamic stress-relief phenomenon.

normal joint accepts its loads can, if changed properly, produce a loading distribution that exceeds the limits of the ability of the normal adaptive mechanisms (of graduated flexibility) to compensate for. As an example, this can occur in knockknee (genu valgum), where the lateral half of the knee takes more vertical compression load than it can accept* and still provide durable function; consequently and after some years of functioning in that situation, that half of the knee joint may break down (see Fig. 18.07) and some orthopaedic surgeon then has an opportunity to help the patient by doing a "varus proximal tibial osteotomy." It also occurs

---

* Some due to transfer from the medial side, and some arising as flexural moments in a cantilever bending arrangement.

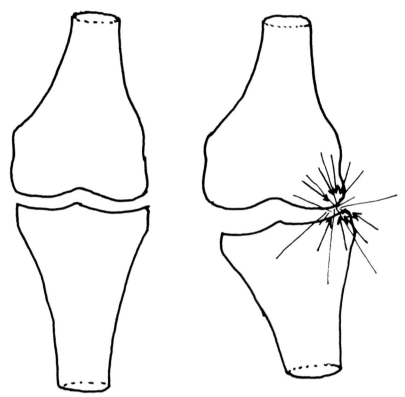

Figure 18.07. In a knee (or other ginglymus) normally aligned relative to all of the loads it carries, essentially equal unit loading exists on both sides (because the lateral condyle has less tibial bearing area I assume it carries less total *time-averaged* load than the medial). But when, as on the right here some malalignment accentuates unit loads on one side at the expense of the other, a bearing failure can ensue on the overloaded side. Such lateralization can follow *anatomical* malalignments or, as we will describe in the next chapter, purely relative ones due to abnormal dynamic forces traceable to altered patterns of muscle contraction. While observation establishes these cause-effect relationships beyond reasonable doubt, we still do not understand well the process of the subsequent breakdown of the joint.

in temperomandibular joints (214) as a result of altered muscle contractural patterns.

Surgeons sometimes unwittingly cause such phenomena. Examples: An adult undergoing corrective valgus osteotomy for severe genu varum due to rickets. The postoperative knee alignment pleases both surgeon and patient—but five years later the latter now has pain in his ankle which grew properly aligned *relative to the knee deformity* and now, postcorrection, itself lies in excessive valgus as the patient walks. Or, a hip operation which translates the upper femur medially (such as a MacMurray osteotomy) produces a relative knee valgus leading to lateral compartment overload during subsequent function. We will say more of such matters in Chapter 19.

7) THE LUBRICANT PUMPS: At least four quite different kinds of synovial fluid pumps exist which seem important in maintaining adequate supplies of synovial fluid between the articular cartilage surfaces. Two relate to the wedge-incongruity referred to previously, the other two to anatomically based facts. We discuss them in order of their probable importance.

(*a*) *Wedge-flow effects*: When compression loads transfer across a moving joint, they tend to squeeze some of the synovial fluid out from between the articular surfaces. Were this lost lubricant not replaced or compensated for by some means, after a while a dry joint would develop leading to surface contact and accelerated wear. But in this regard, motion in joints differs in an important way from motion in machine journals. A joint moves only so far in one direction; then it must move back. In other words, joint motions have the reciprocal property, where machine journals usually rotate continuously in one direction. This has two interesting effects.

On the backward or recovery phase of a joint's motion cycle, the synovial fluid squeezed out and left behind (see below) the trailing joint margin during the first part of the motion cycle, then becomes trapped in the advancing peripheral wedge between their peripheral regions, so the leading edge of the joint then tends to climb up or ride or float on that reservoir of lubricant. As Figure 18.08 illustrates, one function of the wedge-type incongruity consists of maintaining bearing flotation, in the presence of continual loss by sideways squeezing out of the volume of lubricant lying between the articular surfaces. As one moves towards the left in that

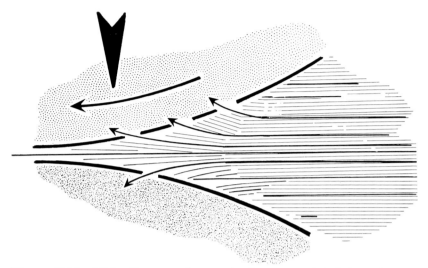

Figure 18.08. This diagrams the "wedge-flow" synovial fluid effect in mammalian joints. Seen in sagittal section, the upper articular surface here moves towards your left on the stationary lower. This drags synovial fluid from the right towards the left and into the wedge-shaped opening between them (exaggerated here as to its angle and depth). The constantly decreasing volume of space lying between the articular surfaces as one enters the wedge more and more deeply from right to left, must act to compensate for some of the fluid lost by squeezing out sideways, here both towards and away from you.

It must follow then that on the left side of the close contact region, a negative hydrostatic pressure or vacuum-like force must arise, which must tend to suck synovial fluid into that wedge. Clearly such an effect provides good preparation for lubricating the return or reciprocal motion of the joint.

drawing, the volume of fluid between the surfaces, decreases, so that as one approaches the region of closest contact, each progressively smaller region requires progressively less volume of fluid to maintain good hydrostatic pressure, and so good bearing flotation. Clearly for this mechanism to function properly, the angular rate at which the wedge closes towards the left sets some limit to the acceptable rate of lubricant loss, beyond which contact and bearing seizure will occur. Clearly too, the more viscous the lubricant, and the more it adheres chemically to the articular cartilage, the more tenaciously the lubricant will remain where it can minimize wear.

(*b*) *The Negative Pressure Effect*: The second aspect of the wedge-flow effect occurs at the trailing edge of the joint. As a given region on the trailing edge falls further and further behind the region of closest contact, a larger vertical gap separates it from the other, opposing side of the joint because of the wedge. Since only a small amount of fluid can get to it through the surfaces under close contact, a negative hydrostatic pressure must arise in this trailing wedge. Such a vacuum must tend to draw fluid in from any available source. And a very good such source constitutes any fluid squeezed out laterally or sideways to the direction of motion by the compression load on the joint.

Figure 18.09, bottom, illustrates these effects.

(*c*) *The anatomical "pump"*: When some synovial fluid does squeeze out sideways from between the moving surfaces of a loaded joint, the anatomy of the local soft and hard tissues usually returns that fluid to the joint. That occurs because the sides of most joints lie against overlying fascia, muscle bellys, ligaments, fat pads and tendons, all of which exert centripetal pressures that act to prevent lateral pooling of the lubricant and tend to force any fluid arriving there back into the center of the joint where it is most needed.

(*d*) *The Bernouilli-Contour Effects*: Recall from Part I of the book that when a fluid moves rapidly between two surfaces it exerts less transverse pressure upon them than when it moves slowly, other things remaining equal. In fact, that pressure changes as the square of the velocity change. Thus doubling the flow speed tends to cut the transverse pressure to $\dfrac{1}{2^2} = \frac{1}{4}$. Here an anatomical property of most rapidly moving heavily loaded joints appears: their contours arrange things so that the relative speed of articular motion in the middle, most heavily loaded region of the joint, exceeds that on either side. Think of the hip extending during the act of running: that perimeter of its ball which lies on a section through its middle and parallel to the motion of the shaft, moves considerably faster (by $2–5\times$) in terms of cm/sec than those perimeters lying in the same plane but close to

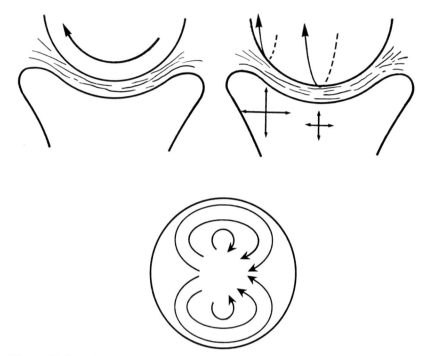

Figure 18.09. The "contour-Bernouilli" effect appears in diagram above. Because the surfaces at the center of the joint move significantly faster than those at the margin, the lateral fluid pressure at the margin must exceed that in the center. However, except for conditions of light loading, it probably does not play a major role in keeping the central regions supplied with lubricant, by resisting lateral expression or squeeze.

At the bottom, looking down onto the top of the tibial aspect of the knee, the lines trace out the suggested flow or "stream lines" of synovial fluid movement (due to the wedge-flow and negative pressure effects) as the superimposed femoral articular surface moves from your right towards your left.

the lateral and medial sides (and so nearer the axis of rotation) of the femoral head, as illustrated in Figure 18.09. Then the hydrostatic lateral pressure tending to extrude synovial fluid sideways from the central perimeter must fall below that along the slower moving peripheral ones. The greater peripheral pressure must then tend to force peripheral fluid in between the faster moving regions. Whether this probably minor effect, which I term the Bernouilli-contour effect, becomes large enough to significantly oppose the squeezing effect of vertical loads at feasible joint speeds and working loads remains to be seen.*

8) VARIABLE VISCOSITY: Synovial fluid has the non-Newtonian property, in the sense that as the speed of joint shearing motion increases, the drag of the synovial fluid increases but, proportionally speaking, less so. In other words, its viscosity varies reaching its highest values in slow moving joints and its lowest ones in fast moving articulations. This permits transferring large loads across rapidly moving joints without generating too much shearing drag on the cartilage, and without generating too much heat. At the same time it serves to reduce and minimize starting friction (we might more properly speak of starting wear), and to provide an effective boundary layer-like form of lubrication at low joint speeds.

Note: The viscous drag on any joint due to the viscosity of the synovial fluid can be found with this relation

$$F = \eta\, PVA(h)^{-1} \qquad\qquad Equation\ 18.01$$

Where F equals the drag, V the velocity of the two articular surfaces relative to each other, A the area of that fraction of the surfaces actually carrying the load, h the mean thickness of the synovial fluid film between the articular surfaces, eta the coefficient of viscosity per unit film thickness, and P the total normal compression load on area A.

III: BIODYNAMICS

1) THE SELF-REPAIRING MECHANISM: All bearings show surface wear, whether made of living materials or inanimate metals, and this remains true no matter how efficient the lubrication and wear minimizing mechanisms (136). Furthermore, it holds as true for animal joints as it does for the bearings in man-made machinery. In tackling that problem, en-

---

* The effect probably will prove minor in joint function, for in the hip as an example it can cause a pressure difference on the order of $50 \pm$ gm/cm² between center and edge of the ball-socket joint. But this seems rather small, in the face of the 50,000 gm/cm² normal load carried by that joint. Any one interested can work this out for himself, using equation 4.06 from Part I.

gineers took two different approaches. One, they tried to use bearings large and massive enough that their service life exceeded the expected useful life of the machine. Often this meant going from journals to more expensive ball—or roller—bearings. And two, as a more economical approach they designed the bearings to permit easy replacement by new ones after sufficient wear had arisen to impair reliable function.

But nature compensated for wear in our joints by another means entirely: she provided self-repair mechanisms of impressive efficiency and sensitivity which affect the cartilage, its bony backing and the synovial fluid. Thus for the chondral element, a gradual continual slow production of new cartilaginous matrix substance occurs throughout life, and in effect it somehow repairs or replenishes the worn articular material, so one may legitimately term it a self-repair mechanism (176). Readily available clinical evidence suggests that some kind of feedback mechanism exists which relates and controls these processes, for wear and repair usually match each other so well and so regularly over the whole life span of a man that it becomes stochastically unreasonable and illogical to assume it arises from perfectly acting, predetermined and casually unconnected processes. Failures in this self-repair mechanism really occur rarely.* When for whatever reason, repair cannot keep up with wear, then the joint begins to show varied evidence of excessive wear. For example, its radiographically apparent cartilage space begins to narrow. This leads eventually to a bearing failure (i.e., a traumatic or degenerative arthritis). Note that the microscopic debris of the normal wear process usually appears in centrifuged normal synovial fluids.

As for the bone element, deterioration of a joint with use and age does not confine itself to the articular cartilage alone. It can also affect both the backing (i.e., the subchondral bone) and the synovial fluid, although in different ways; see Figure 18.10. In animal joints, repair of most forms of use derived damage to the subchondral and deeper underlying

---

* On the order of less than one major failure per 1,000,000 joints per year of service life.

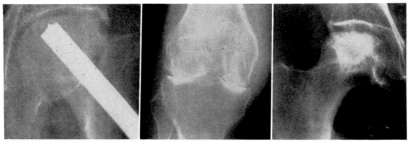

Figure 18.10. *Left:* About two years after reduction and nailing of a transcervical femoral fracture with a triflanged Smith-Petersen nail and a Thornton side-plate combination, this femoral head began to "settle," due, not to the nail lying too close to the joint but to a clinical syndrome termed "aseptic necrosis" and, as to its pathophysiology, badly misunderstood by our profession at this writing. But the fracture did ultimately cause this situation, which bothers the patient because the mechanical incongruity has begun to "batter" the well-innervated bony backing, and somehow to irritate the synovial lining of the joint.

Middle: This knee of an adult male has developed rheumatoid arthritis. Its bearing failure began, at least in the overt sense, as accelerated wear of the articular cartilage, so that now subchondral bone rubs on subchondral bone.

Right: Another adult hip which has developed the syndrome named "aseptic necrosis." Note: unlike the middle situation in which the Babbitt went first, here the "backing" goes first, and all subsequent deletory changes derive from that fact.

trabecular bone derives from the BMU based bone remodeling mechanism referred to earlier and described in some detail in Volume III of this series.

As for the synovial fluid, deterioration of its organic fractions (whatever its nature) probably remains at some acceptable minimum level in normal life and aging, by virtue of a relatively rapid turnover of its constituent dissolved organic molecules, a turnover effected by mechanically circulating the fluid between the joint surfaces and the synovia by means already described (31).

2) Nutrition: For proper function as a biological Babbitt, the articular cartilage needs its cells, called chondrocytes, in a viable and healthy state. We have clinical proof of this in the form of biological bearing failures following diseases—such as an infection—which kill those cells. Over the

next six to twelve months of use, the joint cartilage space progressively narrows and disappears. This remains true even though we cannot as yet name with assurance those specific properties of normal articular cartilage that its cells maintain.

The articular chondrocytes receive their nourishment from the synovial fluid, which transports nutrients from the synovia to the cells as it circulates because of the joint's motion (31). In the reverse sense, synovial fluid also carries waste products from the chondrocytes to the synovia. Both nutrients and waste products must traverse the distance from chondrocyte lacuna to synovial fluid by diffusing through the cartilage substance, and here mechanical straining of that substance in shear and compression during normal function may act as a kind of facilitating physical pump.

The synovia has many blood vessels and nerve endings, as do also the subchondral bone, the underlying trabecula and the cortex. The number and diverse origins of the vessels in these structures make it very unlikely that closure of any single vessel can do significant harm to a joint by causing an infarct (for the relevance of these remarks, see discussion on aseptic necrosis in a later chapter). We have stated already that cartilage contains neither vessels nor nerves.

Summary: The joint properties most important in subserving its major second order function, durability in time, include smooth geometric contour and distribution of compliance; a longitudinally graduated compliance in compression, maximal at the joint surface and minimal at midshift; summation of that compliance over the bone's whole length; turnover of the articular cartilage substance (probably by local biochemical processes); a mechanism which repairs fatigue-like and other damage in the backing material; chemical turnover of a non-Newtonian lubricant; and pumps of several kinds which act to keep lubricant in the bearing area.

IV: TENDON SHEATHS

Tendons which run in a straight line from their muscle to the structure they act upon, lie embedded in loose fatty tissue without a specific gliding mechanism. The fatty tissue accepts elastic distortion from motions of the tendon readily enough that no lubrication problems arise, and no mechanical harm to either tendon or its enveloping connective tissue arises either.

When the line of action of a tendon changes, as when the flexor tendon in the hand curves from palm to the distal phalanx, a tendon sheath surrounds it, as shown in Figure 18.11. As bearings, these sheaths seem similar in principle to cartilage-covered joints. Their prime function consists of redirecting the tendon's pull, and one finds a definite, tunnel-like sheath only where this redirection occurs. Like joints, these sheaths have a synovial membrane lining their internal surface, which supplies synovial fluid to act as a lubricant. The tendon has a smooth external surface and its fibers align parallel to its directions of motion. The lubrication mechanism can break down when some surface irregularity arises in the tendon or its sheath, or because of unsmooth gradation in flexibility of the deeper layers of the tendon or sheath. The

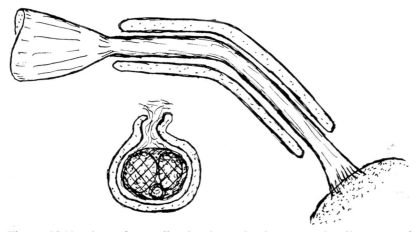

Figure 18.11. A tendon pulley-sheath mechanism, seen in diagram and longitudinal section. Muscle on the left, tendon insertion on the right, and enveloping sheath with an enclosed synovial fluid cavity around it. The cross sectional view illustrates the latter. Note that we rarely find capillaries on gliding surfaces in close contact, or on surfaces exposed to much pressure in terms of unit loads, probably because they prove too fragile to withstand the combination of rubbing and great compression.

tendon sheath forms a closed cavity so the synovial fluid within it cannot escape, and motion of the tendon, as in joints, has the reciprocal property, i.e., first in one direction, then in the opposite, which circulates the synovial fluid effectively. A physical basis also exists for a contour-Bernouilli effect.

Having described some (and only some, alas) of the biomechanical principles underlying the functions of normal joints, let us now turn our attention to selected aspects of reconstructing damaged joints, and see how some of our basic information applies and what new possibilities crop up.

V: BIOMECHANICAL CONSIDERATIONS IN ARTHROPLASTIES

Arthroplasty signifies making a new joint, or remaking an old joint, and a variety of schemes have evolved over the years for accomplishing this. Since we could write a complete monograph on arthroplasties alone, and in fact other authors even have written whole monographs about single types of arthroplasty, we cannot reasonably expect to review the whole problem here. Consequently we will mention several of the procedures evolved over the past, and then pay some particular attention to a class of arthroplasties which depend upon normal reactions and adaptations inherent in our living tissues to generate a new joint.

1) RESECTION ARTHROPLASTY: One of the oldest forms of arthroplasty, this represents the simple excision of the major bony parts of each joint. While this sounds like a terrible thing to perpetrate upon a man, in a variety of circumstances it can still function actually quite well. As an example, we may resect the radial head which constitutes a resection arthoplasty of the lateral compartment of the elbow joint. In some post-fracture deformities and in chronic or persistent radial head dislocations due to a variety of causes, this procedure works quite well. Also, occasions can arise when simple resection of the humeral head will correct disabling shoulder pain and restore useful mobility. Likewise, simple resection of the femoral head and neck (called the

Girdlestone operation after the English surgeon who popularized it) was and remains an excellent hip salvage procedure under particular conditions. While it would seem that such a patient could not bear weight after such an operation, in fact most of them do; the limb shortens sufficiently that the unresected hip capsule plus the "sling" made of the iliopsoas muscle-tendon effectively suspends the upper end of the femur from the pelvis. Also we sometimes resect interphalangeal joints or whole phalanges of toes for a variety of deformities in older patients, usually with excellent functional results, if obtained at the expense of some visible deformity. Thus such a procedure, usually quite acceptable to a patient past age 55 who has already caught her husband and educated her children, may prove less than acceptable to a still unattached cute young thing in her twenties.

2) INTERPOSITION ARTHROPLASTY: A second form of arthroplasty consists of surgically removing the damaged surface layers of the articular surfaces on each side of a diseased joint and then interposing a membrane, frequently of fascia (as the elder MacAusland as well as Potter used to do in Boston) but sometimes of skin cut thin with a special knife called a dermatome (Prof. S. Kono of Japan performed large numbers of these with considerable success), and even on occasion, with artifical plastic mesh membranes, as Drs. J. L. Fleming, J. Devlin and P. Gram once experimented with in laboratory animals at H.F.H. While still done, and while in non weight-bearing joints such arthroplasties often produce quite acceptable function and relief from pain, in the biological and mechanical senses they differ relatively little from the resection arthroplasty, and may not bear up reliably in heavily loaded, weight bearing joints.

3) REPLACEMENT ARTHROPLASTY: In yet a third class of arthroplasties we replace one side of a joint with an artificial implant, a typical example consisting of the Near prosthesis for the humeral head, or the Austin Moore replacement of the femoral head and neck following an intracapsular hip fracture in an aged and/or medically infirm patient. In reality this

usually constitutes a patient salvage procedure rather than a hip reconstructive procedure, because when the latter constitutes the surgeon's major objective, he will usually try to give the patient a chance to keep his or her own hip by reducing the fracture and internally fixing it by some means. See Figure 18.12. The replacement arthroplasty serves currently in patients in whom the major consideration becomes early mechanical mobilization, for example to offset the harmful effects of prolonged bed rest on older patients whose medical and physical infirmities make them unable to walk satisfactorily on one good leg with the aid of a walker, crutches or similar device.

One may do a true (or more extensive?) reconstructive procedure by replacing the femoral neck and ball with the metallic implant, plus resecting all of the damaged articular surface in the socket. However, the postoperative management of these cases differs considerably from that of the acute fracture cases, a matter we go into in more detail below.

4) TOTAL REPLACEMENT ARTHROPLASTY: In this particular era, so-called total joint replacements have become increasingly popular, largely as a result of the pioneering work of the English surgeon, John Charnley, who devised a hip joint replacement system in which a metal ball sitting upon a metal neck and stem, rides within a plastic socket, both stem and socket being affixed to their respective bony parts by a plastic cement which one inserts while still in a pasty state, and then by pressing the implants in on top of the cement manually, ensures perfect adaptation and fit of the cement, both to bone and to the implants. At least in older patients, this method has proven far more successful than many (including this author) had anticipated going in, and one must consider that this and related systems have now become a part of acceptable orthopaedic surgical expertise. Of course, and as always, that acceptance applies within defined limits, limits which only at present begin to come into clear focus.

5) MOULD ARTHROPLASTY: The final type of arthroplasty (considered in a bit more detail than the above) constitutes

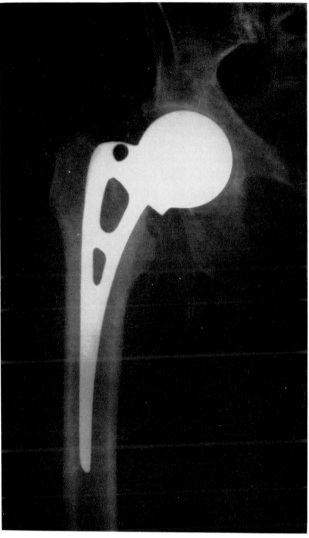

Figure 18.12. This elderly woman sustained a subcapital fracture of this hip treated by replacement of the ball and femoral neck by this Austin-Moore prosthesis. The stem fits within the marrow cavity of the femur. An example of a *replacement arthroplasty,* by means of an *endoprosthesis.* Here this procedure was done not to reconstruct the hip primarily but to salvage a patient who badly needed early resumption of physical function to minimize the probability of developing any one or combination of a host of serious complications of prolonged bed rest and pain in the elderly.

that initially popularized by Dr. Smith-Petersen of Boston for use in the hip joint. Basically in this class of procedures, one resects the damaged layers of tissue from both sides of the joint surfaces, thereby in effect seriously injuring them. One then interposes an inanimate implant which has very highly polished surfaces of smooth contour and regular geometric configuration. This implant will serve as a mould, to which the two living sides of the joint must gradually coapt and to which their subsequent healing and mechanical adaptational processes must adjust and adapt. Hence we will call this class of arthroplasties mould arthroplasties.*

The operative technique used to obtain access to the joint upon which one does a mould arthroplasty does not concern us here (53). Once there, in effect the surgeon will remove the damaged articular and subchondral surfaces down to underlying bare and bleeding (and thus viable) bone on both sides of the joint. He will also attempt to contour those resected surfaces so that they fit reasonably well the contours of the mould subsequently interposed between them. See Figure 18.13.

Subsequent healing and restoration of function in this arthroplasty proceeds through a number of necessary, and conveniently if somewhat arbitrarily designated, stages. They include the phase of granulation tissue, the phase of chondrometaplasia, the phase of biomechanical adaptation and finally the phase of steady state use.

(a) *Granulation Tissue Stage*: Within approximately two weeks following the operation the damaged living bone surfaces on either side of the new joint react to the injury created by the operation to produce a healing tissue growing out of those surfaces and made up of new blood vessels, fibroblasts and other supporting cells. We call this healing tissue granulation tissue. It grows somewhat like a mushroom off the surfaces of the bone, and in the process fills any cavity or fluid-filled dead space that may exist. It will coapt quite accurately to the inanimate and very hard surfaces of the mould.

---

* Their originator thought he would reoperate and remove the moulds after the new living joint surfaces had developed. But it did not work out that way.

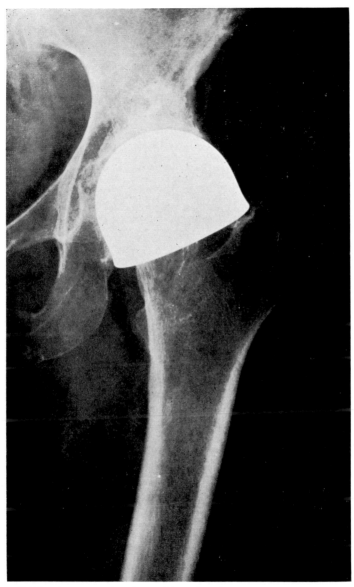

Figure 18.13. An example of mould arthroplasty. Now less popular than during the 1940–50 decades, this Smith-Petersen cup arthroplasty of the hip joint improved a disabling osteoarthritis of that joint. Its success depended upon a realistic understanding of normal hip biomechanics (99,198,212,213,217,227,284,285), and on the articular adaptive and repair-regeneration processes, an understanding we just now begin to visualize in crisp and cogent form, as mentioned later on in the upcoming text. Drs. C. L. Mitchell and D. C. Mitchell (as well as O. Aufranc) have acquired and used exceptionally good biomechanical intuition with this problem and have done large numbers of these procedures, most of which still function quite satisfactorily in the view of their patient-recipients.

For the nutrition and very survivial of its various cells however, *granulation tissue depends absolutely upon the patency of the capillaries within it.* Because of these capillaries' considerable fragility, transmission of compression loads of any magnitude across the new joint during this stage will simply crush the capillaries between the hard surfaces of the mould on one side, and the hard and irregular surfaces of the underlying bone trabeculae on the other. That will then set the healing process back to where it all began, in the operating room. As a consequence, during the first few weeks after such an arthroplasty one encourages active ranges of joint motion within the patient's comfortable pain tolerance, but studiously avoids applying any large compression loads across the new joint.

(*b*) *The Stage of Chondrometaplasia*: Usually by two weeks and often before that period of time, one may begin active, frequent ranges of motion of the joint, arranged so that large compression loads across the new joint do not associate with this motion, as described above. Partly because of the inherent biological response properties of the tissues, and partly because of some stimulus provided to the granulation tissue by this repeated motion, a different kind of cell begins to differentiate within it, the chondroblast. These new chonroblasts then proceed to manufature the organic matrix of a new layer of cartilage on the joint surface, usually termed fibrocartilage. While some dispute exists among authorities as to whether it actually constitutes that or hyaline cartilage, the dispute has academic importance only. By this means, approximately two months later a layer of new fibrocartilage has evolved, largely replacing the preexisting granulation tissue and lying interposed between (and freely moveable upon the surface of) the mould on the one hand, and the underlying trabecular bone firmly affixed to the cartilage on the other. This new cartilage obtains its nutrition exactly like normal articular hyaline cartilage, that is, by diffusion of nutrients brought to it by mechanically circulated synovial fluid. Specifically, its viability does not depend upon blood flowing through any capillaries lying within it. As a result, this new cartilaginous tissue can accept quite large compression loads for brief periods of time without suffering any threat to its viability or to its inherent biomechanical responsiveness. This in fact forms one major anatomical and mechanical fact which makes hyaline cartilage suitable as a Babbitt for human joints: its viability does not depend upon capillaries lying within it, so it can accept large compression and rubbing loads without risk to its nutrition and viability.

(*c*) *Stage of Biomechanical Adaptation*: Accordingly at this stage (i.e., about two months postoperation) one then starts the patient on a program of slowly progressive loading of the new joint, while continuing the active motion program mentioned before. Resumption of full loading must occur gradually over a period of approximately the next four months, and for a good reason, to wit:

At the conclusion of the operation the contour of the new subchondral bone layer does not accurately fit the surfaces of the mould, and the mechanical nature of our surgical techniques and its tooling makes it unlikely that by any practical means we could achieve an accurate fit of the living to the dead in the mechanical sense.* As a consequence, when the patient begins to bear increasing weight upon his new hip joint, at some points along the articular surfaces trabecular bone protrudes higher than at others. Of course the high levels accept a disproportionate fraction of the total loads across the joint, so that unit loads over them can rise ten-fold or more above the average over the whole surface. Tough these tissues may be, but not that tough!

However, if these loads occur intermittently and build up gradually, the underlying bony tissues will then react and adapt to the situation, and in exactly those ways which tend to restore an evenly distributed bony subchondral support to the overlying layer of new articular cartilage. This occurs by complex combinations of bone resorption and formation activities in the underlying trabecular bone, which stress-relieve highly overloaded areas by cutting through their un-

---

* And we do not want to anyway—one must leave room for the granulation tissue layer to develop.

derlying supports with a torch of active osteoclasts, and which build up underloaded areas by deposition of new woven bone. Thus, in response to repeated active motion *and gradually increasing functional loading,* the subchondral bone comes to adapt to the contour of the overlying cartilage and the surface of the joint mould, and with all operationally necessary geometric accuracy. Accordingly by approximately six months postoperative, the new joint has become ready to accept full loads.

(*d*) *Steady State Use Stage:* At this point, orthopaedic practice around the country diverges into two streams.

One group of surgeons believes that patients undergoing such arthroplasties should contrive to do progressive resistance exercises of the muscles actuating the new joint until they regain normal power and endurance. The various means by which one achieves this do not matter here, but it constitutes a repeatedly observed fact that a third or more of such patients develop bearing failures of the new joint within the next five years which require either revision of the original arthroplasty, or performance of a different type of arthroplasty (24).

A second school of thought, to which the author belongs, considers that any new, man-made joint cannot equal in its functional endurance the one originally provided by nature (50). Granted that, then in order to obtain the maximum service life possible out of a man-made one, we should protect it from overload, i.e., from very large loads and from prolonged mechanical demands, throughout its subsequent existence. Accordingly while encouraging patients with such new joints to develop active and painfree ranges of motion and to keep them by means of daily exercises, this school does not require the patient to restore normal power and endurance to the involved hip muscles, and elects rather to let them remain somewhat weak. Recall that the major mechanical loads across our joints constitute muscular forces, not those of gravity (as mentioned elsewhere, gravity simply provides the reactions against which our muscles work—and not the major loads themselves). By allowing the hip muscles to remain somewhat weak, and encouraging the patient to accept gait patterns which protect a new hip from maximal muscle forces, one thereby *reduces the time-averaged unit loads on the interface between the mould and the living tissue*. This definitely promulgates longer service life, for at least in the writer's experience, only some five per cent of mould arthroplasties handled in this way have required later revision.

In performing mould arthroplasties in the past, unit loading factors received relatively little attention, partly because twenty or thirty years ago when this operation had its peak of popularity, we had little awareness of such matters, and partly too because at that time we lacked realistic numerical values for unit loading in a joint, and in the analytical sense at least we tried to swim underwater in a sea muddied by turbulent controversey, conflicting opinions and advice.

Witness: While the complex of programmed activities just described suggests it might proceed quite unreliably in practice, the converse has proven the case: it has been *very* reliable in actual use, and suffered primarily from our own haste when on occasion we attempted to hasten convalescence by shortening the time periods in each stage. This was usually done out of ignorance.

The next section will provide an illustration of one way in which some of the biomechanical principles outlined in Parts I and II of this book could apply to designing a durable total hip replacement.

VI: DESIGN OF A COXENDOPROSTHESIS
(a total hip replacement system)

In the next few paragraphs we will take a kind of bird's eye view of the design of a total hip replacement system, not primarily to tout the design but rather to illustrate the kinds of things one must take into account in doing biomechanical work, and some of the compensations one can find for the problems that arise (102). Now to work.

1) Prime Objective: This has several parts dependent upon the major one: To devise a total replacement for the

hip joint which possesses satisfactory mechanical and biological durability and acceptance. Now, a variety of the thirty-three designs currently in service at this writing (!) have proven acceptably satisfactory. A partial listing would include the Charnley, Charnley-Mueller, Ring, McKee-Farrar, McBride and Bechtol. There seems little point in adding yet another device to that list unless it offers advantages they do not. Which means then that we should examine and identify their limitations—if any and whatever. Providing solutions to those limitations would justify trying to add a thirty-fourth design. Briefly, all thirty-three designs have these limitations, which make it undesireable to implant them electively in most younger patients (at my age that means anybody fifty years old or less).

They provide sliding bearing mechanisms of two or more inanimate parts on each other, so that wear—and service life problems—seem to make it wise to limit them to use in patients fifty-five years of age or older.

In those designs in which a metal part slides on another metal one, sludge production threatens sufficient tissue irritation, given time, to cause biological rejection.

Some of them contain obvious design defects, such as stress risers or other mechanical arrangements which of necessity induce considerable flexural moments in cross sections too small to assure satisfactory durability. And, indeed, some failures of this type have begun to appear.

In those which employ a plastic cement to obtain good fixation of the living to the inanimate, wound infections have proven more likely than with other systems, and thus has led to elaborate and expensive precautions during and after the operation. These infections not only may develop in the days immediately after the operation; they have also become apparent one or more years after it. We say a few words about this problem in Chapter XXIV.

Then we now have our subsidiary prime objectives:

a) To provide enough reduction in wear and sludge, and enough increase in mechanical durability and biological acceptability, to justify a new design.

b) To minimize the risk of wound infection sufficiently that out of the ordinary precautions in this respect prove unnecessary.

2) First Bioengineering Solution: One could go at this problem in a great many ways, but we will follow a particular one, which begins with the basic nature of the bearing mechanism. In industry ball and roller systems provide sufficient reduction in wear to prolong the useful life of machine bearings (over sliding, boundary layer conditions) something like one hundred-fold (range 10X–1000X). If we could come up with a practical rolling design, then increasing the service life to one hundred times the current five to fifteen year value would allow the bearing theoretically to last longer than the lifetime of a man; that would certainly comprise acceptable durability, in this one particular respect of course. Note that if one could devise a reliable and efficient hydrodynamic lubrication-flotation system it would have the same desireable attributes.* And note too this well proven engineering axiom: Simple devices possess greater inherent reliability and durability than complicated ones.

Figure 18.14 shows our simple, two-piece roller bearing, in which a metal ball rolls inside a metal socket. Making the diameter of the ball slightly smaller than that of the socket, say by .0003 in.–.003 in, allows them to touch at only one point or small region. Of course, for this arrangement to work the socket must have the ability to spin, which brings us to bioengineering solution number 2.

3) Second Bioengineering Solution: Most designers of total hip prostheses have made what the writer believes forms a mistake. They believed it imperative to achieve total, persistent and absolutely rigid mechanical fixation of implant to living bone. Yet our total experience over the last thirty years with implants which transfer sizeable mechanical loads to living bone sums up to this simple fact: *they always work loose*. But this need not make them turn out badly, as we shall

---

* Mentioned because it is possible in principle and somebody may actually come up with one in the future.

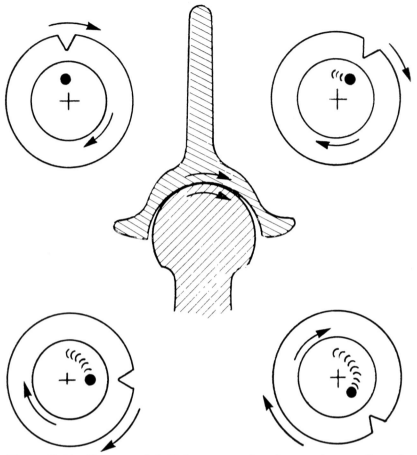

Figure 18.14. Fit a metal ball into a metal socket as shown, allow the socket to spin freely around its longitudinal axis, and press the ball onto some part of the socket's surface other than that over its axis of rotation, denoted by the small cross. Then if the ball has a slightly smaller diameter than the socket the two will meet at one "point"—actually a region of very small area, denoted by the heavy black dot. If the ball then moves back and forth, the load compressing these surfaces together times the distance from dot to spin axis will generate a torque tending to make the socket spin around that axis. Given a coefficient of friction of metal on metal of ≈.2, and of socket in living tissue of ≈.01, and the spinning force combination will exceed by 20× the force combination tending to make the metal surfaces slide on each other, and spin will occur instead. We need not go into why that spinning force probably only exceeds by some 10× the sliding friction of the metal on metal; the major point remains: the outcome does not lie in doubt.

The four views looking up into the socket show how it spins (clockwise here) as the ball (of this artificial hip) moves reciprocally within it.

Note that the above describes the worst case situation. If body fluids between these bearing surfaces provided any effective "floatation" of ball in socket by hydrodynamic means, the mobility and wear situation shown improves, rather than degrades.

see, and it becomes apparent to many investigators of these systems that most of them continue to provide good service even though some loosening has developed.

Given that simple fact, then why not accept it, and furthermore try to turn it to some good use, instead of just accepting it? Which leads to the concepts incorporated in Figure 18.15. We design the socket to lie in a hole reamed in the pelvic bone, and deliberately allow it to move and in the process take advantage of that property of living bone in which it will make a new joint, complete with new cartilage, synovia and synovial fluid, if injured and then subjected to properly staged sliding motion and compression loading programs. We just described this rather briefly under mould arthroplasties. In permitting that motion we make use of it by aligning the spin axis of this socket so as not to coincide with the plane of the hip's to and fro motion during walking, yielding the ball or roller bearing effect opted in our first solution. In this arrangement the mould (made of steel or chrome-cobalt alloy) does not wear because of its immensely greater hardness and resistance to abrasion, relative to cartilage. While the cartilage does wear (as it does too in all normal joints) it has a built-in self repair mechanism just as normal articular cartilage does, so that if its wear rate falls below the compensatory capacity of the repair rate, the new joint should last as long as life.

4) THIRD BIOENGINEERING SOLUTION: To achieve reliable rolling motion of the two parts of this system, and to ensure that the socket does not come out of the pelvic bone, we must give it a defined rather than a free or indeterminate spin axis, as already implied. This is done here by means of the external contour of the socket which has been arranged to ensure rolling motion during walking. The normal tonus of the muscles bridging the hip plus the weight of the body above it should keep it pressed in place, as they do with a cup or an Austin-Moore prosthesis.

As you can now see, the to-and-fro motion of walking makes the metal socket spin to-and-fro, ball bearing fashion, within its living bed of new articular cartilage.

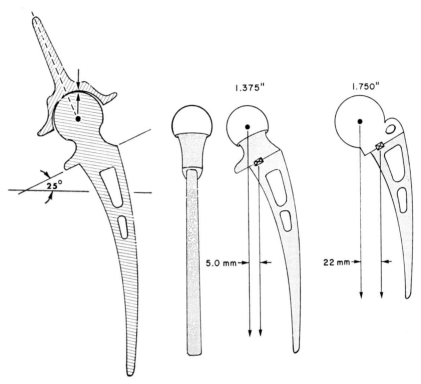

Figure 18.15. *Left:* The left hip seen from the front, showing the socket mating with the ball. The spin axis of the socket, determined by its flange, not its upwards spindle (which serves only to facilitate proper orientation while installing it at operation), lies purposely *not* parallel to the back and forth reciprocal motions of the hip during walking. Thus the spinning torque on the socket equals the total load times the coefficient of friction times distance from spin axis (dotted line) to the metal-to-metal contact point (two vertical arrows). Note that the geometry of the socket provides a simple way to restrain or define the spin axis; the device cannot rotate in any other way than around that axis.

Right: The femoral component by virtue of some design modifications provides three improvements. It reduces the toggling load tending to move the lower stem laterally against the wall of the medullary femoral canal; it further reduces the unit loads arising therefrom on that lower stem by increasing its surface area; it uses a more horizontal base plate to minimize the shearing load tending to make the prosthesis slide down and to the left during weight bearing; and it makes the major hip abductor muscles mechanically inefficient by shortening their horizontal lever arm, thereby reducing the major loading source on the hip: the pulls of those muscles.

5) FOURTH BIOENGINEERING SOLUTION: We now face the problem of the unit loads on the joint metal interface. While we have no extensive body of hard data to go on here we do know several useful things which we can state in verbal fashion, to wit:

Normal peak unit loads on the hip joint approximate fifty to seventy kg/cm^2 averaged over the whole projected area of the ball. But since the outer two thirds of the ball has sloped or slanted surfaces relative to the compression load resultant, it carries that resultant inefficiently.

In doing arthroplasties of all types for some fifty or more years, our specialty has learned this: the lighter the subsequent mechanical demands on a new joint the longer it lasts; the heavier those demands, the sooner it will fail (i.e., by means of pain, loss of mobility, increasing mechanical instability, and yielding of bone before the device in heavily loaded regions).

Accordingly we choose a size (i.e., total diameter) and geometry of the acetabular part of the implant such that it accepts its major loads in a direction normal to its surfaces, and assuming normal hip muscle mechanics it functions then at approximately ten kg/cm^2 unit loading instead of fifty kg/cm^2. Table 18.03 provides some calculated data on this. While obviously estimates, the comparisons provided should retain their sense and validity because most of any errors in the underlying assumptions should affect each case alike. Now we encounter another problem whose solution we can arrange to assist us with this one.

6) FIFTH BIOENGINEERING SOLUTION: It would be nice if we came up with a totally different way of attaching our ball to the femur than the one evolved by trial and error and embodied in the Austin-Moore, Scuderi, Eicher or F. R. Thompson designs. But we do not. Rather we will modify those designs to compensate for two faults which occasionally turn up with them. These include first, pressure of the distal stem against the internal side of the lateral femoral cortex, due to toggling or a torque arising because the center of load transfer at the ball lies eccentric to the center of

TABLE 18.03

UNIT LOADING FACTORS, HIP DESIGNS

Design	Total projected cross section: Area, cm²	Diameter, cm	Effective momentary Bearing area, cm²	Total load 225 kg; Unit loading, kg/cm²:	Total load 110 kg; Unit loading, kg/cm²:
Normal acetabulum	15.7	4.4	5 (36%)	44.	22.
57mm Frost total hip	25.6	5.7	23 (90%)	10.3	5.1
AA Smith-Petersen Cup	17.3	4.7	5 (29%)	44.	22.
Charnley—Mueller and Charnley	28.	6.0	15 (52%)	15.	7.5

This table provides computed loading data for the acetabular bone-implant interface for the four hip situations listed in the left column. The total projected area and diameter form the area and diameter of a plane circle equal in diameter to the greatest diameter of the socket of each situation. It equals the area cast in shadow if one held the device between the sun and a piece of tracing paper. The effective momentary bearing area equals that portion of the projected area which accepts walking loads essentially normal to the surface; in spherical sockets the text takes it to equal approximately ⅓ of the projected area, or slightly more than half the projected diameter. The parentheses express that area as a per cent of the projected (and thus maximum possible) area.

Assuming total loads of 225 kg and 110 kg transferred across the hip, the two right hand columns provide the unit loads on the bone-implant interface, which in the Charnley types constitutes the juncture of plastic cement to bone, (we deal here not with problems of durability and interfaces of inanimate with another inanimate part, but rather with the interface of dead with the living). The writer believes that the success of these devices relative to cup arthroplasties in large part derives from the marked decrease in the unit loading factor their design affords at the animate-inanimate interface (⅓ that of a cup). The system we discuss here improves even upon that by achieving ¼ that of a cup—and indeed of the normal hip.

support by the femur under the medial base plate. The second fault consitutes too steep an inclination of the base plate (see Figure 18.12), which creates a shearing force tending to bring the medial part of the calcar femorale hard enough up against the upper medial stem that it overloads, and the bone gradually crumbles ahead of the prothesis, allowing it to sink gradually into the femur, forming the so-called migrating prosthesis.

To solve this problem we will do three things: broaden the distal stem to provide more cm² of bone-metal interface and thus lower unit loads; align the neck of the prosthesis more vertically to decrease the lever arm of the load which generates the toggling torque to begin with (116); and decrease the inclination of the base plate from ± 40° to 25° from

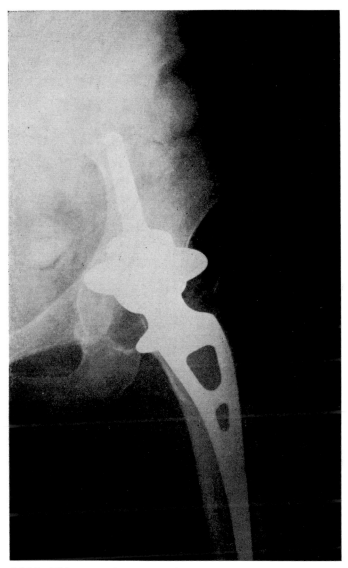

Figure 18.16. This x-ray shows one of the prostheses described in place in a middle-aged male patient. As currently produced the vertical spike on the acetabular component has only half the length shown. Who, not having reviewed this text, would have thought it possible to construct a two-piece roller bearing? Orthopaedic surgery may expect to see much more and probably even better melding of mechanical and biological engineering expertise in the future, to the benefit of our patients and our own feelings of satisfaction. For, while some lay people may find it difficult to accept, the usual orthopaedist gets much greater pleasure out of a good result of some procedure than he does from the fee for it, and public figures who claim otherwise prove thereby, not their courage and interest in the public's benefit, but rather (and at best) their lack of any real contact with main stream medical and surgical practice.

horizontal so the load transfer at this bone-metal interface will remain essentially normal in orientation under normal working loads. Figure 18.15 right diagrams some of these design features.

7) SIXTH BIOENGINEERING SOLUTION: We have to choose the material of which we will construct the device. Here we only have two reasonable choices (no other materials have had as much testing in actual use or proven as satisfactory) : the chrome-cobalt alloy systems, and the 316 stainless steel. Either would serve very well, and the actual choice was based upon considerations lying completely aside from biological and mechanical acceptability.

8) SUMMARY: Thus we evolve a new total hip replacement system which has actually proven quite satisfactory in use. Figure 18.16 shows one in place in a patient of Dr. Kent Wu. It has simplicity—only two parts; mechanical durability—probably greater than the adult human life span with probability on the order of $p = .95$; no greater risk of would infection than during an ordinary Austin-Moore replacement prosthesis for an acute fracture; biological acceptance, for it uses a single material of established and quite satisfactory acceptability; and biomechanical acceptance, in that its unit loading factors, geometry and manner of function remain compatible with a variety of the biomechanical "yeas" and "nays" that we have accumulated from actual surgical experience.

VII: CONCLUSION

The facts that the mould arthroplasty technique works at all, and that the cellularly driven and biomechanically purposeful events described herein occur naturally, repeatedly and consistently when one performs a mould arthroplasty and manages it properly during the convalescent period, indicate that even in adult life the body's mesodermal tissues still possess all of the responsive and adaptive potential required to generate new joints of acceptable mobility and durability. It follows as night the day that an almost certainly fruitful area for future research in this whole field constitutes learning how to control the proliferation and differentiation of the cell lines responsible for these phenomena, and to do so sufficiently reproducibly that we can make patients with damaged joints regenerate new ones made entirely of their own living materials. While possibly still visionary in that no immediate threat looms on our therapeutic horizon that such an expertise will descend upon us tomorrow or even in the next decade, it has become abundantly clear from past basic biological research that it does exist as a real possibility. Therefore it constitutes a legitimate and, ultimately, almost certainly productive and therapeutically worthwhile line of biomechanical research.

Let us now turn our attention from bearings, to supports and levers and divers other things, by looking at bones, and bones plus joints, at the organ and higher levels of biological organization. Again we must select examples that illustrate generalities because the vastness of the subject and the limitations of your author require it.

But first, test questions please!

QUESTIONS: CHAPTER 18

1) What does the concept of graduated compliance signify relative to joint design?
2) How can a common identical building material provide structures of widely differing bulk stiffness (or compliance if you prefer), and at the same time constant or varying total strength?
3) a) Name the primary function of a joint. b) And of its lubricant. c) And of its cells.
4) Basically, how did nature solve the problem of maintaining accurate alignment of the joint surfaces?
5) The text proposes what as a major function of articular menisci?
6) How many separate lubricant pumps do we identify in a human joint?
7) What basically accounts for the high reliability and long service life of mammalian joints?

8) A biomechanical research group has gone to extraordinary lengths to determine the precise combinations of sliding, rotation, translation and moment to moment changes in the center of rotation occurring in the natural knee joint (81). In designing a total joint replacement for a knee (or hip, ankle, shoulder, elbow, interphalangeal joint or whatever) another group has gone to equally great lengths to reproduce them exactly in the inanimate replacement device. Evaluate this strategy.

9) In some contemporary total hip and knee replacement endoprostheses, a plastic cement serves as a filler, or grouting lying between the implant and the bone. What major role or purpose does it probably subserve?

10) The designers of systems such as those in the above question intended the cement to anchor the implant securely and immovably to the bone. a) In the light of what you have learned in these five volumes, evaluate this objective. b) What design-oriented conclusion might one draw from the evaluation? c) What seem to emerge as the major immediate problems in designing such devices?

11) a) Describe the major objection to total joint replacement systems in which one metal part slides on another. b) Give two ways of correcting the problem which should allow a metal on metal device to provide satisfactory service.

Chapter 19

Some Relations between Musculoskeletal Structure and Mechanical Function

I: INTRODUCTION

1) THE MINIMUM STRAIN PRINCIPLE: One simple design objective crops up time and again throughout the architecture and functions of the bony parts of the adult skeleton. Let us call it the principle of minimum strain, meaning: the structure and manner of use of the musculoskeletal system tend to reduce flexural unit strains of lamellar bone tissue, to or below some minimum level (92). This comes about because mechanical loads so control the bone modeling processes as to size, shape and locate a bone in tissue space in the way which most efficiently minimizes flexural strains. Of course, achieving this implies an underlying condition: that muscle contractions correctly time, synergize, and gauge as to magnitude of contractile force, and as to stereotyism of pattern, so as to use the actual strength of bones in the most efficient way. These matters appear described in some detail in Volume IV of this series, to which the interested reader should refer (99).

But to illustrate briefly here for the benefit of nonorthopaedic readers what this principle means, we will describe a few specific examples of it in action. These will include the narrow waisted shape of bones; the longitudinal geometry of the human clavicle and femur; some aspects of the function and structure of the knee; and the lumbar spine. We will consider first the apparent reason for the narrow waisted shape of most bones, one which produces a kind of static and inherently arranged minimization of flexural strain of its cortex. The other situations will illustrate how muscle usage under the control of the nervous system provides a dynamically determined but otherwise similar minimization of strain and flexural deformation.

Before the description, consider two traps into which earlier analysts of such matters inadvertently fell (including your author), and which delayed effective understanding of the principle of action involved. These traps constitute the trivial case and the time averaging property.

2) TRIVIAL AND MEANINGFUL CASES: If you determine the distribution of mechanical stress in the massive frame and running gear of a locomotive induced by the engineer's weight in his chair in the cab, and compare that with the distribution of structural strength in that gear, you will find that no design-meaningful relationship between the two comes to light. A poor scientist could infer that from this that he had not used a good enough computer, or sensitive enough measuring instruments, or the right kind of instruments, or the right kind of scientist, and so he would apply for another grant, more and better equipment and more and different highly trained people (170) to solve this pressing but frustrating problem (!) .

Of course, like the reader at this juncture, a good scientist might suspect he had made a more basic if simpler error, one in his investigative strategy, not his tactics (See Volume II) , and would soon realize that he had studied a trivial case, in which the two parameters compared really had no important connection for one to discover. To understand 99.99 per cent of the locomotive's design he should compare stress to strength distributions within it as it pulls a train; after all that constitutes the locomotive's basic *raison d'etre*.

The point of this paragraph: Many biomechanical analyses of the human frame done in the past actually chose trivial cases for study so nobody should find any surprise

or mystery in the fact that little or no common sense understanding of skeletal architecture evolved therefrom.

3) THE TIME AVERAGING PROPERTY: The mechanisms—
whatever their basic nature—which guide skeletal growth
and architecture to conform to the skeleton's mechanical
force milieu do so in a very particular way: the architecture
conforms to all of the separate mechanical loads it carries
averaged over some period of time. In Volume III, we
named such a characteristic response period of a dynamic
system sigma (σ), and for skeletal architectural modeling
purposes its value ranges from approximately four to six
months in an infant to longer than our three-score and ten
life span at skeletal maturity.

Remember then in trying to develop good biomechanical
thinking habits and intuition: *analyze meaningful situations* (117), and *think in terms of averages over considerable
chunks of time,* when relating loads to skeletal architecture.

II: FLEXURE-DRIFT LAW

1) THE NARROW WAISTED SHAPE: Let us first define
the *flexure-drift law,* as follows:

*A series of similarly aligned dynamic flexural strains
cause all of a bone's surfaces to drift towards the concavity
that arises as the strains develop* (92,101).

Thus, on a surface which typically becomes more convex
(than originally) under such conditions, a surface stimulus
of some kind arises which makes osteoclasts progressively
remove bone from it (causing, technically, an osteoclastic
drift), as repeated passes with a carpenter's spokeshave
might cut down the edge of a board. On the opposite surface
which becomes more concave (than originally*), another

---

* Note: The original shape of the surface does not matter. It is the kind of
change it undergoes that matters and only two biodynamically effective ones occur:
convex-tending, and concave-tending.

surface stimulus of some kind makes osteoblasts deposit new bone on it, building it up layer by layer (causing, technically, an osteoblastic drift).

Note: This flexure drift law applies only to the portions of a bone lying between its articulations and/or apophyses. The growth in length and the modeling of growing chondral tissues follow a different "conductor," described in Volume II.

(*a*) With this simple cause-effect rule (or principle of action) in mind, consider the closed container shown in Figure 19.01, with walls made of an elastic solid and a cavity filled with a less compressible fluid-like material (actually, here, trabecular bone inside). If it originally had straight sides when it carried no superimposed compression load, then a weight (such as body weight) added on top of it would load the side walls in compression so they would shorten slightly. But decreasing the height of the container also decreases its volume, causing the incompressible fluid within to push outwards on, and thus to tend to bulge outwards the walls of the container, even though minutely.

(*b*) According to the flexure-drift law, if the cortical wall of the vertebral body (the container we actually analogize here) tends to bulge out as we stand up, both its internal and external surfaces should begin to move or drift towards the concavity, i.e., towards the center of the vertebral body. They would do so until the narrow waisted shape develops.

(*c*) *Flexural Neutralization*: At this point an interesting further development arises. Due to its new, inwardly convex shape, any further vertical compression loads placed on top, and carried in part by the cortex, now tend to make the wall bend even further inward, i.e., to exaggerate the inwaisting. Obviously that cantilever arrangement flexural tendency acts in the opposite sense to the aforesaid bursting force. And I proposed in 1964 that the actual inwaisting of real vertebrae (and of all other bones) represents just that shape (acting in conjunction with the compression compliance of the

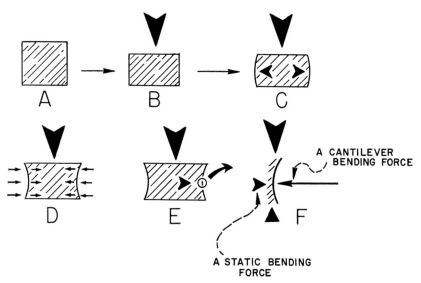

Figure 19.01. The *flexure-drift law* as a determinant of the inwaisting of bones, here a vertebral centrum. See the text. Understand the following about the relationship between the flexure-drift law and bioelectrical effects at bone surfaces: The flexure-drift law represents an operational rule or principle of action based upon clinical observations. It works consistently and repeatedly, and that observation and relationship in no way depends upon or becomes threatened by the bioelectric activity and the experimental findings related thereto. Many workers suspect the bioelectric activity relates somehow to the cellular control that causes the bone surface drifts inherent in the flexure-drift law; they include Brighton, Friedenberg, Fukada, Shamos, McElhaney, Becker and Bassett. But the research goal in this field represents finding out if the electrical facts can account for observed flexure-drift relationships in the living, *not the converse.* (Reprinted by permission of author and publisher, ref. no. 101.)

trabecular mass within) which causes these two different mechanical sources and arrangements of flexural strain to cancel out. Let us call that the flexural neutralization principle, and observe that it requires as an essential element in its behavior a component of uniaxial compression acting on the bone, in addition to any flexural loads. And, in point of anatomical fact, all inwaisted bones in mammalian skeletons do carry such an end-loading compression component. Figure 19.02 shows the finished vertebra.

Given the above, then one can show that behaviorally speaking such a system must constitute a negative feedback system, in which excessive flexure forms the specific error it detects and controls, and it must act to reduce unit flexural strains and stresses (or moments) throughout the compacta towards some minimum (and common) value.*

Note: It has been shown that when lamellar bone undergoes flexure parallel to its grain the outer surface of the concave tending side develops a negative electrical charge, that of the convex tending surface a positive one (29,82,105). Considerable interest has arisen in this phenomenon because of the obvious possibility that those voltage potentials (See Appendix 6,7) provide the signal that stimulates, coordinates and regulates the cellular behavior responsible for the consistent accuracy of the flexure drift law (92,99). Orthopaedists should hear more on this in years to come.

Of some parenthetical interest here, we now have available the information that in living sheep during ordinary walking and breathing cyclic strains arise in the vertebral central cortex on the order of $20-50 \times 10^{-6}$ mm (L. E. Lonyon, J. Biomech. 5:277, 1972). In other words, perfectly ordinary activities cause measureable dynamic strains in the living skeleton.

Having outlined what happens within a vertebra, next we will show how external forces acting on a whole bone achieve dynamic flexural strain equalization and minimization, first for a typical long bone, and then for a typical joint.

2) FLEXURE DRIFT ACTIVITIES IN THE CLAVICLE: Two things put the writer on to the principle just described. One of them appears in Figure 19.03, which you might cogitate on briefly and then move on.

---

* Although they certainly need not always become zero or remain minimal or equal at all instants in time; do not forget the time-averaging sense in which this principle surely acts, as some of its earlier critics did.

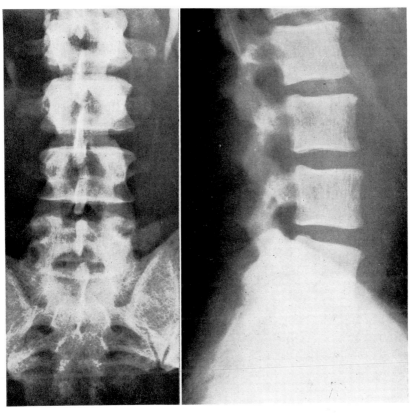

Figure 19.02. AP (i.e., anteroposterior) and lateral (right) views of the lumbar spine of a human adult. It reveals the cortical inwaisting of the vertebral centra described in the text. That inwaisting characterizes the architecture of all modeling dependent bones in all known species, from predinosaur ages of the history of evolution right up to now.

The upper left of Figure 19.04 shows a view of a man's clavicle as one might see it while standing above him and looking down. It exhibits an S-shaped curve. The succeeding diagram at (B) illustrates that the clavicle normally carries a uniaxial compression load component, arising as the sum of the pulls of several powerful muscles which we need not name here.

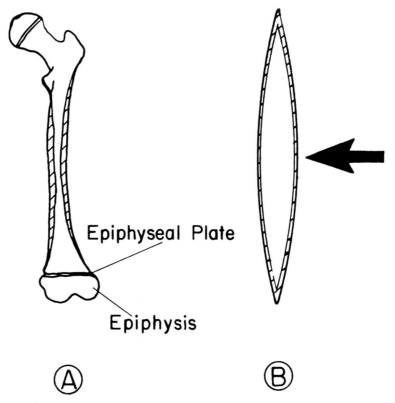

Epiphyseal Plate

Epiphysis

Ⓐ　　　　　　　　Ⓑ

Figure 19.03. Like most of yours probably, my anatomy professors spoke of bones as pure *beams* loaded primarily in flexure, and at the time there seemed little reason to ponder that matter in favor of more obvious and pressing things, such as formaldehyde and phenol, common femoral arteries, lobes of the lung, and finals.

But an introduction to mechanics while teaching at Yale University School of Medicine taught that the ideal shape for pure beams constitutes that shown here on the right. Clearly the shape of a typical femur then had to mean that either He made a mistake in design, or we made one somewhere in its analysis. Having acquired at least some (even if not nearly enough) humility by then, the latter possibility was pursued first, which brings us to this chapter. (Reprinted by permission of authors and editor, ref. no. 68.)

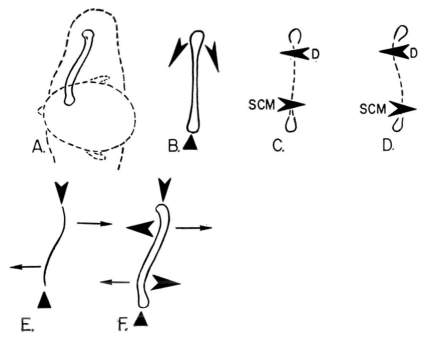

Figure 19.04. Here we see the flexure-drift law producing grossly visible structural adaptations in the human clavicle as seen from above. See the text. And keep in mind that this form of behavior of surface drifts becomes inapparent only in special circumstances, which include during active repair and in the presence of changes and activities set off and guided by local disease. (Reprinted by permission of author and publisher, ref. no. 101.)

In addition, from the view in which we observe this clavicle, two muscles apply dynamic flexural load components to it whenever they contract, and of the static bending arrangement. The deltoid (D) tends to strain the upper half of this clavicle in flexure convexly towards the reader's left, each time it contracts, while the sternocleidomastoid muscle (ScM), acting on the lower half tends to strain it in the opposite manner. Of some interest, at birth the infant's clavicle usually has an essentially straight shape. Shortly after birth however he begins to use the muscles which actuate the shoulder girdle and the forces described above then develop repeatedly and consistently on the clavicle. According to the flexure-drift law, all of the affected surfaces should then begin to move towards the concavities arising during stereotyped series of dynamic flexures, which represents posteriorly for the upper half of the clavicle, and anteriorly for the lower half. In a relatively few months these patterned drifts produce the normal S-shaped curve of the clavicle already shown at the upper left, and again at the lower right.

At this juncture, the uniaxial compression component now has the effect of tending to make each of these curvatures worse each time the compression end load develops on the outer end of the clavicle. Note that these loads have the cantilever arrangement shown at (D) in Figure 19.05, that they tend to accentuate the normal anatomical curvatures, and simultaneously they tend to neutralize the bending actions of the static flexural arrangement forces due to direct muscle pulls. And I propose that the stable shape of the

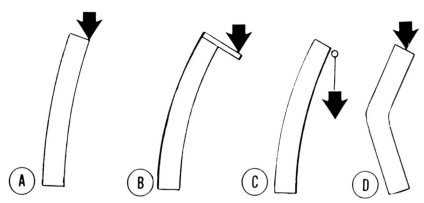

Figure 19.05. To review matters, we see here four mechanical arrangements for inducing flexure in a beam—or bone—by the cantilever arrangement. The one on the right analogizes the seemingly purposeful effects of long bone curvatures in skeletons of all bony vertebrates. An end load on this shape tends to make the flexure worse, and nature deliberately uses the moments generated thereby to cancel or neutralize other but oppositely acting moments and flexural loads, thereby to achieve time-averaged normal loading at any cross sectional level of minimum cross section area.

clavicle (and any other normal long bone from rib to femur) represents that in which the amount of flexure generated by the one mechanism essentially equals and so cancels that generated by the other. Again, *do not forget that the time averaging property applies here,* and it means that all of the loads of all types applied to the clavicle over a period of many months, become time-averaged by the system, which then adopts that architecture which in essence cancels out all opposing (and also time-averaged) forces. Or in different words, it requires repeated flexures to actuate this system, as clearly stated in 1964, and apparently rediscovered recently by Chamay and Tschantz.*

Nearly all normal gross long bone curvatures in all mammals, upon proper analysis of their dynamic musculoskeletal functions, will prove to have their origin in the phenomenon just described above with the clavicle, taken only as a typical case. Examples of such bones would include the ribs, the bones of the pelvis, the ossicles of the inner ear, the fingers, the hip joints, the vertebral arch and the leg.

Note: Other causes of abnormal curvatures can arise in a variety of bone diseases, so the flexure-drift law does not account for all curved bones; just most of them.[†]

Volume IV described several additional examples and effects of the flexure-drift law in action.

3) THE BONE MODELING BARRIERS: The flexure drift law applies only to lamellar bone surfaces directly covered by overlying soft tissues, and bones so characterized constitute the bone modeling dependent class of bones listed in Table 13.05.

The drift law *does not apply* under the following four circumstances:

(*a*) *Where cartilage covers a bone surface.* Thus all joint surfaces, and the attachments to bone of tendon, lig-

---

* Chamay, A.; Tschantz: J. Biomech. 5: 173, 1972.

† The exceptions arise when the direction of epiphyseal growth no longer parallels the long axis of the shaft, introducing thereby a curvature at the end of the bone but one which subsequent bone modeling activity (following the game rules just described) smooths out.

ament and fascia, and the bone on either side of epiphyseal plates (and apophyses) remain locally immune to the flexure drift law and, rather, obey the chondral growth/force-response characteristic described earlier (see Figure 19.06). Note that all sesamoids in growing children lie completely embedded in cartilage and so their external surfaces obey the chondral modeling law, not the bone's flexure-drift law. Sesamoids form examples of bone modeling independent structures listed in Table 13.05.

(b) *Where teeth cover bone.* They too prevent the flexure-drift law from acting on the facing mandibular and maxillary surfaces. But in edentulous patients those surfaces can then become competent in this respect, and this probably plays a role in causing the recession of the alveolar ridges in edentulous patients, a problem which taxes the therapeutic expertise of our friends in the dental profession.

(c) *Bare bone.* Where a bone lies bare in the floor of wound it does not display modeling activity, and for obvious reasons—no cells can live on a bare bone surface, and only cells can produce these drifts.

(d) *At implant-bone interface:* Between a plate and the underlying shaft, or between the surfaces of a mass of bone cement and the underlying bone, modeling does not occur. Note that both inflammation (and its attendant resorption) and repair activities can still occur at such interfaces.

III: NEUROMOTOR RELATIONS

Having looked at lamellar bone architecture in action in response to mechanical factors, and defined the principle of action which applies to lamellar bone architecture generally, let us now turn attention to a higher level of integration and the major source of those mechanical factors, muscle contraction, and again with two specific examples obtain some ideas that apply generally to musculoskeletal functions.

1) The Femoral Shaft:

(a) Figure 19.07 shows from the left side the left femur of a man running upstairs, and in the act of down-

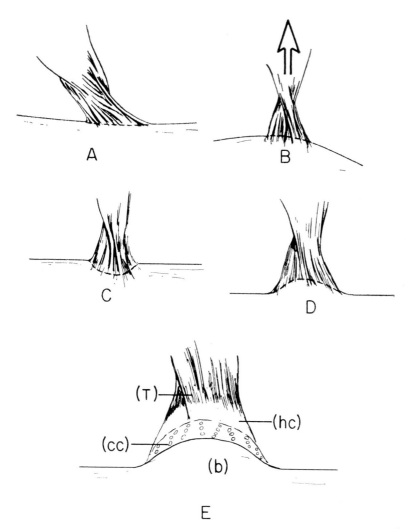

Figure 19.06. A tendon attachment diagrammed at A. At B, we see the type of local flexural deformation a pull on the tendon causes, and at C, the local modeling response if the flexure-drift law applied there. But actual tendon insertions appear as at D. Why? Because a layer of hyaline cartilage (hc) covers the bone surface in the region of the tendon insertion as shown at E, and that not only inactivates the flexure-drift law on that surface, it now grows according to the chondral modeling law described earlier. *b*: bone. *cc*: calcified cartilage. T: tendon. (Reprinted by permission of author and publisher, ref. no. 92.)

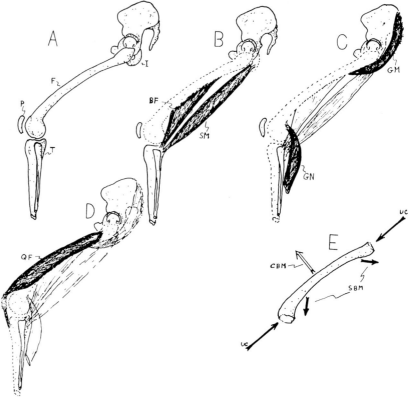

Figure 19.07. Some anatomical and functional relationships in the human thigh. We envision the left one from the left side as the subject climbs a stair. See the text.

thrust with that limb. To push his body upwards, muscle forces must (and do) extend both hip and knee. At first glance it would seem that they must create a tremendous bending force on the femur, one tending to make it bow convexly on the posterior surface of the shaft. Let us see.

(*b*) At (B), we see the action of three of the four hamstring muscles* as darkened muscle masses. While they extend the hip, they do so somewhat like a chain brace without creating significant anteroposterior bending moments in the bone. Like a walnut between the jaws of a nut cracker, they load it for practical purposes in uniaxial com-

---

* Semitendinosus, semimembranosus, biceps femoris.

pression, through the knee joint below and the hip joint above. In this figure the short head of the biceps femoris, with its fleshy origin on the shaft of the femur, does add a backward bending tendency to it.

At (C), the gluteus maximus also tends to bend the femur more convexly posteriorly, and the two gastrocnemius heads add a similar flexural load to the lower end of the bone, so a total of four muscle attachments contribute dynamic flexural loads tending to bow the femur backwards.

At (D), four other muscles which function as a unit (so anatomists gave them one name: the quadriceps) tend to bend the femur oppositely to the tendencies of the gastrocnemius, short head of the biceps and gluteus maximus.

(*c*) For this dynamic muscle system to work, i.e., for it to minimize large net flexural loads on the femur, the muscles involved must all contract in the proper phase or time, and with forces of the proper relative magnitudes (137). And they actually do. Partly this arises because the anatomy and function of the lower limb has arranged matters so that the act of thrusting away from the ground requires that hamstrings and gluteus maximus contract to extend the hip; that the quadriceps contact simultaneously to extend the knee; and that the gastrocnemius contract to aid in extending the ankle. And partly too it arises because the nervous system controls and synchronizes these separate muscles in exactly such a way as to form an integrated, smoothly coordinated system. *That control possesses the property of stereotypism,* meaning that all the muscles involved contract in the same pattern of synergy and relative amplitude every time one thrusts off the ground. *The lamellar bone architecture adapts to just that stereotyped pattern.*

(*d*) Note that the direct forces bending the femur backwards (the static bending arrangement ones) slightly over-cancel those which tend to bend it forwards.* As a

---

* In most quadrupeds these forces do cancel so the femoral shaft has no longitudinal curvature when seen from the side. And of some interest, the right and left bones of one individual—tibias for example, or femurs, display strikingly similar properties (246).

TABLE 19.01
MECHANICAL PROPERTIES OF THE BODY AND ITS SEGMENTS

Body or Part	Mass as % whole body	Center of gravity as % of segment length proximal-distal	Mean density
Head and Trunk	55	60–40	
All limbs	44	—	
Arm	3	43–57	1.07
Forearm	1.8	43–57	1.12
Hand	.7	51–49	1.15
Thigh	10.5	43–57	1.05
Leg	4.7	43–57	1.09
Foot	1.6	44–57	1.09

result, human femurs have some anterior bow, as shown in the figure. The large muscular uniaxial compression load components acting parallel to the long axis of the femur generate from that bow an indirect bowing tendency (i.e., cantilever arrangement bending moment) of large enough magnitude to neutralize any excess of posteriorly bending forces. Table 19.01 provides some data about centers of gravity and masses of body segments on which these muscle forces act.

SUMMARY: The above situation illustrates an important and quite general and consistent principle of mammalian musculoskeletal biomechanics:

The muscular and neural anatomy, its manner of use and the bony architecture, all* combine, to produce time averaged minimum bending forces on long bones. Or if you prefer, to minimize strain energy. *The nervous system simply has to form an essential element in this relationship,* for it determines and coordinates all of the muscle forces, and thus establishes the stereotyped patterns of muscular function required for any system with as long a sigma value as this one has to work effectively. This situation also reemphasizes another equally general principle or rule of thumb:

The normal bowing of certain bones (ribs, radius, vertebral processes, femur, tibia) exists to generate cantilever arrangement flexural moments (arising from the uniaxial

---

* That is, the relative timing and force of various muscle contractions averaged over time does effectively neutralize all flexural loads and moments.

compression components) which tend to neutralize opposite, static arrangement bending moments created by flexural loads applied directly to bones, usually by muscles. In other words, the curves of a woman's bones prove just as functional and necessary as, in a different way, do certain other non-linear aspects of her anatomy.

Note: Gravity enters into the above relationships, not in the direct and obvious sense (i.e., as body weight on the femur for example), as much as in providing some of the reactions of bodily parts and regions that muscle forces must act on in order to effect acceleration and deceleration of the body's mass against the pull of gravity. Since the muscles usually have to work at a mechanical disadvantage to accelerate the various masses of the body, the absolute values of the muscle forces easily exceed those of gravity, by *on the order of 2X to 4X*. Hence the features of muscle anatomy and function, not gravity, dominate bone architecture, and the alignment of the gravity gradient and other gravitic concerns play a very minor direct role in that regard. This should prove of some value to future astronauts living in free-fall situations for any length of time (but they will have to do so for longer than one $\sigma_r + \sigma_f$ before we can know this for certain; see Volume III). Of course other things than purely biomechanical concerns operate too, such as age and disease as the cited references imply (232,236,267,269,277, 278), but we deal with the biomechanical ones.

Parenthetically, for any older reader who finds he still must doubt the simplistic accuracy of this concept of architectural functional relation and believes a femur must withstand far more flexure than uniaxial loading in normal use, ponder these demonstrated facts: at age twenty-five years it requires a uniaxial compression load of 5000 kg to make a male femur fail, yet it fails in flexure at only 280 k side load: a difference in load capacity of about 20:1 (293). Do you believe our Maker so lavishly supplied uniaxial compression strength if it were unnecessary?

Next, we will analyze some dynamic forces that occur at the knee.

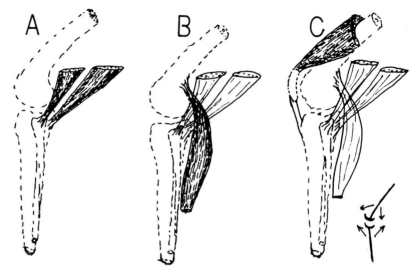

Figure 19.08. A slightly enlarged view of the knee in the previous problem. See the text.

2) THE KNEE: Figure 19.08 shows a sketch of the knee from the side, in the same situation as described in the previous section. Note that biomechanically *the knee and the elbow serve the main purpose of altering the total lengths* of the lower and upper extremity respectively. By this means they also lessen the true muscle energy and power required at any one joint to position and move these extremities in space against the inertial reactions involved.

At (A), note that the hamstrings try to pull the tibia backwards on the femur, and to bow the upper end of the tibia backwards.

At (B), note that the two gastrocnemius attachments also tend to bow the lower end of the femur posteriorly.

At (C), note that the infrapatellar tendon, because of the pull of the quadriceps muscle applied to it, exerts a component of forward pull on the tibia which balances out some of the posteriorly directed component the hamstrings. It forms no accident that as the knee flexes more and more, the posteriorly pulling component of the hamstrings increases in proportion to the anterior pulling component of the infrapatellar tendon (as the quadriceps elongates its maximal contractural force increases, while as the hamstrings shorten their maximal force decreases, the force-length relation described in an earlier chapter). Consequently these forces show some tendency to balance out in any position of the joint, provided they both operate at the same time. And the anatomy and function of a normal knee cause exactly this to occur, for in thrusting away from the ground as an example, the knee extensors (quadriceps) and hip extensors (hamstrings) must contract at the same time.

The quadriceps muscle also tends to bow the femur anteriorly by virtue of its broad, fleshy origin (i.e., attachment) on this bone. This cancels some of the posterior bowing tendency of the gastrocnemius. Now it would seem that if the knee lay flexed to a right angle, the posterior bowing force of the gastrocnemius of the lower femur would prove more effective than the opposite one of the quadriceps, to give rise to a resultant and considerable unbalanced posterior bowing force in the lower fifth of the bone. This probably does occur because normally an anterior femoral bowing occurs in this region which, by virtue of the large uniaxial compression load component acting on all weight bearing long bones, would generate an anterior cantilever arrangement bowing force tending to neutralize the gastrocnemius induced flexural load. Note too that with the knee in the right angle position the gastrocnemii lie in a shortened state, and so cannot develop a maximal contractile effort, and equally cannot make full use of their better mechanical advantage.

The above two examples of analyzing the minimum flexural strain principle in action apply quite generally throughout the human body, from the hip joint to the ossicles of the inner ear. Consequently let us now ascend one more level of organization (or degree of complexity) and analyze a problem dealing basically with the function of the trunk.

3) THE LUMBAR SPINE

(a) *The Dissection Room Approach*: Figure 19.09 shows the lumbar spine from the side of a man lifting a weight with his arms. How does the anatomy and its usage relate in this situation? At B we see the kernel of the static older anatomical idea of this function. It includes the lever arm of the back extensor muscles, which equals the distance between the two arrows, or about an inch. The lever arm of the weight in the arrangement shown equals about twelve inches, for a twelve times greater mechanical advantage than the muscles, as indicated in C.

Were the above analysis realistic, then a man lifting a 100 pound weight should develop a 1,200 pound compression load across the intervertebral discs, to which one should add the superimposed weight of the body plus the additional muscle pulls required to stabilize the spine side-to-side. We could conservatively set the total of these loads at 1,500 pounds. Since the intervertebral lumbar disc has a cross sectional area of about 2.5 square inches, the compression unit load should equal 1500/2.5, or about 550 psi on the disc in this situation. And since most men in real life can lift 500 pounds or more in this way, their discs (according to this analysis) should be able to carry 7,500 lbs., or 3.75 *tons.*

In the light of such an analysis, the following facts become significant: (1) Professor Alf Nachemson has actually measured the intradiscal pressure in live people performing such actions, and found values less than half those calculated above (206). (2) F. G. Evans (among others) has shown that the unit compression strength of a mass of vertebral cancellus bone approximates 600 psi (73); see Table 13.07, leaving much less than no factor of safety in any such analysis. Since we do not regularly break our backs by lifting 500 lbs, clearly the above analysis must contain some error. And it does, as follows and as D. Lucas, and V. Inman's and other groups have pointed out (197):

(b) *The Dynamic Approach*: The above analysis omitted the thoracoabdominal wall and its contents. And the reader can confirm for himself that whenever he lifts anything heavy (over 75 + lbs) in the way shown in (A), his abdominal muscles tighten. For a very heavy weight he even holds his breath while the muscles on the chest wall tighten too (try it). Why?

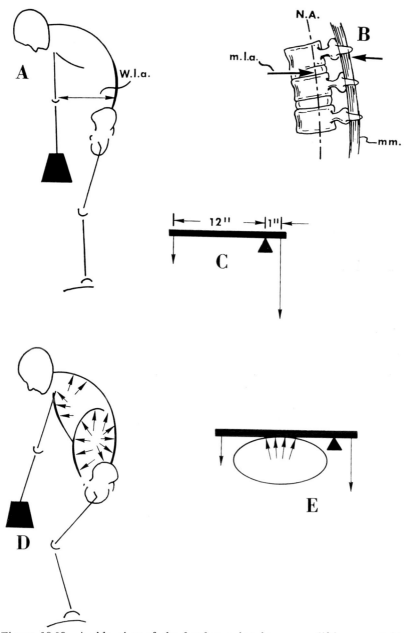

Figure 19.09. A side view of the lumbar spine in a man lifting a weight. It illustrates at the top left the simplistic mechanical approach most of us originally had in mind in analysing this problem, and at the bottom the more accurate approach required by actual measurements by Swedish workers of intradiscal pressures in subjects doing such activities. See the text. (Reprinted by permission of author and publisher, ref. no. 94.)

Think of the abdomen and chest as balloons or airtight bags, and the ribs and spine simply as stiffeners in their walls. When the belly muscles tighten, this increases intraabdominal pressure. Since the viscera act like an incompressible fluid under these conditions they develop an internal hydrostatic pressure which acts in all directions simultaneously, including upwards, as in (D). As a result, the balloon in front of the fulcum in the spine holds up or acts to float some of the weight the man lifts, so his spine and its muscles need to carry only a part of it. Note that the pressure within the thoracolumbar cavity also tends to develop a tension load tending to elongate the spine, a component which must subtract from the total compression load it carries. Thus a more realistic diagram of the mechanical factors involved in heavy lifting appears in E.*

This and the previous situations should suffice to give some hint at least of some of the unexpected nuances and shifts in emphasis one finds in the mechanical functional realities of living bodies when we compare them to our own machine—and structural—design practices. In this area we can make this general statement or rule: When an analysis leads to nonsensical or paradoxical results, it left out something important (but probably unperceived and/or unrecognized) at its outset.

4) DYNAMIC STABILITY: Now let us ascend yet another step in functional organization to gain perhaps even further insight into the manner in which the central nervous system controls some of the mechanical functions of the body.

Review briefly everything you did with your hands in the previous year. No matter how diverse the tasks they did, the power they expended, their location in the space around you, or the directions in which they exerted pushes and pulls, you probably not only did not tip over and fall, you find some humor in the very idea. But think: How would you, as an engineer, design a platform or backup for the human hand

---

* This perhaps shows that calling a man a windbag renders him a compliment on his strength, and that some politicians could be very good weight lifters.

which could do the same variety of things, provide equal mobility and yet never tip over, or weigh more than you do, have as much versatility and flexibility of motion in limb and trunk, and lie on as narrow and shifting a pedestal as the foot?

We achieve the stability we have, not by providing a fixed wide base, but rather by opting for a small base, and then providing means to position and orient it in space

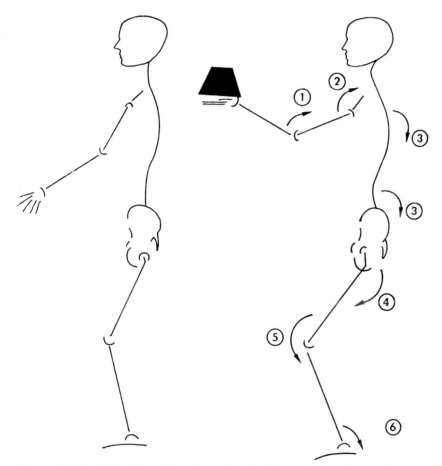

Figure 19.10. A brief analysis, from the left side only, of the muscle contraction patterns required to lift a weight by hand. It reveals that the nervous system must constitute a major factor in determining muscle activity patterns. See the text.

quickly and precisely, using a negative feedback positional control system (163). Our sensory system's apparatus provides the necessary data concerning our body's location in space, our orientation in the gravitational field gradient, any motion and change of it (i.e., acceleration), any muscle power exerted, and any goings on in our environment. The nervous system then does the necessary computing with that information, sends out the necessary control signals and monitors their effects. How, roughly, does this work?

(a) In Figure 19.10 left, a man stands at ease. On the right, he lifts a weight upwards with one hand. In order to do this (check the following on yourself) the following must occur: (1) Elbow flexor muscles must contract to lift the hand. (2) But this also tends to depress the whole extremity at the shoulder, requiring contraction of the shoulder flexor and elevator muscles. (3) This tends to bend the body forwards, and preventing that requires contractions of the back's extensor muscles. (4) Now he has stabilized his trunk, but his hips tend to flex to fold him over like a hinge. The hip extensors contract to prevent this. (5) That makes the knee tend to flex which would cause a fall, and quadriceps contraction opposes it. (6) Now the whole man tends to tilt and fall forwards at the ankle, so the muscles pulling on the Achilles tendon must contract.

(b) Were we to analyze the same situation as seen by standing in front of the subject, a different group of forces or falling tendencies would present themselves, they too would extend from the hand to the floor, but they too would all correct in the same way. Such corrections normally remain entirely subconscious (i.e., automaton determined) so that we live almost totally unaware of them. But in certain neurological diseases, such as tabes dorsalis or spastic diplegia or multiple sclerosis, the nervous system can lose some of its ability to do this, requiring the patient to concentrate consciously on maintaining balance to avoid falling in such situations, and to minimize clumsiness. Figure 19.11 abstracts the automaton concept.

(c) Thus, in order to lift up on something, or exert any

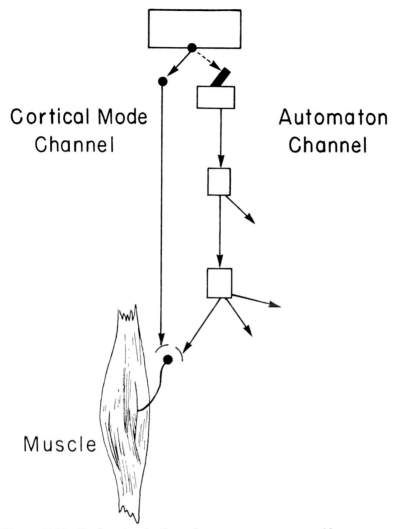

Cortical Mode
Channel

Automaton
Channel

Muscle

Figure 19.11. In functional effect, the nervous system provides two means for controlling muscular action and activity patterns. One, a direct routing, we may call *cortical control* (left), and it allows one to make any single muscle contract independently of all others and at will.

The second means, termed the *automaton*, provides unconsciously patterned and integrated activity of groups of muscles without conscious attention, in large part according to inherited patterns, and it constitutes the most important mode of CNS control of body function in biomechanics. When the "mode switch" functions properly one can switch at will from one to another mode, and one can retrain the automaton to produce new and novel patterns upon command. When the mode switch malfunctions, various types of neurologic disorders can ensue, only one of which represents spasticity. (Reprinted by permission of author and publisher, ref. no. 96.)

other kind of force with the hand (or elbow or head or foot) many, many muscles in the body must contract in addition to the prime movers to provide dynamic stability to the many joints between the foot lying on the floor, and the hand doing the work. These muscles must all contract at the right time (i.e., in proper phase) : their pulls must correctly proportion (i.e., occur in proper relative amplitudes) ; and the CNS must continuously monitor, detect and correct the unavoidable errors in the system before they cause a failure or error— such as falling down. Thus a single command by the conscious mind becomes converted largely within the automaton, into an avalanche of innumerable specific orders, shown in Figure 19.12.

The principle of dynamic stability in musculoskeletal function allows a minimum of structural mass and motive power to provide a nearly infinitely adaptable range of function. It achieves this by using muscles, bones and joints to make a pyramid of dynamically powered and stabilized platforms extending from ground to hand (290) .

The preceding sections gave merely a glimpse of the principles which underly the precision and beautiful exactness with which the functions of muscles, bones and joints match their structure and relationships. For example, they reveal that the patella forms neither a useless nor an incidental structure; dividing the origins of the hamstrings between the femoral shaft and the ischium was not haphazard; and arranging the function of the limb so that in running all joints extend simultaneously while rotating oppositely in sense was not an accident.

Each part demonstrates that shape, size, location, attachment, and is made to junction, so that the bending moments and other stresses in long bones and joints become minimized.* Thus, as Rybicki *et al.* demonstrated in a particular case of hip joint function, the muscles not only use most efficiently the bony strength available to them; they also pro-

---

* This leads one to suspect that in some developmental abnormalities, disturbances in relative muscle power could cause a skeletal abnormality. Stanisavljec has found such a change in infants with hip dysplasia (253) , and they have been long known in postpoliomyelitic states [Fleming (43) ; Crenshaw (30)].

THE COMMAND AVALANCHE

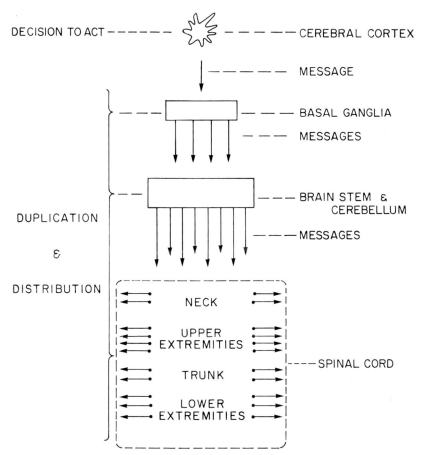

Figure 19.12. Once one consciously commands a general musculoskeletal act, that order usually passes down to the automaton within the CNS, which computes the necessary subordinate orders, passes them down to further computing centers and finally causes an avalanche of ultimate detailed orders. While the diagram omits it for clarity, these outflowing messages associate with inflowing ones which allow the CNS to monitor the actions it has ordered and, thereby, to detect and correct errors before they exceed trivial magnitudes. (Reprinted by permission of author and publisher, ref. no. 96.)

tect it by contracting in those patterns which minimize strain energy, exactly the same thing but in different words as minimizing flexure. (Rybicki *et al.*, J. Biomech. 5:203, 1972).

The use of dynamic forces to balance out bending moments behaves in a highly reliable fashion and rarely becomes disordered. Great reliability of some function usually means one or both of two things: (a) Very simple mechanisms control it, and/or (b) its ability to function does not depend on any single part.* (Wiener (287) ; Ashby (19)) These ideas suggest a negative feedback loop in the musculoskeletal system which detects excessive strain in bone and converts it to signals for changes in muscle function which will relieve the strain. We already know that no single cell proves essential for normal musculoskeletal function. That is, no single nerve cell, muscle fiber, Haversian system, chondrocyte or trabeculum proves essential. In fact, as we age we lose a sizeable fraction of our skeletal and CNS cells without any major deterioration in function or control happening (at least at my age one fervently hopes so—). We can even lose entire muscles, nerves, tendons, or bones, with only minor impairment of function.

Rule: In the normal skeletal system then, we can state a rule of thumb:

The distributions of structural strength in tissue space reflect the distributions of loads averaged over time.

Observe that this really constitutes the minimum strain principle, but rephrased in the analytical focus of another objective: strength.

Certainly the stretch-hypertrophy rule, the chondral growth/force-response characteristic and the flexure-drift law, separately and in concert, imply exactly such a relationship. Many if not most authorities on such matters could accept such rules as reasonable premises; the writer firmly believes in their essential correctness, having had more time

---

* A "part" here would be one muscle cell, one neuron, one bone cell, one tendon cell, one cartilage cell, or the extracellular products made by some of these cells. Many cells all doing one job (as in the nervous system, or in a muscle) create reliability through redundance (239) . That is, there are so many more cells than actually needed at the average moment that thousands, hundreds of thousands of them can die without impairing the function they supply, as an entity, to the body.

to evaluate them in clinical situations than anyone else to date, and having found them to function with uncanny accuracy and impressive consistency. We lack the space to provide a comprehensive analysis of numerous other particular situations but we will consider one more below for it carries a worthwhile if simple lesson.

Thus:

5) LOAD-STRENGTH RELATIONSHIP: The accompanying illustration in Figure 19.13 shows an anteroposterior x-ray view of a normal hip joint. It demonstrates the apparent densities of the subchondral bone on the femoral head and and the adjacent socket. The subchondral bone represents

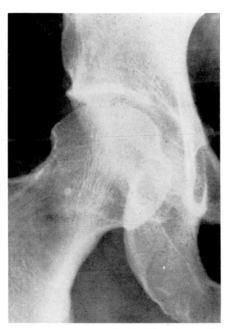

Figure 19.13. Note in the AP x-ray of this hip, the radiographically denser subchondral bone in the socket as compared to that of the head (this is a perfectly normal adult hip joint). It seems obvious that whatever mechanical load one subchondral bone layer carries, that on the facing side must carry too. Or at any moment they must equal each other. Yet the acetabular subchondral bone still shows much greater density than the femoral head. If skeletal mass does in fact reflect biomechanical demand, and in near direct and equal proportion, then how come? See the text!

that immediately adjacent to the clear space occupied by the radiotransparent articular cartilage. We call that space the cartilage space of the joint. Now in a normal skeleton the amount of calcium in the path of an x-ray beam reflects, and essentially in direct and equal proportion, the amount of bony tissue in that path. Since an ordinary x-ray represents a gamma ray shadowgraph of heavy metal atoms (here, calcium atoms), furthermore one not photographically reversed (i.e., the x-ray forms a true negative), the whiter regions on this x-ray have more bone lying in the path of the x-ray beam than less white regions.

Then it should follow that the acetabular subchondral bony layer contains significantly more bone than the comparable layer of the femoral head, and direct quantitative histological examination of these two regions confirm that in a decisive manner.

Obviously as this patient stands upon this hip the loads carried by each of its adjacent subchondral regions must equal each other. Which leads us to the question: Does that not become inconsistent with the above stated strength-load rule? How can the rule remain true in the face of this obvious radiographically demonstrated fact? Furthermore, one which you will find duplicated in all metacarpophalangeal joints, talo-navicular joints, ankles, elbows, knees, shoulders and many others?

The resolution of this apparent inconsistency has a lesson in it concerning the ways in which we habitually think, for the paradox here lies not in nature but in our own initial and frequently even subconscious assumptions.

As this patient walks, runs, climbs, swims, sits and sleeps during the span of an entire year the hip moves through a wide range of motion. During those motions widely varying parts of the surface of the femoral head accept loads from the acetabulum, *but the same part of the acetabulum usually transmits them.* Thus when averaged up over the whole year, all the loads transferred across the hip moment by moment transfer more consistently across a given region of the socket than across any equivalent sized region of the head.

Recall, in case you forgot (and if you are like most people new to this field you did, so you travel in a good company), that in its architectural responses to mechanical loads the skeletal tissues adapt to time-averaged loads, not instantaneous ones. Thus the x-ray findings remain quite consistent with our previously defined ground rules for bony biomechanical adaptations.

Others interested in this whole field will find with increasing regularity and frequency that where some apparent conflict arises between a factual natural situation or phenomenon and the skeletal tissue modeling laws I have described, that a hidden assumption in our thinking processes, not a flaw in the laws themselves (actually, principles of action), lies at the root.

IV: CHONDRAL MODELING FACTORS

Volume II described the general aspects of chondral modeling activity in enough detail that here we need only a reminder of its manner of behavior, plus analysis of a situation in which a not-so-obvious dynamic factor interacting with the principle of action it represents can cause what amounts to a deformity in our eyes but not in the eyes of nature. Recall that chondral modeling signifies those architecturally aimed modifications of cartilage growth patterns which have as their role or purpose in the scheme of things permitting and ensuring good biomechanical function. Then let us consider two limb alignment problems based upon chondral modeling behavior, one normal in any sense, and one abnormal in the ordinary medical sense.

1) Normal Knee Alignment: As the particular case of the general problem whose biomechanical determinants confront us in the office every week, let us look at the alignment of the hip-thigh-leg system as one sees it from the front. A number of behavioral properties it demonstrates (both in health and disease) serve to illustrate some of the biodynamic principles that determine the responses of growing chondral tissues to mechanical forces in action, and they also can serve

orthopaedic surgeons in the clinical sense of helping them to diagnose the causes of malalignments of joints, and to choose effective modes of treatment thereof.

To begin, note that as one bears weight on the lower extremity, and as seen from the view described and shown in Figure 19.14 the transmission of mechanical loads from the main body mass to the floor through the lower limb commences at the middle of rotation of the hip joint, that is, in the center of the femoral head. From thence the weight bearing line must pass down the femur and across into the tibia through the middle of the knee joint. And in turn, the loads on the tibia must then transfer to the floor by passing through the middle of the ankle joint. The accompanying sketch illustrates this normal situation and two possible malalignments of the centers of these three joints with respect to each other. One can see that in the normal situation on the left, with the knee fully extended, a *straight line will connect the centers of the hip, knee and ankle joints.* However when the knee develops a certain amount of valgus (the middle situation), one then finds the center of the knee joint comes to lie medially to this line, and the originallly even partition of the total load across the knee between its two condyles now lateralizes to overload the lateral condyles relative to the medical ones. Should this occur in a growing child, the curve of the chondral growth/force-response characteristic shown earlier in Figure 14.02 illustrates that longitudinal growth on the lateral side of this knee should accelerate slightly, and that on the medial side decelerate slightly, because the malalignment has introduced small torques or bending moments which tend to disturb the normal situation of equal unit loading on the two femoral tibial condyles, towards that in which the medial condyle bears a lesser fraction of the total than the lateral. With further growth, this situation would then automatically lead to correction of the malalignment and that correction would cease as soon as equal distribution of the loads on the two sides of the knee had developed.

Should a varus deformity arise as on the right, then the

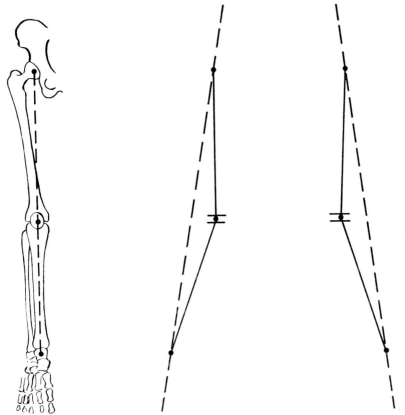

Figure 19.14. *Left:* AP view of the pelvis, and right femur and tibia and associated joints seen from the front, illustrating the normal (i.e., usual) alignment: A straight line runs from the center of the hip to the center of the knee and extends through the center of the ankle joint.

Middle: When too much angulation convex to your right exists, the knee has excessive *valgus* and, other things remaining unchanged, the lateral half of the knee now carries too large a fraction of the total load crossing the joint.

Right (still the right lower limb) : We call the reverse angulation *varus,* or genu varum, and this overloads the medial or right side of the knee, other things such as muscle contraction patterns remaining equal.

However: When these malalignments remain minor in degree, the chondral growth/force-response characteristic responds in its negative feedback mode to restore the proper alignment. Only when the malignment overloads growing cartilage on one side of a growing joint onto the descending limb of that curve (see Figure 14.02) does it then become worse with continued function because now the response characteristic has moved over into the descending limb where the positive feedback response mode lies.

converse behavior would ensue and, equally, lead to auto-correction of the varus.

In both above situations, loads remained to the left side of the peak of the curve in Figure 14.02, so the negative feed-back response mode ensued.

Accordingly, we may accept as a premise that not by accident in normal people do the centers of these three joints really align in the manner described. In fact *the feedback between chondral growth and mechanical forces acting on the growth planes require this mode of alignment.* A similar analysis would apply to the alignment of any other ginglymus or hinge joint in the body, including particularly the elbow joint, ankle joint, and the interphalangeal joints of the hand and feet.

Note: This idea allows a clinician to determine with good accuracy whether a knee has normal alignment or not. Simply lie the patient supine, patella pointing upwards and with a string or tape stretched taut and centered at the upper end over the middle of the femoral head (it lies halfway between the anterosuperior spine of the pelvis and the pubic spine) and its middle over the middle of the patella, see if the lower end lies over the middle of the ankle. The amount by which the ankle lies medially (varus) or laterally (valgus) to it defines with much more than the clinically necessary accuracy the amount of malalignment of the knee, and thus how much correction it requires at osteotomy, should you contemplate one.

Question: If so, then what happens to a knee which does possess an element of valgus or varus at the time of skeletal maturity?

Since no further chondral growth occurs after skeletal maturity that deformity should persist throughout the remainder of adult life. And clinical experience reveals that it does and that at least some of these joints subsequently do get into trouble. The affected patients begin to experience pain, usually on the overloaded side of the joint, pain related primarily to mechanical use, worse on heavy than upon light demand, and relieved by mechanical rest. These symptoms, which often may not appear until after age fifty (and may begin with a very nocturnally as well as day time painful, degenerated meniscus), gradually associate with progressing radiographic changes consisting of narrowing of the cartilage space on the affected side of the knee, and the development of bony spurs at the margins of the articulations. Often some palpable evidence of crepitus or grating also develops as the affected joint moves, particularly when it carries a respectable load. Thus we have clinical confirmation that the departures from the normal alignment described above can lead to a kind of bearing failure which clinicians have termed degenerative arthritis or osteoarthritis. And we now have additional confirmation, consisting of the fact that when one does a high osteotomy of the tibia to correct the malalignment of the knee and in fact restores the normal alignment as defined and described above, such patients become almost uniformly happy with the symptomatic results thereof. Indeed they have proven so uniformly happy that one suspects the few failures may represent an incorrect preoperative diagnosis, leading to the performance of an operation which perhaps the patient really did not need.

Question: Then does a malalignment of the knee, for example a few degrees of varus, necessarily imply an unequal distribution of the loads of body weight and muscle forces across the two sides of the knee joint?

To this question, the negative answer, with explanation next.

2) ADAPTATIONAL MALALIGNMENT: While such a malalignment certainly can signify or associate with lateralization to one or the other side of the knee of a major fraction of the body weight transmitted across it, equally in some other patients who during growth have or acquire abnormal patterns of muscle contraction around the hip, the varus may simply represent a predictable and necessary adaptive phenomenon which acts during growth to maintain a normal distribution of such loads on the two sides of the knee. In order to understand how this can come about, progress from the static abnormal situation shown on the left of Figure 19.15;

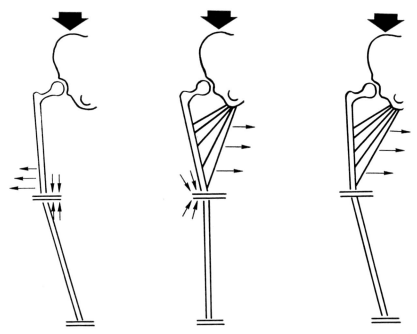

Figure 19.15. *Left:* Given excessive bowleg or *genu varum* (an anatomical alignment error) but *normal muscle activity patterns,* and the chondral growth planes on the medial side of this knee joint can overload in compression. During growth this will retard longitudinal growth on that side relative to the lateral to create a self-aggravating situation. In adult life it can cause a degenerative arthritis of the medial half of the knee requiring surgical interference.

Middle: Abnormal adductor contraction patterns can cause overload of the lateral side of a knee perfectly aligned in the statistical sense of anatomical "normal." If this happens in a growing child, the negative feedback mode response of chondral growth will lead to the development of compensatory varus as shown on the right.

Right: But in adult life after these adductors have become weak—or little used because one spends too many waking hours sitting down and writing legends for book figures—the varus can then become a *functional alignment error* which leads to medial joint compartment breakdown.

So we must distinguish between alignment errors in the anatomical or purely morphologic sense, and those in the purely functional sense. A given error can represent both, or only one of these, and either one at that.

now add to it an assumed overactivity of the adductor muscles, one which arises during each stance phase of gait. By overactivity we mean relative to all of the other muscle contractions that occur around a hip during gait, and relative to the normal pattern, meaning the normal ratio of the adductor/abductor: flexor/extensor contractions, and their synergy. In the situation of the overactive adductors then, clearly during the stance phase of gait these muscles apply a dynamic, adducting force on the knee which has two components. One, the vertical component, acts in line with the shaft of the femur and therefore does not tend to generate valgus or varus. The other component, a horizontal one directed medially, tends to pull the knee medially during each stance phase against the inertial mass of the hip joint above, and the friction of the weight-bearing foot on the floor below. In other words, the horizontal component generates a static bending arrangement torque or moments around the knee which adds a tensile load to the medial compartment and a compression load on the lateral compartment. When one adds these loads to the other and much larger uniaxial compression forces of body weight acting across the knee, the resulting situation becomes one of a larger total compression load on the lateral side of the knee than on the medial (not an actual tension force on the medial side). The middle diagram of this figure illustrates this situation. Given the chondral growth/force-response characteristics described previously, *and assuming these loads remain within the physiologic range of the growth/force-response curve,* the initial reaction of the growing chondral planes to this middle situation should follow the negative feedback mode, i.e., one should find slight *overgrowth of the lateral side relative to the medial side,* which would tend to make the knee grow into a little varus. In this situation, a now new and strictly cantilever arrangement torque, or accentuation of loads on the medial side at the expense of those on the lateral (which occurs when the malaligned knee carries body weight), then acts to neutralize the strictly dynamic, static arrangement and opposite sense lateralization. Accordingly one can easily conceive that in some such patients a certain amount of varus (or valgus) at the knee might reflect the perfectly normal function of a growing joint adapting its architecture to a statistically abnormal childhood pattern of muscle contraction in order to achieve, and then maintain, a desired situation: equal unit loading on both femoral and tibial condyles.

And in fact the author believes that at least some cases of symptomatic knee varus and valgus seen in adults in our clinic represent the consequences of exactly such situations (258). Then why do they hurt? Probably they get in trouble simply because with aging the patterns of muscle contractions tend to alter, the offending group such as the adductors tend to become weaker, and the varus (or valgus) which effectively equalized the loads (rather than the alignment) in the two compartments in young, growing, healthy, and muscularly vigorous individuals, now constitutes an overcorrected situation for older, weakened and much less active muscles. Under these circumstances the superimposed body mass then becomes the predominant factor, the medial side of their joint line space consistently becomes overloaded, and it then begins to break down.

As indicated above, comparable reasoning also can apply to the case of mild genu valgum, although seemingly less frequently.

Now if the adductor overactivity referred to above became large enough to load the lateral side of the growing knee into the descending limb of the growth response curve in Figure 14.02, i.e., into the pathological range of compression, medial growth would exceed lateral and a valgus deformity would ensue. And we see just that in spastic children with overactive adductors, a phenomenon which led to the workable diagnostic and therapeutic rationale of handling that problem presented in Volume I of this series, as well as in a series of articles in Clinical Orthopaedics written with A. Majestro, J. Conrad (51), R. Ruda and G. Hoover.

Remember: The same kind of dynamic imbalance can lead to two different types of chondral growth-based deformities, depending upon the magnitude of the imbalance. When the imbalance lies still within the physiologic range, a negative feedback response mode will follow: but when in the pathologic range a positive feedback response mode will ensue.

Clinicians have not thought much about such matters to date and accordingly we lack a large amount of relevant data, including experimental studies of normal and abnormal subjects, which would substantiate (or demolish) the above reasoning. The text presents it because the writer's clinical experience has left little doubt that such things do occur, and when people begin to look for them in children by systematic means, they will find them.*

V: BIOMECHANICS OF TENSION TRANSFER ATTACHMENTS TO BONE

Reflect a moment: no vertebrate could live a moment in a competitive environment, nor could the whole phylum have evolved successfully out of earth's ancient seas, had nature not found effective and efficient means to attach a variety of structures to hard skeletal tissues *so they could transfer tension loads to the skeletal members.* With every breath and spoken and written word, every gesture and physical act, every mouthful of food and child conceived and born, we demonstrate our totally unconscious yet absolutely reliable dependency upon these tension transfer mechanisms. Man has not yet succeeded in duplicating them or finding effective substitutes for use in the human body, and in truth only now do some of us conceive this as a nontrivial problem,

---

* Let me lean on this a bit harder: You clinicians may rest assured that the analytical processes and results described in this text work in clinical practice, and consistently so, for they have been tested 10 years in exactly that milieu in this institution and displayed those clinically necessary properties. Consequently do not be thrown off by any squeals (or grunts or brays or moos) that may assault you, claiming to find some theoretical or evidential flaw lurking in these principles of action. As a clinician, I am willing to leave all such noise to others because regardless of how one may reword the essence, it does work in the clinical action, and consistently so, and repeatedly so, and that is all our patients really care about when they accept our advice and ministrations.

find some challenge in it, and envision some merit in solving it.

So let us take a brief look at nature's solution with our biomechanical eyes and see what we find.

1) THE TENSION TRANSFER MECHANISM: While we cannot foresee accurately how our successors may ultimately succeed in attaching living tendon, ligament and/or fascia to inanimate bone replacements, or the converse problem of attaching inanimate replacements for the former to living bone,* we might again profit by examining and trying to understand the way in which nature seems to have solved this problem, for solve it she has. And if we wish to produce functional and durable inanimate replacements for such structures (which by that definition must prove acceptable to living skeletal tissues in the mechanical sense), it could well turn out that we must follow her ways, whether we like it at this point in time or not.

So in a biomechanical context let us examine certain structures called Sharpey's fibers first, and something I will name the tension transfer fanout second.

2) THE SHARPEY'S FIBER MECHANISM: The greater trochanter of the femur has attached to it a variety of tendons which transfer to it the tension loads generated by a powerful group of muscles, which include the gluteus minimus and medius, tensor fascia femoris, internal and external obturators and the pyriformis; also two relatively weak gemelli. At maximum effort in a human adult these muscles can exert a total contractile force exceeding 2000 lb. f., i.e., more than a ton.

Question: By what means does nature transfer this respectable load from tendon to bone?

As the drawing in Figure 19.16 shows, if one makes undecalcified, histologic sections of this region cut parallel to the orientation of the collagen fibers in the tendon, he will find

---

* The author suggests respectfully that we should take our cue from the salamander and concentrate on learning how to make the living system regenerate its own missing parts. This no longer seems an impossibly visionary challenge.

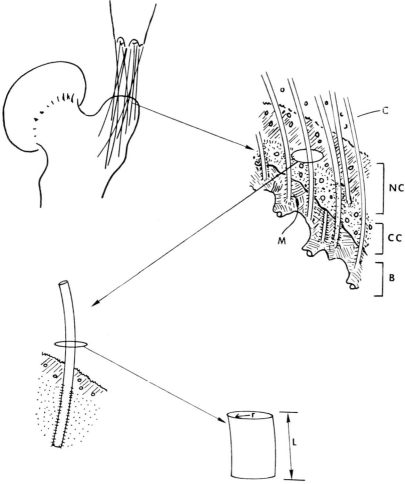

Figure 19.16. This drawing illustrates the Sharpey's fiber tension-transfer mechanism. See the text.

collagen bundles of these tendon fibers (c), continuing through the layer of unmineralized (nc) and mineralized (cc) cartilage (the latter designating the mechanical interface between bone and tendon), and right down into the underlying lamellar bone (B). As these fibers enter and come to lie in the mineralized cartilage and bone they become encrusted and embedded with mineral salts too (M), the same mineral found in all calcified skeletal tissues. And above the mineralized zones as well as within them, these collagen fibers also lie embedded in mucopolysaccharides which, as with man-made polymers, attach by some type of chemical bonding to each other, MPS to collagen. Now, within the mineralized bone these collagen fibers change their name to become "Sharpey's fibers" but that name change should not conceal the mechanically important fact that they remain the same continuous fibers as they enter the bone that they constituted in the tendon itself.

Thus we have a mechanical arrangement in which the total tension load on a given collagen fiber transfers partly to the mineralized cartilage (a thin layer) and mostly to the underlying bone (a thicker layer). This transfer occurs through its outer, cylindrical surface as a shearing load. Thus the mineral salts deposited thereon must respectably boost the shearing strength of the union between the two, over that which would exist without them, and this seems to analogize the particle reenforced materials described briefly in an earlier chapter in Part I of this book. We might compare this mechanical situation to a knitting needle embedded in jello. Without some mechanically interdigitating mechanism which locks them together in shear, it should prove quite easy to pull or pluck the needle out without disturbing the jello.

Observe that the deeper the penetration of a given collagen fiber into the bone, the greater the cylindrical surface it exposes to the embedding bone medium for transfer of that load, and so the smaller becomes the shearing load on any particular square micron of that surface, and so the greater the strength of the whole bonding mechanism. Since almost all Sharpey's fibers lie embedded in bone to depths and lengths many times the diameter of the individual fibers, each presents a large cylindrical surface area to the bone over which transfer of the uniaxial tension load they carry will occur. One can in fact formalize this arrangement with some simple equations. As the drawing illustrates at the lower right, let r signify the cross sectional radius of a typical Sharpey's fiber, and L its length embedded in mineralized bone. Then the surface (S) presented to the enveloping bone for bonding and transfer of the tension load on it must equal the area of the wall of a cylinder, or:

$$S = 2 \pi r L$$

Now earlier we described a stretch-hypertrophy law. You may have to ponder the matter a moment to realize that one of its necessary behavioral consequences implies that the time averaged load on any tendon determines the latter's cross section area, i.e., that a normal tendon's cross section area reflects in some direct and proportional way the loads it typically carries and transfers to its insertion. If true (and I have little doubt about that as a proposition for it also works in clinical and operating room situations, although nobody has yet done the experimental studies which could verify it) then another anatomical property of tendon insertions becomes biomechanically meaningful, one which relates to the collagen fiber's surface-to-volume ratio within the bone.

To illustrate, assume first an unreal case: we have a perfectly solid, nonfibrillar rod of tendon of one cm outside diameter which carries a time averaged unit load of one kg/mm² on its cross section. This equals a total time-averaged load on the tendon of one kg/mm² × (cross sectional area of a cylinder one cm in diameter expressed in mm²), or 1 × πr^2. And:

79 mm² × 1 kg/mm² = 79 kg total load on the tendon.

Assume furthermore that a length of approximately seventy-five microns (i.e., 0.075 mm) of this tendon lies embedded in the bone, so the total outer cylindrical surface it presents to the bone, to transfer to it as a shearing load this 79 kg, equals 2 π rL = 2 π 5 × .075 or 2.3 mm². This provides a unit loading in shear on that tendon's outer surface where it bonds to bone of 79/2.3 = 34 kg/mm². But since bone has an ultimate strength in shear of only 5 kg/mm², clearly such a bond could never hold—even below average muscle contractile forces could break it or pluck it right out of the bone more than six times over.

Accordingly nature did not do it that way. She broke the grossly solid tendon up into lets say one hundred thousand separate collagen bundles. These one hundred thousand bundles still have the same total cross section area, that is, 0.79 cm² or 79 mm², and they still carry the same total load, although each fiber now carries only 1/100,000 of it or .00079 kg = 790 milligrams force. But they now have an enormously increased total cylindrical bonding surface area in contact with the bone, one which has increased from the 2.3 mm² total in the spurious example above, to a figure some 3160 times larger: 7,300 mm². The unit shear loading on the surface of each fiber has now reduced to .09 kg/mm². Now let us take into account the fact that while the shear strength of solid bone may equal some 5 kg/mm², the shearing strength of the anchorage of Sharpey's fibers in bone probably equals only one fifth of that, or about one kg/mm². Then the bonding strength between bone and tendon fibers still exceeds by some ten times the strength needed to do the job. And given that under maximum, momentary effort the total load on a tendon probably exceeds its time-averaged value by some five times, and the bond still remains at least two times stronger than required, i.e., it has a safety factor of two (strictly an order of magnitude estimate because we lack good measurements of the total number of Sharpey's fibers for given tendons, and of their actual shearing strengths in bone).

Consequently, and conceding the uncertainties deriving from lack of accurate numerical measurements, the major concern about the strength of tendon-to-bone attachments clearly becomes, not whether the muscle will pluck its tendon's individual fibers out of the bone by the roots as it were, but whether the bone itself has enough strength to carry the total load transferred to it by the mechanically highly efficient Sharpey's fiber mechanism. And that brings us to the tension transfer fanout.

3) THE TENSION TRANSFER FANOUT: For some generations of man our anatomy texts have provided us with nice little red (or blue) circles delineating the attachment on the

greater trochanter of the gluteus medius tendon, or to their own respective bones, the flexor digitorum longus, or pectoralis major, or peroneous brevis, or tendoAchillis, or any other tendon. The medical student may gain the impression therefrom that these small regions of bone (usually a cm² or so in size for the hip abductors) accepts the entire load of that muscle's contractile force. But think a moment: that muscle can exert an effort in excess of 450 kg/f, an effort resisted only by the bone's total shearing strength on the cylindrical perimeter of that one cm² area which attaches it to the rest of the trochanter, as shown at the lower left of figure 19.17. The total load of 450 + kg/f must then transfer as a shearing load to (assuming a 1mm thick bony cortex) and area equal to the cylindrical area of that tendon attachment through the depth of the bone. Thus:

$$S = \pi \ DL; \text{ now convert to mm:}$$
$$S = 10 \times \pi \times 1 = 31.5 \text{mm}^2.$$

The unit shear stress then equals

$$450/35 = 12.9 \text{ kg/mm}^2$$

But at the most the shearing strength of that bone (given favorable orientation of its grain) equals only 5kg/mm², so only a forty per cent of maximal effort should pluck the bony anchorage right out of its bony surround, i.e., cause an avulsion fracture of that region of the trochanter.

Of course the problem here lies in that pretty red (or blue) circle—it does not accurately represent the manner in which this tendon attaches to the femur. As Figure 19.17 reveals and as any surgeon who exposes this (or any similar) region can readily affirm at a glance, the fibers of that tendon fan out over the entire trochanteric region, and even extend downwards onto the external fascia of the quadriceps muscle. This fanout distributes the muscle's whole load over a quite wide region of the upper fifth of the femur, and allows it to dissipate in a much larger volume of cortical bone than that small plug mentioned earlier. Of course, Sharpey's fibers provide the ultimate bony anchorage of the vast majority of that load.

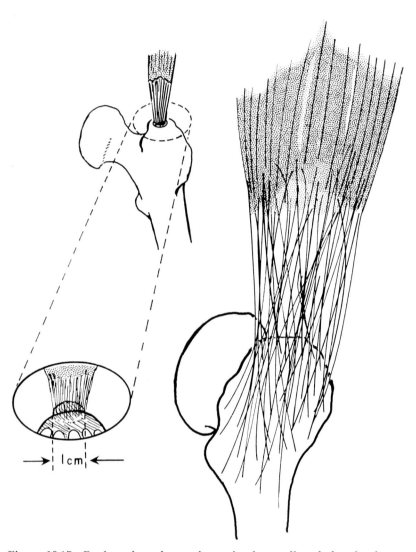

Figure 19.17. Real tendons do not insert in the small and sharply circumscribed regions of bone illustrated on the left. Rather a large fan-out of collagen fibers distributes the tension load widely over the bone and even over adjacent fascia, so that the Sharpey's fiber mechanism functions far below its safety limit. Neat, eh?

Note bene: The Sharpey's fiber biomechanics, and the tension transfer fanout, characterize all ligamentous, fascial and tendon attachments to bone. Sharpey's fibers also secure all fleshy muscle attachments to bone. Such attachments would include those of the quadriceps femoris, anterior tibial, interossei of the hand, coracobrachialis and erector spinae in the back. The greater the total tension loads transferred thereby, the greater the fanout. And we find simple but unequivocal proof of these matters in two circumstances: avulsions of tendon attachments from bones by active muscle contractile forces occur rarely; and avulsion fractures of the greater trochanter, on the rare occasions when they do occur, seldom displace upwards very much for the aforementioned fanout of collagen fibers bridges the fracture line, usually does not rupture because of its greater compliance, and so usually limits the upwards excursion of the trochanter.

Note too: The fanout obviously further multiplies the safety factor of the Sharpey's fiber mechanism by reducing, below the levels assumed above, the actual loads carried by the typical individual collagen fiber.

Growth and Post Surgical Adaptation: The Sharpey's fiber arrangement begins to appear in the fetus, and persists throughout growth largely because bone growth consists of increasing the external bone diameter, in the process of which collagen fibers of already attached soft tissue structures simply became engulfed by new osteoid, like an upward jutting tree stump by a rising tide, and then become mineralized and thereby locked in. One may suspect that the mineralization process does actually provide the shear-locking mechanism and strength which secures Sharpey's fibers in any bone.

As for the origin of the tension-transion transfer fanout, when a surgeon transfers a peroneus brevis tendon to the midfoot to reenforce weak ankle dorsiflexors, initially all of the contractile force of that muscle becomes applied to the quite small region of the foot where the surgeon drilled a hole to insert the tendon's end. But after the patient leaves the operating room and for the next year or so, the local fibrous tissue undergoes considerable rearrangement by biomechanically oriented cellular activities, so that by the end of that year *a new and naturally made tension transfer fanout has come into being.* Surgeons can see such new fanouts very clearly if they later have to move the tendon attachment again to improve the side-to-side balance of the foot. Probably this reflects some aspect of the stretch-hypertrophy law in action again.

In other words fibrous tissues still possess in adult life the inherent reponse characteristics needed to reestablish effective tension fanout mechanisms, and will do so consistently in response to the appropriate stimulus—which probably forms intermittent tension loading. This response characteristic reactivates to achieve its basic biomechanical purpose: to distribute a concentrated tension load over a large surface and volume of bony tissue.

QUESTIONS: CHAPTER 19

1) An expensive analysis of femoral stresses induced by a 70 kg load sitting directly on the femoral head fails to explain its architecture. Why?

2) a) Define the flexure-drift law. b) Name its most important limiting condition. c) What inactivates it?

3) Define the principle of flexural neutralization.

4) Lifting a weight with the hand requires only contraction of the muscles that flex the elbow: True?

5) A physician in your hearing claims that external rotation splints applied to the feet correct tibial rotation deformities by deforming the bone plastically in torque. Evaluate that idea.

6) A shoe salesman has convinced a mother that high top shoes will prove necessary to support her infant's feet, and that failure to use them will harm their development. a) Is this true? b) You tell her this and she clearly does not believe you (many humans have an oft repeated tendency to prefer to believe absolutely in the nonsensical rather than in the correct!). What should you do, as a physician now, not a biomechanician?

7) A nine month old youngster, brought to you for advice, has approximately 45° of internal tibial torsion, concealed from casual inspection when he stands by moderately severe pes planus which, as usually proves true, associates with considerable forefoot abduction.

   a) A lift of 1/8 inch on the lateral heel does exert an external rotational force on the leg during walking. Would it therefore correct the tibial rotational deformity?

   b) How might you correct the tibial rotation?

   c) What penalty or trade should you expect to have to make if you correct the tibial rotation by external devices?

   d) A Fillauer splint holding the feet turned out 60° past neutral typically leads to no visible correction in a four month old after four months treatment, but to better than one-third correction in an eighteen month old. Why?

8) A prestigious laboratory reports out living animal experiments involving implantation of small electrodes on the periosteal surface of a long bone. A direct current of several microamperes was passed through them for several weeks and in the region near the negative one some woven bone was deposited, while near the positive one some local resorption and tissue irritation developed. Evaluate such an experiment in the following respects:

   a) As a model of bioelectric control of bone architecture, attempting to explain osteoclastic and osteoblastic drifts.

   b) As a model for stimulating bone repair where it has previously proved incompetent due to a biological failure.

   c) As a model for stimulating bone repair previously incompetent due to a technical failure.

   d) As to the physical reasonableness of the experiment.

   e) What did the experiment teach us about the determinants of bone architecture and bone healing?

f) Assume this experiment was published ca 1970. Given the relevant material published up to that time, were the strategic defects of the experiment a necessary consequence of our collective ignorance, or (to be kind) due to an oversight in not taking into account available and pertinent information?

g) What comprised the basic strategic flaw in the experiment?

9) The accompanying Figure 19.18 illustrates on the right an internal rotation of the distal relative to the proximal end of the left femur. Assuming this deformity must develop by altered patterns of chondral modeling during growth, and that the bone architecture simply follows

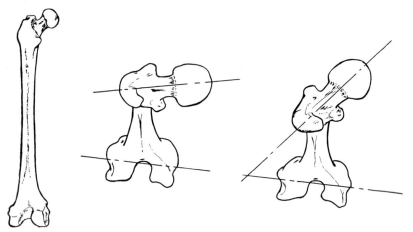

Figure 19.18. *Right:* An internal rotation deformity of the lower end of the femur relative to the upper (or if you prefer, an external one of the upper relative to the lower). The left normal views shown for orientation. See text.

In clinical practice we usually see such problems as results of overloading chondral growth planes into the region of the descending limb of the growth/force-response curve. While they might also occur as functional adaptations to muscle activity patterns lying still on the ascending limb, and so constituting negative feedback adaptations, none of us have thought much about it and so we do not have pertinent clinical facts to evaluate the idea. Perhaps some young reader of these words will obtain them for us all. (Reproduced by permission of editor and author. H. M. Frost, *Clin Orthop, 79:* 44, 1971.)

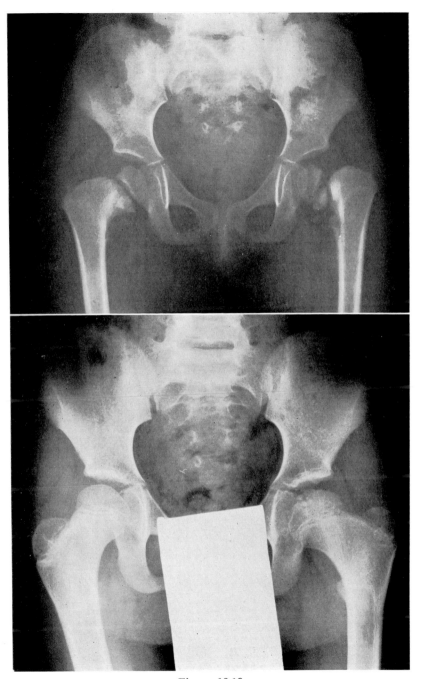

Figure 19.19

the chondral leader, conceive of some plausible causes of this deformity which do not involve any inherent abnormality in the responsiveness of the bone's tissues.

10) To the hips in the accompanying Figure 19.19, apply your previously acquired expertise to:
   a) Give the diagnosis.
   b) Postulate a reasonable biomechanical basis for the disease.
   c) Explain the obvious cure of it shown in the lower cut.

Chapter 20

Fatigue Failures in Biological Structural Materials

FATIGUE FAILURES OF biological structural materials* do occur, but before we discuss them let us establish certain points to put the subject in context.

First, such failures occur seldom (fewer than one per million structures per year of service life), a rarity emphasizing the exactness with which the design of our bodies has achieved dependable and durable musculoskeletal function. And while our clinical and scientific interests in these failures lie far out of proportion to their numerical frequency, they do not lie out of proportion to their ability to teach us useful things about normal human physiology.

Second, the spontaneous fractures and ruptures that we will describe usually favor selected regions within the body's anatomical structures. The rest of the body's structural regions rarely seem to suffer such problems, probably because mechanical load-carrying ability does not constitute one of their important functions. And while some systemic disturbances may play a causal role in fatigue failures of biological structures, some local factors must play causal roles too.

Third, distinguish between mechanical fatigue failures of intact structures or organs on the one hand (rare in the human body), and mechanical fatigue processes of structural materials on the other (all known structural materials, both living and inanimate, exhibit susceptibility to them).

---

* To repeat, these materials include lamellar bone, hyaline cartilage, and tendon, the latter serving as representative too of ligament and fascia.

I: BONE

Five recognizable kinds of structural (as opposed to material) fatigue failures occur in bone, speaking now from the clinical standpoint. These include (*i*) those that occur in the presence of expanding bone lesions, called pathological fractures; (*ii*) those that follow making a hole, notch or other stress riser in a bone (usually in the course of an operation) ; (*iii*) sudden complete spontaneous fractures with no externally obvious cause; (*iv*) a group of incomplete fractures known variously to clinicians as stress fractures, march fractures and fatigue fractures, which may or may not associate with some unrecognized underlying bone disturbance; (*v*) and pseudofractures, or Looser's zones of transformation, which occur in bone of abnormal quality and abnormal biologic competence,[118,282,255] and which we characterized briefly in Volume III.

In further detail then:

1) PATHOLOGICAL FRACTURES: In these fractures, an expanding lesion exists, usually inside the bone, often a metastatic malignancy in adults and a unicameral bone cyst in children[7]. When such a lesion expands faster than the normal strain-responsive adaptive mechanisms (the modeling process described earlier) can correct the bone weakening caused by the cortical thinning, a complete fracture following a trivial loading can ensue eventually. Presumably microscopic cracks arise in the affected region[95,98,226], and propagate through its substance faster than the local remodeling process can repair them. One or more of these cracks then probably progresses to the point where so little intact material remains that eventually a minor load, such as might occur while simply turning over in bed, completes the failure as a fracture (J. Dorgan, A. Haddad, J. W. O'Meara and J. Kelley once shared with your author at Worcester, Massachusetts, a certain puzzlement over the phenomenon in a scoliosis patient in whom a tibial cortical graft had led to a spontaneous fracture six weeks later while still bed ridden in a plaster cast). Often for some weeks before such a fracture the pa-

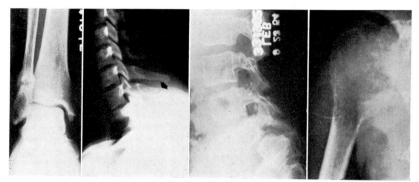

Figure 20.01. *Left:* A healing stress fracture of the distal fibula. No underlying injury. Patient of Dr. J. L. Fleming.

Second: A stress fracture of the spinous process of the seventh cervical vertebra, known as "clay shoveler's fracture." No direct injury.

Third: A spondylolisthesis of L5 on S1 vertebra, usually due to a stress fracture of the pars interarticularis acquired during early adolescence. Patient of Dr. C. L. Mitchell.

Right: A pathological fracture of the right humerus due to a very aggressive giant cell tumor of bone arising within the humeral head in a 17 year old girl.

tient may have minor, vaguely localized aching in the affected part of the body. See Figure 20.01.

2) FATIGUE FRACTURES CAUSED BY STRESS RISERS: We have long known that a notch made in a bone by a saw cut, drill or osteotome may in six to eight weeks lead to a spontaneous fracture, and C. O. Bechtol once published excellent studies of this process (28). This also follows drilling a small hole for a pin or for a bone screw, and not as much difference appears between small and large drill holes as intuition might lead one to expect. These fractures occur because the ends of the saw or osteotome cuts, or the drill holes themselves, form stress risers in which tiny cracks start and then propagate through the bone* until what remains fails suddenly and completely. Such fractures commonly exhibit the spiral form, less often the transverse (44). Possibly from the standpoint of the stresses involved, a stress riser in a bone may function somewhat as a line defect (i.e., dislocation) does in a metal. That is, it may prestress or strain the material at the bottom

of the crack or crevice so that external loads, by simply adding further stress, can more readily exceed the rupture strength of the material in the local area; and it allows the crack to propagate in step-by-step fashion so that a very low level of mechanical power insertion (in the form of cyclic mechanical working) can, if given enough time, cause failure of even massive structural members.

One can minimize the chance of such a fracture developing after taking a rectangular or triangular graft from a long bone, by drilling large diameter holes (3/16 inches or 1/4 inches) at the angles and cutting radially into them, as shown in Figure 20.02. The large hole, having a large radius of curvature, concentrates the stress less at its surface than a small hole or a sharp notch cut by a saw.

Stress fractures can also follow the use of dull drills, probably because the bone around the drill hole becomes cooked by the heat generated by the drilling. Cooked bone cracks easily and until local but slowly developing biologic processes have removed it and replaced it with living (and mechanically competent) bone, it has no living mechanism within it to detect and correct such defects (57).

One can often (but not always) prevent this kind of structural fatigue failure by enforcing eight to ten weeks of mechanical immobilization and deloading of the part after making the defect. Bechtol showed in dogs (and clinical experience confirms in man) that such a time period usually suffices for the repair process to correct the stress riser. Only if some impairment of the repair mechanisms exists does it take longer to correct such a defect. Examples of actual such impairments can occur in bone previously dosed heavily with x-rays, in some cases of late lues, and in some patients with diabetes mellitus.

3) SPONTANEOUS FRACTURES: These form a group of sudden, complete structural failures in which no universally recognized underlying condition has received recognition (74,

---

* The essential feature in this situation: the microcracks propagate faster than the biological system can detect and repair them.

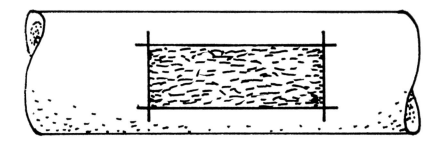

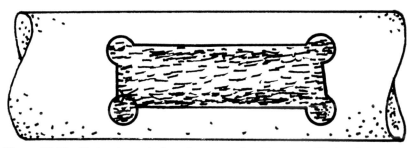

Figure 20.02. *Top:* A cortical graft removed with an oscillating bone saw in which corner cuts extend beyond the graft donor site. The corners of these cuts serve as stress risers, and within 8 weeks can lead about one time in four (i.e., with probability = 0.25) to a fatigue fracture, even if the limb was casted and totally protected from weight bearing from the day of the operation.

    Below: Drill holes at the corner help this situation (probability of fatigue fracture now: p = .05) by stress-relieving the corners with notches of much greater radius, even though intuition tells one this should make the problem worse, not better. Fickle girl, that intuition . . . (Reprinted by permission of author and publisher, ref. no. 94.)

76) . As an example, a man may suddenly fall in the middle of a normal step because his hip fractures. Or a vertebra may suddenly crumble, or a patella break in half, following some quite ordinary act. A predisposing factor may sometimes consist of some degree of skeletal osteoporosis, a condition in which less than a normal amount of bone exists so that unit stress levels within the remaining bone tend to have higher than normal values (247,249) (see Volume III) .

    Evidence accumulates suggesting that these spontaneous fractures in reality comprise fatigue failures, which arise because the biological mechanism that normally detects the microdamage that probably leads to them, has become somewhat deaf. Volumes III and IV take this matter up in some detail. Interestingly, while the biological system may become deaf to the microdamage that precedes the fracture, it usually reacts quite normally to the macrodamage constituting the completed fracture. Exceptions to this occur in several kinds of osteomalacia, in which both micro- and macrorepair processes demonstrate marked impairment.

In skeletal regions which contain much or primarily cortical bone, one factor predisposing to such fractures probably forms the presence of regions of a special type of dead bone called micropetrosis (84). Lacking living cells, this micropetrotic bone also should lack the biological ears which can detect microdamage and lead to its repair before it reaches a dangerous level. Another and peculiarly dynamic factor, found especially in some kinds of osteoporosis and osteomalacia, consists of a decrease in the speed at which the remodeling BMU can repair a microdamage process (i.e., it represents a prolonged sigma value; see Volume III) to such an extent that the microdamage progresses through the bone faster than the pursuing repair process. Thus it enlarges steadily, and presumably could continue, until a complete failure occurs. The macro or gross healing process usually proceeds normally after such a complete failure (which usually is a crumbling or vertical squashing of the bone). However, when radiation damage exists in the tissue (159), or if it has become osteomalacic, the gross repair response can become as defective as the microrepair mechanism. Other conditions in which we see an impaired ability of cells to detect and/or correct microdamage include Cushing's syndrome especially of the exogenous kind; severe hepatic cirrhosis; tertiary lues; radiation necrosis (43,49), osteomalacia (175), osteogenesis imperfecta (46) (brittle bones); osteopetrosis (177), and fragilitas osseum (a newly recognized children's disease entity mentioned in Volume III and reported by B. Braiker and D. Lucas at the Bone Symposium, Henry Ford Hospital, June 1972).

4) STRESS FRACTURES: In these affections a normal person develops gradual pain and dysfunction, plus local swelling and warmth, arising in some bone. For one to four weeks, x-rays usually show nothing. Then a tiny, usually transverse crack appears, accompanied by a periosteal cuff of callus, followed in two to four months by good clinical healing, disappearance of all symptoms and signs,* and resumption of normal function. These constitute fatigue failures which seldom progress to gross displacement and/or angulation. They commonly follow a period of unaccustomed strenuous activity, such as long marches by recent draftees, or an orgy of golf played by normally city-bound older women. They occur in children as well as adults (and in the former initially may cause one to suspect an underlying malignancy). These facts and the numerical rarity of such fractures suggest that perhaps the microdamage repair process in these people remains normal in kind but reponds too slowly to cope with the new mechanical situation the patient finds himself in (see Figure 20.01).

The lack of angulation and displacement in this group arises partly from the fact that because of pain early in the development of the lesion they favor and protect the part in the mechanical sense. But why this group hurts so much during the early stages of the underlying processes, while the group of spontaneous, complete, sudden fractures above hurt so little, lacks any proven explanation.

5) PSEUDOFRACTURES: Probably these phenomena, described in Volume III, arise initially as stress fractures but they do so in diseased bone in which both the microdamage detection and the macrorepair mechanisms have become impaired by the disease. The disease usually forms an osteomalacia, or occasionally Paget's disease of bone. Since the macrorepair mechanism has also become defective, pseudo-

---

* In medicine, a symptom represents a subjective phenomenon, something the patient reports to the physician, pain forming an example. A sign signifies something objective and observed independently by the physician, such as local redness or swelling.

fractures may persist unhealed for years, and cause pain and impaired function until one corrects the underlying biochemical disease.

6) ASEPTIC NECROSIS: HISTORY: This term arose in the early part of this century to signify death of the femoral head by infarction following an intracapsular hip fracture in which nonunion of the fracture occurred, and in the process sufficient motion at the fracture line persisted as to prevent complete reinvasion of the marrow space of the infarcted head by granulation tissue arising from the living tissues in the fracture surface of the distal fragment. The treatment of these fractures in the 1920's had not evolved to a satisfactory state, so that most of them went on to nonunion. Upon removal at the time of surgical reconstruction a year or more postfracture, histologic examination of such ununited femoral heads often revealed a biological desert, consisting of dead bone trabeculae and empty, avascular intertrabecular marrow spaces. Often a region of partial reinvasion by living tissue would appear here and there, and it would gradually replace the infarcted bone and bone marrow, a process dubbed creeping substitution by Dr. D. Phemister of Chicago.

The term aseptic necrosis coined to identify this situation rapidly became generalized by orthopaedists to other, seemingly analogous situations such as osteochondritis dissecans, Osgood-Schlatter's disease (in fact and in most instances not an aseptic necrosis at all but a type of "tendonitis" of the infrapatellar tendon insertion, analogous to so-called "tennis elbow" or "lateral epicondylitis"), Legg-Calve-Perthe's disease, Kohler's disease, Kienboch's disease and others.

In the mid-thirties, Smith-Petersen developed his technique of closed reduction and internal fixation of these hip fractures with a triflanged intramedullary hip nail, and by *ca* 1950 numerous orthopaedists had added sufficiently to that basic technique to raise the rate of union of these fractures above eighty per cent. For that and other reasons, orthopaedists then had the opportunity to follow large numbers of united transcervical hip fractures for long periods of subsequent time. And in that process another entity appeared with increasing frequency and gained recognition as such. It went about like this (Figure 20.03 shows an example) :

The fracture united soundly—usually within about five months—and the patient resumed walking.

Typically within the next one to four years some of the patients then experienced recurrence of pain in the affected

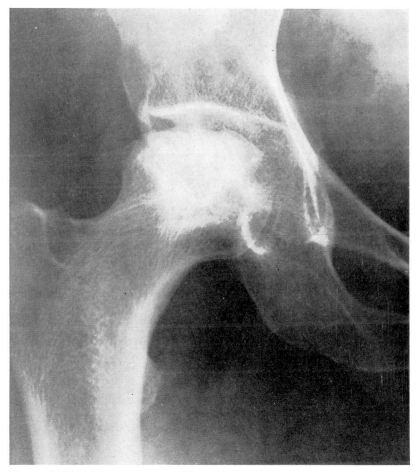

Figure 20.03. An example of idiopathic aseptic necrosis of the femoral head in a young man with no history of injury, corticosteroid treatment, alcoholism or allied conditions. Note the conically separated denser mass of bone at the dome of the head, the flattening of the dome arising because it has "settled," the preserved articular cartilage space and the normal appearance of the adjacent bony parts.

hip, with accompanying clinical signs of irritability of the joint (meaning pain at the extremes of motion and upon rapid motion even without any load across the joint). This happened to some twenty per cent of those with fractures through the femoral neck (transcervical fractures), thirty to thirty-five per cent of those with fractures at the juncion of neck and head (subcapital fractures), and five per cent to ten per cent of those with impacted fractures.

X-ray changes in the hip accompanied the symptoms and signs, and consisted of an initial separation of the subchondral bone from the underlying trabecular support and/or the appearance of radiolucent and radiodense regions within the head. These changes—if untreated—would gradually progress until a large, conical portion of the head separated from the remainder. This portion always lay beneath the articular region of greatest load transfer across the joint. With continued function the head would then begin to crumble and collapse (and then resorb) before the hammer of the acetabulum to the point that in some patients the entire head eventually disappeared. Throughout these developments the cartilage space of the hip joint remained fairly well preserved, a phenomenon that distinguishes this condition from other arthropathies in which articular cartilage breakdown and/or wear represented the initial and causative event in a degenerative joint disease.

This entity also became dubbed aseptic necrosis of the femoral head, and it was assumed *ca* 1950 that it accurately implied a dead head, due to its infarction at the time of fracture, and that it differed in no material way from the situations Phemister had studied and described a generation earlier. In passing, an exactly similar thing happens to about thirty per cent of adults who sustain a traumatic dislocation of a hip joint.

Furthermore, about the same time orthopaedists began to see an exactly similar syndrome on clinical and x-ray grounds, but arising in seemingly perfectly healthy patients without any history of trauma, mostly in men in their 40's, and you will find an example in Figure 20.03 (This entity now goes under the name of idiopathic aseptic necrosis) (138) . And then they noted the same syndrome to occur in association with treatment by adrenal corticosteroid hormones, and finally in alcoholics. Everybody simply assumed that these new entities also represented infarction of the head by some means and so tagged them with the same name, and began (and still do) to look for the cause of the assumed embolic process that led to it.

The writer's own concepts of this disease faithfully copied the above dogma until 1958. At that time a femoral head, resected at femoral head replacement arthroplasty for an idiopathic aseptic necrosis, was studied in the HFHOR laboratory, and to our quite considerable surprise it proved very much alive, not dead. The original trabeculae, original meaning those present before the process began, remained alive and populated with healthy looking osteocytes, proving no previous infarction had occurred. In addition very active reconstruction of the trabecular mass was in process with greatly increased bone resorption and formation. The only dead region in that head constituted the conical portion referred to above, lying in the dome of the head and obviously dead because its mechanical motion in that bed had disrupted its blood supply. But before dying it too had undergone considerable and quite active reconstruction,* indicating that its death formed the end result of earlier processes, not the cause of the later ones.

Here, we can shorten the remainder of the story and summarize our findings in thirty-one cases of aseptic necrosis of the femoral head in which we obtained the involved head at resection arthroplasty. Table 20.01 lists the relevant data which, by way of verbal summary, add up to this (91) :

At the time of the onset of the clinical syndrome of aseptic necrosis, all of these heads had living marrow tissues, regard-

---

* We need not describe here the histopathologic features which allow one to make with such laconic assurance what might otherwise seem overly cavalier statements. Given the proper methods of examination, an up-to-date knowledge of bone physiology and pathology, and one can determine such things beyond any reasonable doubt (167) .

TABLE 20.01

DATA ON ASEPTIC NECROSIS OF FEMORAL HEAD

Type of Aseptic Necrosis	Number of Cases	Original massive infarct occurred	Original trabeculae alive	Marrow tissue alive	Bone resorption increased	Bone formation increased	Dead conical portion	Hot fluorine scan
Postfracture	11	+ (11)	0 (11)	+ (11)	+ (11)	+ (11)	+ (8) 0 (3)	+ (5)
Post dislocation	1	+ (1)	0 (1)	+ (1)	+ (1)	+ (1)	+ (1)	—
Idiopathic	9	0 (9)	+ (9)	+ (9)	+ (9)	+ (9)	+ (6) 0 (3)	+ (4)
Poststeroid Rx	6	0 (6)	+ (5) 0 (1)	+ (6)	+ (6)	+ (6)	+ (5) 0 (1)	+ (2)
Radiation necrosis	1	0 (1)	+ (1)	+ (1)	0 (1)	0 (1)	+ (1)	—
Sickle cell anemia	1	0 (1)	+ (1)	+ (1)	+ (1)	+ (1)	+ (1)	—
Alcoholism	2	+ (1)	0 (1) + (1)	+ (1) 0 (1)	+ (1) 0 (1)	+ (1) 0 (1)	+ (2)	—

A summary of the histological findings in 31 femoral heads removed at surgery because of aseptic necrosis. All were examined in the HFHOR Laboratory by the author between 1958–1972, inclusive, and by Dr. P. Sarnsethsiri in 1972. The clinical type (as recognized conventionally in 1972) appears in the left column. The parentheses opposite the plus or minus signs in the remaining columns list how many of the cases in that row displayed the feature named in the heading at the top.

Note: Histological and radiobiological examinations by various people indicates that, given adequate reduction and fixation of the fracture, the dead soft tissues between the infarcted trabeculae in the post fracture and dislocation cases become essentially fully replaced by new, living tissue, *and this occurs within three months of reduction.* The new tissue arises at the distal extent of the infarct from the healthy distal fragment held in contact with the proximal one, and invades the neck and head in the cephalad direction. Thus by the time any clinical and x-ray evidence of the onset of the clinical syndrome of aseptic necrosis may develop, the marrow spaces of the head have regained their viable state and have remained in it for many months.

Code: +means the phenomenon existed, 0 that it did not.

less of the type of aseptic necrosis. And of them all, only the post fracture and post dislocation cases showed clear evidence that massive infarction of the trabecular bone (and so presumably of the marrow tissues too) had occurred at some much earlier time. In all of them very active reconstruction of bone was in progress in the head except for the conical portion if loose and mechanically detached from its bed (the usual situation), and the postradiation case and one alcoholic case.

Yet in terms of their clinical and x-ray signs, and their progression over time, *these all formed a common behavioral entity.* Clearly the common denominator in this syndrome cannot constitute massive infarction, whether by trauma or embolism, even though in a selected few of them it seems equally clear that an original massive infarct did form a precipitating cause.

How to reconcile these seemingly conflicting facts?* The following hypothesis, first formulated in 1964, now appears substantially correct, and has found some support from observers such as W. Zinn of Switzerland and Wm. Massie of Lexington. Thus:

Fact: in human adults trabecular turnover within the femoral head proceeds much more slowly than in the supraacetabular trabeculae or in the femoral condyles, vertebrae, ribs and so on. Do not know why (that is a good subject for study) but the fact is clear, based upon histological studies of over one hundred such heads in the HFHORL.

Fact: microdamage normally occurs in the capital trabeculae (86,91). Hypothesis: the bone remodeling mechanism usually repairs it, and the sentinel which detects a need for it and semaphores that need to the competent cell populations in the marrow spaces forms the osteocyte.

---

* We need not take the time here to list the numerous publications over the past decade which reflect unquestioning acceptance of the old dogma that these heads crumble because they are dead at the time of crumbling. That simply affirms what we already know: it proves much harder to remove an old mistake from our literature than to inject a new one into it.

Hypothesis: Then removing those osteocytes by killing them as must follow any massive infarction (hip fracture or dislocation), or making them deaf to the microdamage as corticosteroids seemingly can do, or making the marrow tissues blind to the semaphore (mechanism unknown to this author), would allow microdamage to propagate faster than its repair, and to the point that it becomes gross or macro. And at that point the normal macrorepair process starts up, and tries to repair the damage.

Fact: The active reconstruction found almost uniformly in these heads reflects a macrorepair activity—as do the uniformly hot radioactive fluorine scans done by Dr. L. Z. Shifrin on a series of such cases at Ford Hospital, and hot strontium scans obtained in such cases by other investigators at other centers. In fact these scans prove uniformly hot, even when done on such early cases that diagnostic radiographic changes have not yet arisen at the time of initial scan.

Hypothesis: But that repair activity always lags behind the damage production *as long as the patient continues to bear weight,* so the head can completely crumble.

Discussion

One might suspect that if any truth lay in the above statements, then simply by deloading the hip long enough the repair might catch up and the future prospects of the hip materially improve. And exactly that does occur, as I have found in my own practice, and Dr. Wm. Zimn of Switzerland has observed in his own and in that of some of his colleagues. If one deloads such a hip (by making the patient use crutches and totally remove his weight from the affected hip) for six to twelve months, something changes within it, for he can then resume weight bearing without developing further crumbling or collapse. The remaining problem we face in such a patient constitutes a mechanical arthropathy due to the altered contour of the subchondral bone of the head, and possibly to irregularly distributed subchondral mechanical compliance of the bone supporting the articular cartilage. But one has gained in this process, because if this secondary arthropathy should require subsequent surgery, enough head remains that an arthroplasty of any kind, or osteotomy or hip fusion, will heal and turn out as well as if the aseptic necrosis never had existed.

Let us summarize the above as verbal equations, thus:

ASEPTIC NECROSIS

Failure to repair microdamage ———→
accumulation of that damage

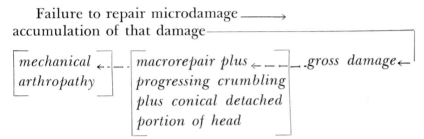

and as to the causes of the failure to respond to microdamage:

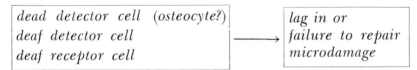

Finally, one might suspect that if the above held true then in some instances this process, i.e., an initial imbalance between microdamage production and its repair such that the latter "leads", might arrest itself before enough damage develops in the subarticular support to cause any serious future problems with joint function. In fact we do occasionally see such cases in the clinic based upon radiographic changes observed incidentally within the head.

This interesting entity then illustrates several clinically useful points. First, it exemplifies how a gradual change in the character of our clinical experience may conceal from us the emergence of a new pathophysiological entity. Here we mistakenly assumed that the truly and massively dead—and aseptic—heads of prehip nailing times also constituted the living but crumbling heads of posthip nailing times. Second, it illustrates how intimately mechanical and biological factors entwine in our bodies and how unrealistic it proves to try to explain such penomena solely upon mechanical, or upon biological, grounds. Third, it demonstrates how easily one may make an honest error of interpretation, and how much more difficult it can prove to correct it later. Fourth, the curious predeliction of this entity for femoral and humeral heads, and on occasion the condyles of the femur, implies that some underlying local factors must exist which predispose them to this development. The fairly impressive reduction in histologically detectable evidence of trabecular bone remodeling in these regions in normal adult people lends some solid support to that idea and it begs study and explanation.

II: FIBROUS TISSUES

As for tendons first, clinically, two major groups of spontaneous tendon ruptures arise: (a) one which occurs in seemingly healthy and normal adults, usually men; (b) another that occurs in the presence of some local abnormality.

1) SPONTANEOUS TENDON RUPTURES: With no warning at all and in an apparently healthy person, a tendon may rupture under a perfectly normal load. This variety usually affects men between the ages of thirty to fifty years, and shows a predilection for the tendoAchilles, the suprapatellar, the supraspinatus, the long head of the biceps brachii and the extensor pollicis longus tendons, and the chordae tendonae of the heart values. At operation to repair such a rupture we usually find gross evidence that the tendon had undergone deterioration for at least several months previously and the findings of microscopic examination of the tissue usually confirms this. Occasionally such failures will occur where tendons turn corners in special tunnels. The major tension and compression stresses and strains arising in such situations appeared described earlier in Part I.

Again in such situations that evidence strongly suggests (to this author at least) that a microdamage sensing mechanism has become impaired. As held true for spontaneous and stress fractures of bone, once the tendon rupture becomes complete, the gross or macrohealing mechanism usually then reacts normally.

To detect microdamage, a biological structural material must be alive and this holds as true for tendon as it does for bone. Perhaps for this reason attempts to make new ligaments out of free tendon or fascial grafts (i.e., grafts completely detached from their blood supply) often do not succeed. If subjected to normal loading immediately after completion of the primary healing process (some six weeks time), such grafts tend to stretch out progressively and so to fail within a few months of the operation.

2) PATHOLOGICAL TENDON RUPTURES: These occur in regions where some recognizable underlying disease exists. It may consist of rheumatoid arthritis in which the disease process simultaneously weakens the tendon and impairs its microdamage repair faculty, or it may arise from a fracture-related roughening of some bone surface over which the tendon must move, or numerous other but individually less common conditions. At operation, such tendons usually show extensive local abnormalities which clearly required weeks or months to appear, and so predated the moment of final, complete rupture. Significantly however, the gross healing process usually behaves normally after one repairs them (if such repair remains anatomically possible).

3) FASCIA: About the only examples of fascial fatigue failures I know of include (a) those of the iliotibial tract, which functions in part as a tendon (the tensor fascia femoris and gluteus maximus muscles exert pull on it), and (b) a local relaxation of that fascia that envelops certain muscles, allowing them to bulge locally when the muscle contracts. Accordingly we name them muscle hernias. Both of these conditions arise uncommonly as true fatigue failures, and occur more often as acute injuries with adequate and immediate causes.

4) LIGAMENTS: Fatigue failures of ligaments rarely occur, with one special exception. This consists of the annuli and posterior longitudinal ligaments of the intervertebral discs of the cervical and lumbar spine (203–206), where failures can

allow protrusion of the intervertebral disc material, commonly called disc herniations or, by the laity, slipped discs (106,129, 130). The total vertical load on a human midlumbar disc when recumbent runs around twenty-five kg; it rises to some 100 kg when one stands up, and to 215 kg when lifting a modest weight (25 + kg), according to studies by Prof. A. A. Nachemson (205,206). Also, the menisci of the knee often demonstrate considerable fatigue-like damage in older patients, even when they have no history of injury, or signs or symptoms of mechanical joint disease.

In rheumatoid arthritis and less commonly in some other kinds of arthritis one may find abnormal joint laxity caused by a slow elongation of the joint's ligaments. Such laxity can also develop when the bony support to the articular cartilage collapses (due to injury or disease) or wears down, regardless of the reason.

III: HYALINE CARTILAGE

Unfortunately, we know little about mechanical fatigue of cartilage, which means it should form a fruitful subject to study. Very likely, much of the vertical chondral fibrillation seen in early degenerative joint disease (i.e., chondromalacia) represents a kind of chondral fatigue damage, as could the occasional separation of fragments of joint cartilage from the underlying subchondral bone which form a kind of abortive osteochondritis dissecans, and a very troublesome one to diagnose because the x-rays of such a joint look quite normal (the cartilage remains radiotransparent). But we remain unsure of this, and these (and other) changes in joint cartilage may represent the consequences of phenomena we have not yet recognized and which do not fit into our present conception of mechanical fatigue failures.

IV: MUSCLE

A muscle may rupture through its belly spontaneously, and with no premonitory warning, in an apparently healthy person. However, this fatigue failure arises more in the fascia that surrounds and invests the muscle and its numerous individual cells (i.e., perimysium) than in the muscle fibers themselves. These ruptures often develop only part way through the muscle, rather than completely, giving rise to the so-called charley-horse (a term whose etymology must be fascinating) and, in the calf, to the usual case of so-called plantaris tendon rupture, in actuality a partial rupture of the gastrocnemius or soleus muscle bellies. The muscles most often affected include the biceps brachii, the soleus, gastrocnemius (where as just noted the condition is usually misdiagnosed as a plantaris tendon rupture) and the hamstrings.

Curiously, voluntary muscle seems nearly immune to the structural weakening effects of those local processes which can impair bone and tendon strength, because muscle rupture occur less commonly than bone and tendon ones.

QUESTIONS: CHAPTER 20

1) a) What makes a bone as an organ virtually immune to fatigue when as a material bone lacks that property? And a joint? And a tendon attachment? And a ligament? And a muscle? And an artery?

2) What must the self-repair faculty have to operate efficiently?

3) Using your general knowledge of medicine, evaluate the proposition that embolism by intravascular fat globules causes those forms of aseptic necrosis of the femoral head not associated with fracture, dislocation or irradiation.

Chapter 21

Biomechanics of Fractures and Bone Healing

I: CLASSIFICATION OF TRAUMATIC FRACTURES

FROM THE CLINICAL standpoint, we recognize the following types of fractures: (1) greenstick fractures; (2) undisplaced fractures; (3) displaced fractures; (4) pathological fractures; (5) spontaneous (i.e., fatigue) fractures; (6) fatigue fractures. Types (1) through (3) come in a limited number of patterns, which we will present separately in a biomechanical classification. The different ways in which bones break derive from (a) certain differences in their physical properties in children and adults, adult bones becoming more brittle and thinner of cortical wall; (b) their essentially brittle nature regardless of age-related differences and (c) their longitudinal grain.

1) GREENSTICK FRACTURES: (See Figure 21.01 left). These occur in three patterns: The infraction or torus signifies a slight crumbling of a metaphyseal region without rupture of the periosteum. It usually represents a buckling failure in longitudinal compression. The tension greenstick fracture follows excessive bending, a tension rupture occurring on the tension side and a permanent set arising in the compression side. This forms the commonest kind of greenstick fracture.

In general, greenstick fractures occur in children and reflect the fact that children's bones have significantly less brittleness and more compliance than adult bones.

2) UNDISPLACED FRACTURES: These represent situations in which enough energy or work was absorbed in making the fracture to effectively dissipate practically all of the injuring impulse. Thus the surrounding soft tissues sustain little dam-

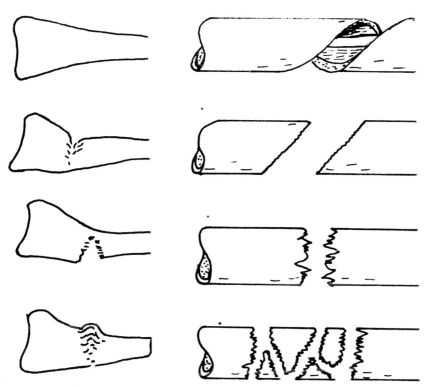

Figure 21.01. Diagrammatic classification of acute fractures.

Left: The greenstick types, top representing normal, next down, the so-called torus (a cortical failure in compression); next down, the greenstick in which a permanent set has developed in the intact upper cortex, and bottom, the infraction, the commoner type of buckling in compression.

Right: Top: the spiral fracture, nearly always due to overload in torque with failure along the line perpendicular to the tension resultant. Second down: the oblique, usually due to combined uniaxial compression plus flexure. Third down: the transverse, usually due to pure flexural overload. Bottom: comminuted, and usually due to considerable direct violence which causes shearing and flexural loading.

age and the bone fragments tend to remain in place with normal positional relationships.

3) In Displaced Fractures: The above does not hold true, and the excess of the injuring impulse dissipates in displacing the fragments at the expense of tearing and otherwise

damaging (sometimes badly) the enveloping soft tissues after the fracture occurs.*

Pathological fatigue and spontaneous fractures: We discussed these already (previous chapter), and understand that no fracture arises truly spontaneously.

4) MECHANISMS OF FRACTURES: A bone breaks fairly (but not wholly) consistently in response to a given kind of loading, so one can usually deduce the mechanism of injury from the x-ray appearance of the fracture. The fracturing force may act indirectly on the bone, or directly on it (i.e., by impact). Fractures usually occur primarily as failures in tension, with the exceptions noted previously. In unusual circumstances, failures in compression or in shear can happen (See Figure 21.01).

(*a*) *Torque*: Twists cause spiral fractures, in which the fracture line usually takes one complete turn around the circumference of the bone and lies at 45° to its longitudinal axis and/or grain.

(*b*) *Static Bending*: This causes a transverse, angulated but often undisplaced fracture.

(*c*) *Cantilever Bending*: This usually causes an oblique fracture, the plane of the obliquity bearing a predictable relationship to the direction or eccentricity of the injuring force.

(*d*) *Avulsion Fracture*: A tendon or ligament may pull its bony attachment completely off from the main part of the bone causing a fracture whose surface plane lies essentially perpendicular to the tension load which caused it.

(*e*) *Uncomminuted Fracture*: This signifies that a single fracture line exists, and thus only two fragments. The injuring force dissipated nearly completely in making that one fracture.

---

* We also call fractures simple or closed if the skin remains intact, and compound or open if the skin has broken so the fracture communicates with the outside world. This classification is not important biomechanically.

(f) *Comminuted Fractures*: This signifies two or more fracture lines, and so three or more fragments. Commonly more violence (i.e., energy) and brittleness associate with this kind of fracture than with the uncomminuted ones.

5) ENERGY ABSORPTION IN FRACTURE SURFACES: In order to fracture a bone in tension or compression, it must accept a load which then induces strain within it, and when the strain reaches some maximum permissible limit which induces stress to the breaking point (approximately 12,000 psi in tension) the bone substance then tears apart. Clearly one square cm of such fracture surface would on the average require a particular amount of work put into it to make it break, so that equally clearly the more square cm of fracture surface appear in a particular injury, the greater energy dissipation the fracture surface represents. Thus, comminuted fractures which present a large total area of fracture surface, represent structural failures occasioned by the absorption of much more energy than a single transverse fracture.

In the absence of direct studies of the phenomenon, one must assume that in compact bone and trabecular bone of similar unit materials' properties the energy absorbed in producing one square centimeter of fractured bone surface remains equal. However, children's bones probably dissipate a greater amount of energy per square centimeter of fracture surface than older bones.

II: BIOMECHANICAL ASPECTS OF FRACTURE HEALING

We previously mentioned the fracture healing process which, to briefly review it, involves the steps of mesenchymal cell stimulus and proliferation, production of new osteoblasts and bone, and replacement. The physiology and problems of fracture healing also relate closely to those involved in bone grafting too, so this makes the problem doubly interesting and relevant. A verbal equation—diagram will clarify the essential relationships of the fracture healing process as follows, using numbers in parentheses so we can identify particular links in this chain of cellularly driven events later in the texual discussion:

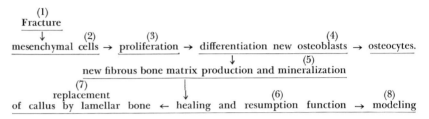

We need not discuss all of the biological and allied problems that can arise in this process, so after some general observations about them we will proceed to consider the biomechanical ones.

Technical and biological failures of bone healing: Record then that prior to *ca* 1940, by far the most nonunions of fractures seen in this country arose from mechanical failures or errors in treatment which caused malfunctions in the chain of events at the #6 "healing" stage in the above expression. Accordingly we will call them technical failures (not at all implying any necessary negligence or wrong doing on the part of the doctor, please note). But since 1940 an impressive improvement in fracture treatment expertise has eliminated most of these nonunions, leaving as a proportionally much larger remainder what formerly proved a trivial fraction of failures of the healing process. This fraction arises in the first four steps in the above relation and henceforth we will term them biological failures. And since the whole process forms a kind of biological chain, *a break at any link can and will abort the whole process.* Volumes II and III of this series discussed these biological failures and we will say little about them here other than that they present peculiarly biological problems, little studied or discussed in the orthopaedic literature to date, which focus upon cellular proliferative and differentiative phenomena and the matter of intercellular communication (115, 120,127,266,272). Our legitimate concern in the remainder of this section will form the technical failures which we did not discuss in any depth in earlier volumes. Let us begin by looking at fracture healing with respect to reduction, and also with respect to motion.

1) REDUCTION: In general, the more perfectly reduced (i.e., set) a fracture, the more reliably it will heal, or the greater the probability that it will heal; and the less perfectly reduced, the less reliably (or probably) it will heal. Obviously there exists some degree of perfection of reduction beyond which further improvements can only trivially improve the healing reliability; equally a degree of imperfection exists such that making reductions worse cannot further impair already hopelessly poor healing. Then the middle ground, the region where things change most quickly, will concern us here. And we can categorize its problems quickly and concisely, understanding that what follows represents approximations based upon a great deal of clinical experience, but not accurate measurements determined under controlled laboratory conditions. From the standpoint of their effects upon union we need consider only these aspects of reduction: distraction, displacement and alignment.

(a) *Distraction*: When fracture fragments lie in direct contact with each other the maximum probability of union exists (i.e., $P > .98$). As they distract, this probability decreases, becoming $P \approx 0.5$ when the gap separating the two ends equals about half the diameter of the bone at that region, and becoming $p < .05$ when this gap exceeds the bone diameter as shown in Figure 21.02. This long known effect of distraction does not even today have an obvious explanation, but on clinical, radiographic and histologic evidence it clearly represents some block somewhere between stages or links #2-4. Accompanying this decline in probability of union, an increase in the average time for union to occur appears.

(b) *Displacement*: When the two fragments lie in direct opposition and in perfect register the maximum probability of union exists ($P > .98$), and as one then begins to displace them laterally upon each other, still maintaining direct contact, this probability remains unchanged until only around twenty per cent contact remains, when it begins to fall, lying below P

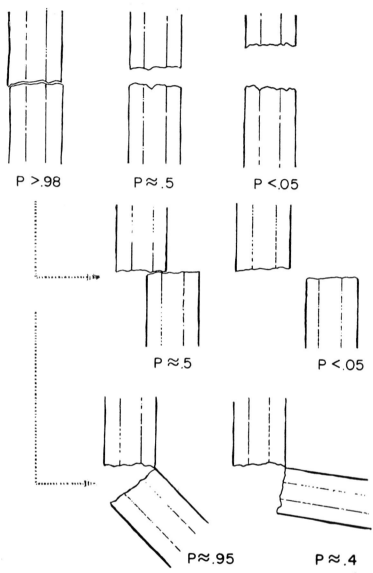

P >.98   P ≈.5   P <.05

P ≈.5   P <.05

P≈.95   P ≈.4

Figure 21.02. The top row diagrams effects of distraction upon fracture union, the p values indicating the probability of union occurring successfully in each situation. The second row diagrams the effect of displacement, and the third of angulation.

The drawings do not illustrate overriding of the fragments; when good side-to-side contact persists this may not prove very deleterious, although it certainly can cause objectionable shortening of the affected bone. In the femur of young children, we usually want some overriding however, to compensate for the longitudinal overgrowth that usually develops in the next 1.5 years as a result of the "regional acceleratory phenomenon."

$= < .05$ when the displacement has exceeded total displacement by approximately twenty per cent, as the second row in Figure 21.02 illustrates. As displacement approaches and exceeds $\approx 80\%$, a prolongation in union time also makes itself apparent.

(c) *Angulation*: Even a considerable amount of angulation (i.e., angular malalignment) of the fragments will not of itself materially alter the probability of successful union, although in the presence of more than $45°$ of angulation some delay in union may occur, a delay however based more upon biomechanical factors than upon biological ones.

2) MOTION: Just as positional factors can affect the probability of fracture healing (or of one not healing), so can further factors which relate to motion of the fragments relative to each other.* And as one might suspect, the harmful effects of one class of factors can augment those of the other in its affect on the probability of healing and, probably, upon its rate. The motion effects include shear, flexural and pistoning.

(a) *Shearing motion*: This probably forms the most commonly deleterious factor acting on fracture healing, for when the two fracture surfaces move upon each other in shear often enough that motion prevents a continuous mass of callus from consolidating around, embedding and uniting the two ends. Thus sufficient shearing motion can nullify the healing efforts of the best biological healing response possible. That shearing may exist as ordinary translation of one fragment on another, (signifying side-to-side motions), or the shearing motion of the cortices of two fragments free to rotate around an internal, longitudinal intramedullary nail or rod.

As to the amount of shear which impairs union, this depends upon how closely the two fragments lie in contact. The closer they lie, the less shearing motion needed to break up union; the greater their separation, the more shear the process can tolerate (although that distraction in and of itself can impair union, as noted above).

---

* We will ignore medical and purely physiological concerns, but not because they lack importance (93,186,208,233).

(*b*) *Flexure*: Angulatory or bending strains per se at the fracture line have little harmful effect upon the healing process until they exceed 20–30° in range, and even then the effect consists more of a retardation in speed of union due to some effect at step #6, than any great increase in the probability that it will fail due to effects in stages before step #6. In fact in some fractures and patients a certain amount of intermittent flexure of the healing fracture seems to evoke more abundant callus that one would otherwise expect to see.

(*c*) *Pistoning*: This signifies intermittently distracting the fracture fragments and then allowing them to come into contact again, and doing this several times a week. This probably impedes healing even more than shear but forms a lesser problem because one cannot ordinarily do this to a conscious patient with a recent fracture. Note however that pistoning does impair the healing process (by some effect exerted on the first four stages of healing that acts to prevent osteoblasts from appearing in the fracture region), especially when it exceeds thirty per cent of the diameter of the fragments.

Let us now say a few words about some biomechanical aspects of the strength of the healing process.

3) BIOMECHANICS OF FRACTURE HEALING: Rather arbitrarily, we generally divide a fracture callus into three different zones, even though the callus really evolves as a confluent mass. Thus, and as Figure 21.03 shows, we identify the periosteal callus, the medullary callus and the intercortical callus. A number of mechanical and physical factors affect fracture healing, given that we define healing here as *that degree of union which allows normal function to resume*. These factors include the following:

(*a*) *Flexural Strength of Callus Zones*: As noted in other parts of this book, the rectangular moment of inertia I_o, and thus the flexural strength of any cylindrical beam, varies as the fourth power of its diameter, so that simply by doubling its cross sectional diameter such a beam will increase sixteen times in its flexural strength and rigidity (!). Consequently, given the choice of taking only the periosteal or only the medullary callus, one should choose the former as mechanically far su-

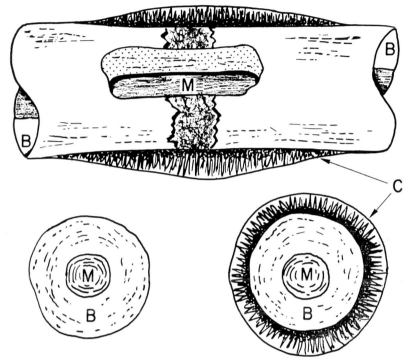

Figure 21.03. We arbitrarily classify the fracture callus into *periosteal, intercortical* and *intramedullary* portions as shown here. Note, below that the total flexural as well as total shear and compression strengths of the periosteal callus must greatly exceed those of the medullary callus on purely biomechanical grounds.

Volume III described a *regional acceleratory phenomenon.* It constitutes a considerable acceleration of all normal turnover processes in the macro region of a major tissue injury or other irritative phenomenon. It affects fibrous tissues and cartilage as well as bone, and it always lasts longer than the time taken for the healing process to complete, or for the irritative phenomenon to subside. It involves the macro region (thus, the whole leg in the presence of a tibial fracture, the whole calvarium with a skull fracture) on a scale and distribution suggesting that the blood vessels and/or sympathetic nerves provide the responsible mediating factor. In an affected region, bone and cartilage modeling phenomena, as well as growth phenomena, usually speed up.

perior to the latter. The figure illustrates this situation, and makes it clear that the above paragraph actually understated considerably the mechanical superiority of periosteal over medullary callus as far as supplying flexural strength goes.

The drawing makes it clear too that intramedullary nailing, which greatly impairs or aborts the production of medullary callus, nevertheless does not really impair the overall fracture healing process *in terms of the clinical soundness of the union achieved,* nor in terms of the time it takes to develop.

(*b*) *Compression and Shear Strength*: Under uniaxial compression loading the rectangular moment of inertia no longer applies, and we deal instead with the total cross section area of the callus. But even on that restricted ground of argument, if one had to choose between a layer of medullary callus or one of periosteal callus, each 0.25 inch thick, one would again choose the former, for as the above drawing illustrates it would provide a minimum of four times more total amount of callus than the latter. And because the shear and compression strength of the fracture callus depend directly upon its total cross section area, the contribution of periosteal union to the healing process would provide a minimum of four times more strength in shear and compression than that of the medullary cavity. For that additional reason we find that internally fixing fractures with intramedullary nails usually permits earlier resumption of function than doing so with bone plates applied to bone's exterior surfaces (but see below).

(*c*) *Bone Surface-to-Volume Ratio Effects*: We can describe two of these. As for the first, use ordinary airplane glue to affix both a one square inch piece of wood to a floor, and a two square inch piece. After equal drying times, now try to pull each of them off. Clearly it should require two times more pull to free the larger piece. While the quality and inherent holding power of the glue in the one equals that in the other, the larger piece with two times more total area has twice the total tensile, shear and compression strength. In this simple physical phenomenon lies a partial explanation for the observed faster healing of metaphyseal fractures compared to diaphyseal ones. Having significantly larger diameters than the midshaft, and since cross section areas increase as the square of such diameters, the metaphyses expose commensurately increased total amounts of surface to a basically constant unit quality fracture healing callus or glue.

As for the second S/V ratio effect, the mesenchymal cells that give rise to bone healing activity lie adjacent to all bone surfaces, and probably in approximately equal numbers on each square millimeter of those surfaces. The total amount of such surface in a fracture through metaphyseal spongy bone exceeds by two to over twenty times that in an equal area of a fracture surface through the midshaft of a bone. Hence another reason for better healing of metaphyseal fractures: a more abundant cellular response arises in them. While the quality of each mm³ of callus at a given time seems identical at these two regions, much more of it in the metaphyseal fracture permits earlier resumption of use.

(*d*) *Torque*: By recalling our brief analysis of torque in a shaft in Part I of this book, it should become clear that here too, periosteal callus provides much greater strength, and sooner so, than can the medullary callus, and too that metaphyseal fractures with larger cross sectional diameters should gain strength in torque faster than diaphyseal fractures.

III: REPLACEMENT AND MODELING OF THE FRACTURE

1) REPLACEMENT OF THE CALLUS AND REMODELING: Once the fracture has healed and function has begun, two further things happen to it before nature has finished with the healing business. The first consists of a gradual replacement of the fibrous bone and cartilaginous tissue within (and comprising) the fracture callus by lamellar bone. This lamellar bone arises by the BMU-based remodeling process described in Volume III, the mechanical grain of the lamellar bone deposited thereby parallels the major compression and tension load resultants on the part, and in a bit by bit or packet fashion the entire fracture callus eventually becomes replaced with it, over a period of about one to five years. Dr. Dieter Wilde of Hannover, West Germany has shown the writer some beautiful preparations of compression plating studies in which the replacement process appeared clearly laid out by means of tetracycline labeling, serial sampling and good experimental design. This newly generated lamellar bone has all of the properties of ordinary lamellar bone arriving by

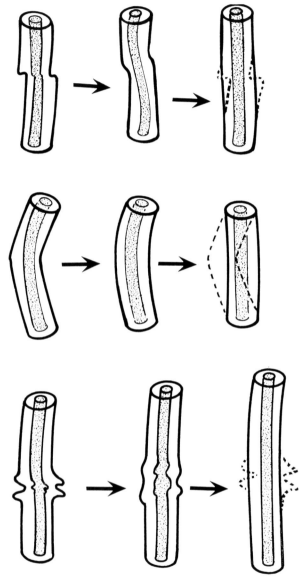

Figure 21.04. These diagrams illustrate the contoural *modeling* that occurs over the one to five years after primary fracture healing, for the cases of malposition top, malalignment middle, and marked contoural irregularities bottom. Exactly the same flexural strains and kinds of drifts that establish normal bone contours during growth cause and control these changes, and their presence even in adults proves that even after skeletal maturity some modeling potential remains, and can reactivate if stimulated appropriately.

any other histogenetic route, and that includes those properties which make it competent in the mechanical and physiological respects. Of some interest, a delay in deposition of lamellar bone during the process, one not accompanied by a comparable delay in removing the preexisting callus, can produce a transitory structural weakness of a freshly healed fracture which will allow it to fail again following trivial injury, or to deform slowly and plastically so that a gradual deformity develops over a period of something like two to three months. While this does not occur very often (and as a result orthopaedists generally have not yet become aware of this as an entity) the author has seen nine examples of it so far, most of which had created situations where the referring physician suspected he lay in legal jeopardy. Given good reductions, all that most of these fractures need to complete healing satisfactorily constituted immobilization in a plaster cast for about three times longer than one would ordinarily immobilize a regular fracture of that particular part of that bone.

2) MODELING: The second thing that happens to the fracture callus constitutes what these texts have named modeling. That means *reshaping the external architecture or contours of the fractured bone.* The drawings in Figure 21.04, and x-rays in Figure 21.05, illustrate the manner in which this occurs. It almost certainly occurs because when function resumes, local flexural loads arise which activate the flexure-drift law to cause osteoblastic drifts to fill up the contoural hollows, and osteoclastic drifts to shave down the sharp exposed contoural edges. This modeling process requires something under a year to complete in a one or two year old infant, and longer than the life span of normal man in a person aged twenty years or more. In other words, the speed with which this modeling progresses declines drastically as we age, and it does not present as a mechanism one can depend upon to produce autocorrection of fracture malunions in children older than about eight to ten years of age.

IV: SOME BIOMECHANICAL ASPECTS OF REFRACTURES

As the drawings in Figure 21.06 show (courtesy of Dr. R.

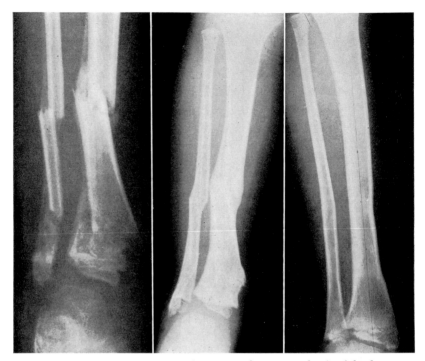

Figure 21.05. *Left:* You see an AP x-ray of a young boy's right leg some two months after a serious injury. Note the multiple deformities.

Middle: Four to five months later.

Right: AP x-ray of both legs, same child, some four years later. Observe how well the bony architectural deformities have modelled out, a process based upon the bone modeling laws described earlier. Now look at the ankle on both original and final films. See it? The boy had a diastasis of the mortise, which allowed the talus to move laterally (or translate as the geometer would say). When he began walking again his ankle loads became concentrated upon a small, lateral surface area, and overloaded into the growth retarding limb of the chondral growth/force-response characteristic curve, the chondral growth occurring in the lateral half of the tibial epiphyseal plate and articular cartilage. Since growth medially was not compromised, this led to progressive ankle valgus, the particular problem for which he was referred to Dr. J. Hohl of this department.

Varadachari of this department), when a fracture heals with a certain amount of offset, as shown in the left drawing, and function then resumes, then stress concentrations under flexural loads tend to develop at the perpendicular sharp angles. Surgeons typically evaluate the clinical degree of healing of a

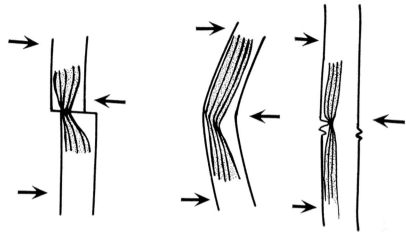

Figure 21.06. When a fracture heals imperfectly reduced, localized stress concentrations arise at abrupt contoural changes just as they might in machine parts. Given the right kind of accidental load (i.e., injuring force), these can lead to refractures of recently healed bones even though the injuring force has a low magnitude and would not cause damage to a perfectly normal bone. But even in adults, and probably potentiated by the acceleratory effect of the regional acceleratory phenomenon, such contoural changes correct by bone modeling activity, which stress-relieves them by increasing their radii of curvature.

fracture, first by the apparent x-ray density of the fracture callus itself, second by the absence of local tenderness over the fracture callus, which implies good healing, and third by the absence of detectable motion or springyness when one manipulates the bones in order to try to evoke either a shearing motion of the fragments or any detectable flexure at the fracture level. The situation such as shown in the left drawing can demonstrate satisfactory healing by all three of those criteria, yet not possess the strength of the normal bone before the injury. Following removal of the cast and resumption of function, if such a patient should slip and fall this otherwise inconsequential load on a humerus or tibia (or whatever) can lead to refracture. We treat the refracture in the same way as the original one, and we have good reason to expect equally reliable healing because the healing of the original fracture demonstrated normal biological competence of the regional tissues.

In the middle drawing, we see a fracture that healed with some angulation. This introduces an artificial cantilever flexural arrangement within the bone, and as a result normal function exposes it to abnormal flexural loads in the manner indicated by the three arrows. Because of the slightly sharp convex left border, some concentration of tension stress occurs at that point, as well as of compression stress at the kink on the concave side. As a consequence, again an injury ordinarily of trivial nature can lead to a refracture.

The drawing on the right indicates that even when the overall alignment of the two major fragments remains anatomic, if sufficient irregularity of surface contour of the fracture exists, the notches can serve as stress risers that can lead to a refracture upon an otherwise inconsequential injury.

Both the first and the third situations ordinarily correct quite well even in adults through the modeling process already described. The middle situation corrects partially in adults by gradual buttressing on the concave side of the deformity by deposition of additional periosteal new bone.

As a consequence of the above, in fracture situations such as these, most orthopaedists advise patients with recently healed fractures to avoid strenuous physical activities for some months afterwards. This of course depends to some extent too upon the patient's occupation, and upon the manner in which he customarily spends his free time. As a biomechanician one worries much less about one of these situations in a musical philosopher than he does in an avid gymnast or a skier.

V: SOME BIOMECHANICAL ASPECTS OF JOINT ARTHRODESIS:

Biomechanical as well as biological principles have a lot to do with how regularly a surgeon succeeds in fusing or arthrodesing a given joint, meaning making the two bones become one solid and mechanically strong structure. And many, many clinicians of wide experience know and understand these matters adequately but our text books—and some of our teachers—do not communicate them effectively to residents. So we will take a look at this problem next, using the following described circumstances as our entry to it.

Fact: Relatively few triple arthrodeses of the foot fail, while a much higher percentage of ankle arthrodeses do, even though each was done with equal technical care.

Question: Why?

The answer illustrates a practical application of some aspects of the biomechanics of fracture healing which we just outlined. Note that biologically speaking, when we do an arthrodesis of any joint we simply try to fool nature into believing that the joint has in fact become a fracture, a situation which she knows demands correction by achieving or reestablishing a solid bony continuity. Let us consider the ankle fusion first.

1) ANKLE ARTHRODESIS: At the conclusion of this operative procedure one has bare bone on the tibial side lying in intimate contact with bare bone on the talar side of the joint, both damaged, both cleared of all articular cartilage but both still viable. We need not here go into the various modifications of technique by means of which one can achieve this situation. One then applies a long leg cast to immobilze the part and waits for some four to six months for bony union to develop, which it usually does. Then the cast comes off and the patient begins to walk. Recall however that histologically speaking, complete healing of this arthrodesis probably will not exist before one year.

As Figure 21.07 illustrates, for the patient to bear weight on the forefoot of the arthrodesed side, the flexural moment created by the load of his body weight (here 150 lb × 6.5 inches) tends to rotate his ankle in that sense which allows the heel to touch the floor, here clockwise. The pull of the Tendo-Achilles opposes that torque but at a mechanical disadvantage. Thus we have:

$$+150 \times 6.5 - \text{T.A.} \times 2.2 = 0$$

Then the TendoAchilles pull must equal 434 lbs f and the total force on the ankle joint equals the sum or 584 lb f. And if the patient very accurately balances the torque arising from body weight with exactly gauged contractions of the muscles pulling on the TendoAchilles, no unbalanced torque arises on

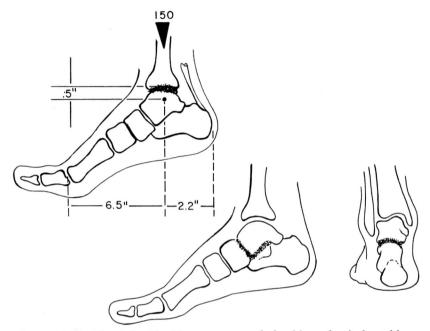

Figure 21.07. The left side diagrams some of the biomechanical problems faced in trying to arthrodese a joint exposed during the recovery phase to large shearing loads, and so exposed because of mechanical factors inherent in the anatomy and function of the part. Here we see an ankle arthrodesis. Measurements from the author's leg! See the text.

On the right, the subtalar portion of a triple arthrodesis. See the text.

the original ankle joint and his ankle fusion holds up just fine.

But, if any imbalance arises from errors in that muscle-force gauging process, then an ankle torque does arise. Let us assume that such an error does develop, consisting of 100 lb f of body weight momentarily not balanced out by Achilles tendon pull. This force then tries to rotate the ankle, *which applies a shearing load in the plane of the arthodesis.* How large might that load be (call it X) ? We can find out by again taking the moments, noting that the plane of the arthrodesed ankle joint lies only 0.5 inches above the axis of rotation of the ankle. Thus:

$$+100 \times 6.5 - (X)\ 0.5 = 0$$
$$X = \frac{650;\quad X = 1300\ \text{lb f.}}{0.5}$$

Now 1300 lb constitutes a large shearing load. Question: In terms of cross section area, how much bone actually carries it? Since the ankle joint has approximate dimensions of 1.75 $\times$ 1.75 inches AP and side-to-side, this equals about 2.7 in^2. But of that only at best fifty per cent constitutes bone, the remainder comprising the vascular spaces between the trabeculae of the healing callus. Thus some 1.35 in^2 carry this 1300 lb load. Since normal lamellar bone has a shear strength of some 8,000 psi across the grain, and solid and completely mature fracture callus probably about 4,000 psi, this should provide a factor of safety of greater than three. That probably explains why most ankle fusions take.

But: any imperfections in the physical fit of the two surfaces which produce gaps between them (inperfections which in fact usually exist), and any small motions during the healing process that delay maturation of the callus (which in fact also usually exist), and any failure to use most of the available 2.7 in^2 of total, gross contact area (which usually happens too), can leave the bony union sufficiently weak at five months post-op that this shearing load of 1300 lb f (which could easily exceed 3000 lb by a single slight misstep on the part of the patient) can break up what union already exists and lead to a pseudoarthrosis. And note: a *single* such misstep can break up the union already there, and perfectly normal function thereafter can cause it to persist in the face of nature's efforts to correct it.

2) Triple Arthrodesis: Here a quite different situation exists, one very much kinder to the patient and his surgeon. The right side of the figure illustrates the joint regions we fuse in this procedure. In the lateral view note first that because the ankle joint remains mobile it becomes practically impossible to develop any great anteroposterior shearing force in the plane of the fusion; motion in the ankle joint simply occurs to stress-relieve or absorb any such load. And if none occurs that can only mean that all the torques acting on it accurately balance out and sum up to zero. Then weight bearing on this situation simply forces the two bones together, a desireable and helpful situation.

In the rear view at the middle, the talus sits on the heel in such a way that only trivial torques in the plane of the paper can arise (the shearing forces they would cause would represent the total superimposed load multiplied by the sine of the angle of the tilt, and sines of angles less than $10°$ (anything greater remains exceedingly unlikely here) equals less than eighteen per cent of the total superimposed load. Note however that in the ankle this same shearing force could easily exceed twice the superimposed load. In the subtalar joint the much larger loads of body weight and muscle pull crossing it simultaneously, act to force its apposing sides together in compression, locking it against shear much as the irregular contours of the calcified cartilage layer lock the articular cartilage to the underlying bone.

Finally, the total surface area of the arthrodesed subtalar joint exceeds that of an ankle fusion by a factor of about two, and it has much better mechanical advantages in resisting the torques acting on it than did the ankle. In fact one can show that in a triple arthrodesis the unit shearing loads acting across the fused subtalar joint rarely would exceed 50 psi, less than $1/20$ that in an ankle fusion.

Thus on biomechanical grounds triple arthrodeses should prove kind to surgeons, for even if sloppily done they should rarely fail to take. But ankle fusions do not so favor us, and demand technically high quality surgery to obtain the maximum percentage of primary takes. Table 21.01 categorizes some of the joints most often arthrodesed, in such terms.

Some simple combination or all of the following factors can serve to increase the probability of a successful fusion across any joint (another biomechanically "tough" joint conquer in this regard: the hip) :

a) Use the maximum surface area of the bone available to you to fuse across the joint. Several different techniques exist for doing this in each major joint, and standard texts describe most of them.

b) Use internal fixation to eliminate shearing micromotions in the plane of the fused joint surfaces during the healing phase. This proves useful because a cast does not—and

TABLE 21.01
JOINT ARTHRODESIS

Joint	Biomechanically favorable situation	Biomechanically unfavorable situation
Subtalar joint	+	0
Ankle joint	0	+
Knee joint	0	+
Hip joint	0	+
Sacroiliac joint	+	0
Spine	0	+
Shoulder joint	0	+
Elbow joint	0	+
Wrist joint	0	+
Metacarpophalangeal joints	0	+
Interphalangeal joints	0	+
Acromioclavicular and sternoclavicular joints	0	+

indeed cannot—completely immobilize any joint in any active person.* Here too, a variety of specific means can serve, including Charnley compression, Steinman pins, Staple fixation and/or screws, various nails and so on.

c) Protect the fusion long enough after the operation to ensure that good quality bone in the mechanical sense has deposited and bridges the original joint. This usually means five to six months in an efficient cast.

QUESTIONS: CHAPTER 21

1) A prestigious group reports upon a complex study of the effect of mechanical compression upon fracture healing. They made a linear cut in a living rat's skull, compressed one end together by means of a silastic rubber band anchored around two metallic inserts implanted on either side of the fracture, some four weeks later gave inorganic and organic radioactive tracers, and then sacrificed the animal.

By comparing incorporations of the two tracers into different regions of the fracture callus, with those in the uncut

---

* A soft, compliant padding of skin, subcutaneous fat and muscle separates the bones from the cast, and as a consequence the bones move around within their rubbery soft tissue environment in spite of the presence of a cast rigidly encasing that environment's perimeter. For such reasons casts provide relatively inefficient fixation of bones and joints. But lest you prepare to sell all your stock in the companies that make it, keep in mind that what fixation they do provide usually suffices quite well.

calvarium on either side, they find increased tracer uptake in the regions of maximum compression and conclude that this force aids fracture healing.

Using what you learned in Volumes II-IV as well as herein, evaluate the following:

a) The choice of model system to study
b) The choice of technique to study this system
c) Their choice of control against which to measure the fracture
d) Their conclusions

2) Refer to the scoliosis x-rays at the end of Chapter 1. Note that in approximately ninety per cent of adolescent girls with idiopathic scoliosis the concavity of the thoracic curve lies to the left; note the further intriguing fact that ninety per cent of these girls are right handed. And, finally, in left-handed scoliotic patients the concavity of the thoracic curve lies to the right in over fifty per cent.

Can you explain this, given the assumption that the underlying pathology represents a softening of the vertebral epiphyseal plates such that they loss much of their rigidity in shear?

Chapter 22

Implants

Most of our implant armamentarium evolved by trial and error, rather than through foresighted planning. And it has had varied sources both geographically and temporally. A man would come up with a basically good idea which lacked something in its concretion. So another man thousands of miles away and years later would modify it, and then another and so on until a reasonably efficient implant came into being. This process of trial and error and natural selection of the fittest resembles rather strikingly the evolutionary processes that led to development of our musculoskeletal systems, and of our minds too.

Doctors S. Romer (223) and S. Jarcho (140) might find this parallel to their interests somewhat amusing. Be that as it may, we will now have a few words to say about the implants we use, and privately applaud some times and cuss at others. Most of these are made out of only two alloy systems: 3-16 stainless steel with added molybdenum, and so nicknamed "SMO"; chrome-cobalt-tungsten alloy (the tungsten greatly decreases the brittleness of the alloy material). In addition to these, other materials find occasional or experimental use and they include titanium, tantalum and zirconium.

Table 22.01 lists some of the materials properties of these systems.

I: INTERNAL FIXATION

Internal fixation signifies attaching two or more pieces of bone together by some man-made device or implant, usually made of a metal or an alloy. Table 22.02 lists some general types of implants in current use, and not confined to those which orthopaedists deal with. Several varieties of each named type exist so we have a large number available and

Orthopaedic Biomechanics

TABLE 22.01

MECHANICAL PROPERTIES OF IMPLANT ALLOYS

Material	0.2% offset stress p.s.i.	Endurance, 10⁷ cycles in air p.s.i.	% elonga-tion at fracture (tension)	E p.s.i. × 10⁶	Ultimate tensile strength p.s.i.
316 stainless steel (annealed)	31,000	50,000	40±	26	74,000
316 stainless steel (cold worked)	100,000	60,000	15±	3.1	125,000
Titanium	65,000	45,000	15±	17	81,000
Chrome-cobalt	65,000	45,000	8±	30	95,000
Chrome-cobalt-tungsten	45,000–190,000	38,000	25±	28	150,000–250,000
Bone (wet, fresh)	10,000–11,000	70,000	3±	2.5	12,000

A listing of some of the mechanical properties of the metals and alloy systems in use for the manufacture of orthopaedic implants. All seem equally acceptable biologically speaking; their relative assets and debits differ in only relatively small ways and complement rather than duplicate themselves.

TABLE 22.02

IMPLANTS

Bone plates	Cardiac pacemakers
Intramedullary nails	Arterial grafts
Screws	Plastic mesh
Pins	Wire mesh
Bone endoprostheses	Monitoring devices
Total joint replacements	Electrical power sources
Wire	Transducers
Sutures	Cardiac valve replacements
Nails	Fluid shunt tubes and valves
Staples	Tissue padding

more come along each year. In the future we may expect that radically different materials will serve to construct such devices.* As to orthopaedic usage, currently we use implants in

---

* They will probably be composite, and involve radically new production techniques. Also an entire science of joining things together has arisen which we orthopaedic surgeons have not yet tapped fully. So far, the materials that the body will tolerate biologically and chemically have not had optimum physical properties. For example, when we wish to join two different structures and to transfer loads across their plane of union, they should have the same Young's modulus and dynamic compliance. If they possess dissimilar properties in these respects, the plane of union becomes stressed too highly and a fatigue failure may develop there. Wet bone has much more compliance than the metals used in our devices currently, and this represents an undesirable feature, one also unavoidable now because we do not yet have better materials.

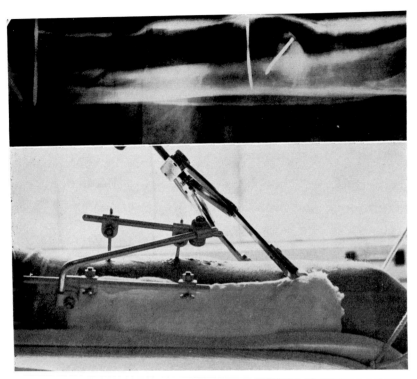

Figure 22.01. Two systems of "crossed pin" fixation of complex fractures. *Above:* Two pins oriented at approximately right angles, lie in each tibial fragment seen here in lateral x-ray view and solidly encased in plaster. Thus mechanical forces transfer from plaster to pins to bone, and if one chooses pin diameters properly to obtain adequate total rigidity of fixation the method works well. The pins come out after bone healing has occurred (94). Dr. Joseph Godfrey of Buffalo introduced the author to this highly useful—and simple—technique.

Below: An exactly similar principle, using specially made parts. This forms the Roger-Anderson apparatus which secures a really smashed tibia in this man's leg, which lies suspended in a Thomas splint. A traction bow (for his accompanying femoral fracture) lies towards the right. As with all other systems, both fixation systems illustrated here have inherent mechanical strength limitations and if the surgeon's demands on them exceed them, the systems will malfunction in a variety of ways. Such problems derive not from the systems but from our failure to learn how to use them properly. Thus the lower system acquired an unjustified bad reputation *ca* World War II time because some surgeons actually made patients walk early on limbs internally fixed thereby, expecting both bone and metal to "take it." Naturally, however, the pins broke, or worked loose in the bone, or both.

six basically different ways to attach two or more bone fragments together:

(a) Bone screws, usually made self-tapping so they cut
     their own threads (Figs. 22.02, 23.03) ;
(b) long stems or rods which fit into the medullary cav-
     ity of the bone, and called intramedullary nails (Fig.
     22.03) ;
(c) tight, circumferential bands such as the Parham
     bands, or circumferential sutures of wire, catgut or
     other;
(d) onlay devices called plates which one attaches to each
     fragment by means of screws and/or bolts (Fig. 22.04,
     22.05) ;
(e) buried sutures;
(f) pins of various designs which one can drill into and/
     or through, and across, two or more fragments (Fig.
     22.01) ;
(g) bolts of several types (Fig. 23.02) .

To repeat an earlier statement: the largest single cause of
implant failures consists of failure to understand the nature of
mechanical fatigue, *and that includes fatigue failures to both
the inert and the living structural materials.* Frequently this
constitutes an inability to manage the patient after implantation in that way which will protect the device from mechanical
failure in an adequate manner until healing of the living tissue
reaches the stage that it can take over its own mechanical
functions.

As now designed, some of the forms of internal fixation in
common use have the disadvantage of inherent proneness to
fatigue failure, and they usually require effective protection
from ordinary mechanical loads until the bone has healed
well enough to bear the loads unaided. In this arena of orthopaedic endeavor, it pays the young resident to try to borrow
some of the biomechanical intuition and horse sense acquired
by many of his teachers with twenty or more years of practical
experience. So many nuances and special situations exist that
a book such as this cannot do justice to the job. Residents of

such teachers may rate themselves as highly fortunate (a partial listing must include B. E. Obletz, G. Marcy and J. D. Godfrey of Buffalo, L. Goldstein, J. Moe, A. Neufeld, G. Hoover, P. MacFarland, D. Lucas, O. Landeros of Chihuaua, R. Wilson and R. Allred).

We will describe next, and briefly, the strain-stress patterns arising in some of the more common devices in current wide use.

1) STRESSES IN SCREWS AND THEIR BONE ANCHORAGE: We use screws often enough in orthopaedic surgery that we all need a clear idea of some of their limitations. Figure 22.02 illustrates two slightly different designs. Their basic design limitation constitutes size. Thus, in designing a machine in which screws transfer loads from one part to another, we obtain the necessary total strength and fatigue protection by making the screws numerous and large enough to reduce unit stresses in each single screw to acceptable levels, and it would take slide rule whizzes such as Doctors Charles Potter and Charles Shock no time at all to match screw holding strength to materials properties and overall loads in such a way as to obtain "four-nine safety", meaning a likelihood of not failing of $p > .9999$, or 9,999 times out of 10,000 usages of such machines. The weakest part of such a type of joining usually represents the screw, not the relatively massive part in which it lies. However we cannot take this approach to its obvious limit very well in bones because when single screws become too large their holes leave too little bone intact to provide good strength and to allow good seating. Also, inserting many screws requires much stripping of the blood-carrying soft tissues from the periosteal surface of the bone, impairing both its viability and its healing ability. These biological considerations force us to make a trade when we use bone screws: we trade strength off for good healing potential.

Metallic screws lying in a bone which secure a plate to the bone, thereby to affix one bony fragment to another, must carry three major types of loads. One represents an extraction force or axial load, tending to pluck a screw directly out of the bone in a direction parallel to the long axis of the screw.

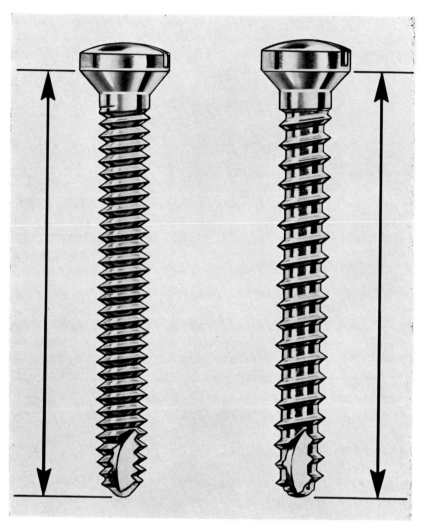

Figure 22.02. This illustrates two current designs of bone screws, the one on the right showing some design changes in the thread roots intended to increase fatigue endurance as well as strength on static testing. At the lower end appear the longitudinal slots which make these screws self tapping (tapping means cutting the threads for a screw in a hole). Other screw designs exist too, both as to size and geometry. All have their places. (Reprinted by permission, O.E.C., Bourbon, Indiana.)

The threads provide the sole resistance to this action. The second represents flexural loads applied to the screw as the plate on one side and the bone on the other attempt to slide on each other in shear. The third represents shearing loads applied directly to the shank of the screw by such loads.

(*a*) *The Extraction Loads*: The total resistance of a screw to an extraction force represents that afforded by each unit area of screw thread in contact with the bone thread, times the total number of such unit areas in the whole screw-bone thread interface. Thus total strength in resistance to the axial load increases as one deepens the threads (but that weakens the root diameter of the screw), as one increases the outside thread diameter (but that makes the screw increasingly bulky), and as one increases the total length of the screw lying in good contact with bone. But as for the latter, the total cortical bone thickness engaging the threads set an upper limit.

As to the state of these matters with contemporary bone screws, when a screw lies across the midshaft of an adult femur the total interface transferring axial mechanical loads from screw to bone provides sufficient strength to those loads that, when loaded cyclically to failure, about forty per cent of the resulting failures arise because of fatigue of the bone threads which, in shearing off parallel to the walls of the screw hole, allow the undamaged screw to extract. About fifty per cent of the failures will occur by breakage of the screw itself, usually in one of the thread roots, and another ten per cent occur by shearing the screw head off transversely to its long axis in the shank.

It follows that the simplest ways to increase the total holding strength of any device attached by screws consist of 1) increasing the number of screws placed in each fragment and 2) increasing the lever arm of the screws by using longer plates.

(*b*) *Shearing Loads*: As a plate attached to a bone by a set of screws works micromechanically by sliding minutely back and forth each time the muscles in the limb contract, these motions parallel or tangent to the periosteal bony surface force a given screw head laterally against the resistance of its bony anchorage. This induces flexural stresses or moments within the screw shank which, at the thread roots, can reach rather large magnitudes. Recall that as one reduces the diameter of a cylindrical rod by a factor of two, the same flexural loads will then generate 2^4 or sixteen times greater flexural stresses in its surface fibers. Hence another reason for not cutting the screw threads too deeply, and, too, a good reason to leave the 0.5 cm or so of the screw shank immediately under the screw head smooth rather than threaded.

(*c*) *Screw head design*: In addition to the above shearing load, a conical shape to the underside of the screw head (shown in Figure 22.02) fits into a matching recess in most plate designs, and this acts like a wedge, developing an axial extraction load on the screw each time the plate works sideways against it. Add to the above the nearly unavoidable alignment eccentricities involved in actually installing plate screw systems, and a basis for considerable prestressing of screw heads can exist at the end of an operation; such prestressing could easily predispose to a fatigue failure.

(*d*) *Role of the bone*: Obviously a bone screw lying across the full diameter of an adult tibia or femur at midshaft has a fairly strong bony anchorage, and if one attempts to extract it by brute force the screw will more likely fail than the bony threads securing it. But if a screw lies in cancellous bone, as it commonly does in fixing a medial malleolus for example, only a small amount of bone actually lies in contact with the screw threads, for as tables in an earlier chapter illustrate, typically eighty per cent of the volume of trabecular bone comprises the marrow spaces which contain only very fragile soft tissues; only twenty per cent of it constitutes bone. As a result if a screw or any other fixation device buried in trabecular bone transfers any unusually large loads to that bone, that small amount of bone at the bone-metal interface can become battered, crumble and leave a screw (or whatever) floating uselessly in an enlarged channel, in contact only with soft tissues and blood. Because screws provide insecure fixation in cancellous bone structures, if one must use them there, then he should provide effective additional protection of the osteosynthesis from mechanical loads during the healing phase (for example by means of a cast).

2) INTRAMEDULLARY DEVICES: While the concept of intramedullary fixation has lain around for a long time (Dr. Ward Plummer of Buffalo reportedly performed an intramedullary fixation of a clavicle fracture with a urethral bougie in the early 1920's), we owe to Kuntschner of Germany during World War II the particular development (in terms of design and use) which opened the intramedullary fixation door to us. More than a dozen different designs enjoy contemporary use. In general these devices should fit the intramedullary canal snugly to control torque and shearing displacement at the fracture or osteotomy surfaces. Yet one usually cannot achieve a snug fit over the whole length of a bone with these devices because the medullary canal varies considerably in diameter at different levels in a given bone, the narrowest part lying in or near its middle. Thus, the choice of the diameter of a rod requires making some kind of compromise, which one can modify on occasion by enlarging the marrow canal with a reamer to achieve better contact along a greater length of the shaft, and thus better fixation. In general, intramedullary rods provide the strongest and most durable of the presently available ways of attaching the two fragments of a broken long bone together. See Figure 22.03. In spite of this, one usually must protect such devices during the subsequent healing phase by putting the extremity in a cast, or keeping the patient on crutches until the bone has healed. Otherwise a fatigue failure of the device can occur, or it can sustain flexural overloads which will deform it plastically, giving it a permanent set. One may have the devil's own time in trying to remove such a device later because its curved portion and its respectable rigidity make it very reluctant to slide out.

Because the outside diameter of the bone greatly exceeds that of an intramedullary rod or nail, the flexural stresses in the surface fibers of the nail will exceed those in the bone (were it carrying the flexural loads), and by more than 27

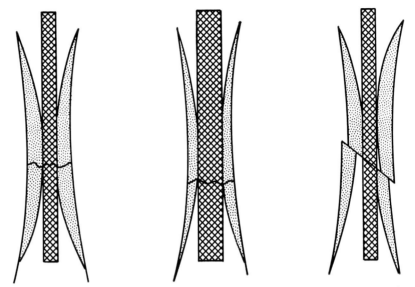

Figure 22.03. A single intramedullary nail can provide solid fixation of a fracture if, first, it has an irregular (i.e., square, triangular or similar shape) rather than a circular cross section so it will control and prevent rotation of the fragments relative to each other. Then in midshaft fractures without reaming as on the *left,* or in fractures modestly distant from the marrow canal's isthmus (or narrowest diameter) in which one enlarges the isthmus past the fracture by reaming it to accept a larger nail as in the *middle,* or in oblique fractures where muscle forces can compress the fragments as on the *right* and, at the expense of a modest lateral translation of one fragment on the other, and perhaps of 1–5 mm of overriding, one can obtain adequately secure fixation and acceptably reliable bone healing.

fold (!) given a one-to-three ratio of their diameters. Given irregular and oblique fracture surfaces, the compression load created by normal muscle tonus across the fracture, plus the geometry of the fracture surface, can lock them together sufficiently well to allow good healing even though the marrow cavity respectably exceeds the nail's diameter.

We not only have intramedullary rods; now we have extramedullary ones too, thanks to Dr. Paul Harrington who devised a system of internal fixation of the spine which serves widely in the surgical treatment of scoliosis. Figure 2.02 in Part I showed a Harrington rod in place in a (now) young woman.

3) Circumferential Band: Put on with special tighteners, these wrap around a spiral or very oblique fracture. While efficient mechanically these devices unfortunately have the disadvantage that they sacrifice a ring of periosteal blood supply which can take a long time to return. Occasionally this allows trouble to develop, such as a secondary stress fracture of the bone. Like most other kinds of internal function, one must protect these devices from large loads until after the bone has healed. In a few special situations they still may serve better than any other available method.

4) Bone Plates: These come in a wide range of sizes and many designs, and serve a variety of purposes. The most commonly used ones include the AO compression plate system, Eggers, Lane, Sherman and Thornton. These devices fit and/ or lie on the external periosteal bone surfaces. Large plates with many screw or bolt holes may prove quite strong on static test, but usually prove somewhat fatigue prone if not protected during the healing process. See Figure 22.04. Large plates have the disadvantage that one must strip much of the regional periosteal blood supply to install them, and their many screws usually seriously damage the marrow cavity blood supply too. In combination these defects may impair healing of the fracture. Also, postoperative infections appear more likely in the presence of large plates attached by many screws, than they do with small and fewer. This probably reflects two things: The larger amount of dead space and devitalized tissue (which cannot well defend itself from bacteriological invasion) associated with the larger devices, and the fact that no modern surgery occurs under truly aseptic conditions so that all of these devices show evidence of bacteriological contamination at the completion of the operation. While small plates definitely prove biologically better than large ones, they also prove mechanically less secure and durable. The choice in a given case must again form a compromise, and in truth too, widely divergent points of view exist on this.

5) Sutures of wire or nonmetallic materials threaded through holes drilled in a bone can serve to hold two or more

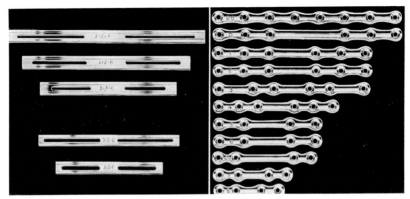

Figure 22.04. Only two of the many available styles of bone plates, and a partial sampling of the size range they cover. On the left the screw holes consist of slots rather than round holes, the idea beneath it being that in the initial phases of fracture healing some resorption usually occurs at the bone ends, leading to a slight (0.5–2 mm) relative distraction and possible retardation of healing. But the slotted plate allows the fragments to slide towards each other under the compression loads of the enveloping muscles, thereby maintaining direct contact.

On the right a more conventional (but biologically and mechanically neither better nor worse) plate design. (Reproduced courtesy of OEC, Bourbon, Ind.)

fragments together. One must protect such a suture from carrying any appreciable loads during the healing period, or it will break by fatigue. This kind of fixation, while relatively flimsy in the mechanical sense, can prove very useful in selected problems.

6) HIP NAILS: A considerable variety of devices have evolved for securing together in the mechanical sense the two major fragments of a broken hip. Figure 22.05 shows only one example. In general these devices should accomplish the following things: provide secure mechanical fixation to the cancellous bone within the femoral head; provide similar fixation to the femoral shaft; and secure mutual fixation or relative immobilization of the two major fragments. This means exposing a sizeable surface area of metal-to-bone in the spongiosa of the head to create a large enough bone-metal interface that neither metal nor bone becomes overloaded in the mechanical sense. If the metal overloads, it bends or fractures. If the bone

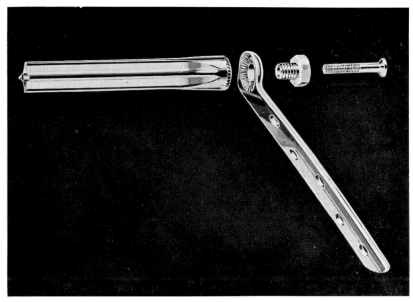

Figure 22.05. A "hip pin," the triflanged Smith-Peterson nail at the top left typically is driven in over a guide wire previously inserted under x-ray control into the cancellous bone of the femoral head. The Thornton side-plate then bolts on to the exposed head of the nail, and in this design a small locking screw with a left-hand thread serves to minimize loosening of the right hand threaded bolt during the bone healing phase (typically some 3–6 months). One then attaches the side plate to the lateral aspect of the femur, as shown in an earlier figure illustrating the Ken nail, to secure the nail to the distal fragment. One-piece devices of similar shape and usage and called Jewett nails and Neufeld nails also enjoy wide favor and use. (Photo courtesy O.E.C., Bourbon, Ind.)

overloads, it crushes or crumbles to create a fluid-filled cavity within which the metal will rattle around, no longer providing the secure fixation the surgeon had in mind when he did the operation.

In addition to fixation to the head, the device must affix soundly to the shaft of the femur. The screw side-plate method shown in the accompanying figures illustrates one way to do this. The Holt nail, I-beam nail, Deyerle method, Badgely and Massie nails and several others also exist. All current methods fall short of the ideal (immediate weight bearing without danger of bone or metal fatigue, of breakage or of plastic deformation) and so require common sense and usually gradual phasing of the return to normal activities.

7) PINS AND BOLTS: We have Kirschner wires (diameter less than 3/32″ and Steinman pins (diameter over 3/32″), some with smooth surfaces and others threaded to provide a nonslip surface, and with a variety of different kinds of points. We also have a bewildering variety of related devices which would include Knowles pins, Webb bolts, pins with graduation marks on them (guide wires) and many other special pins.

8) THE FUTURE: We definitely need much better ways than now available to us to attach and fix two bone fragments together, using a device (s) that has little bulk, resists fatigue well, has adequate strength on static test, and possess a satisfactory level of biological inertness.

None of our contemporary devices are perfect, nor with our present limited knowledge and understanding does it seem likely that any such will appear very soon. Since this is well known, such imperfections may cause, but one cannot blame us for, many of the device failures that occur every year in the civilized world. The majority of failures I have seen arose in one or another way from one common denominator: fatigue. This usually means one or more of several things: (a) an uncooperative patient who would not restrict physical activity as advised; or (b) a surgeon who did not appreciate the role and danger of fatigue in device failures;* or (c) a choice of postoperative care that represented a legitimate and necessary gamble, an optimum compromise between a variety of conflicting factors, but which proved unsuccessful; or (d) the selection of the wrong device for the particular situation in which it was used; or most often, (e) a device which could not provide optimum and necessary strength and endurance because of the limitations imposed on the engineer and manufacturer by our ignorance and by biological tolerance to foreign bodies. It repeatedly disconcerts to find how weak a given system (and this includes both the device and the bone to

---

* This appreciation profoundly affects one's choice of operation, device, postoperative plan and postoperative evaluation and follow-up.

which it may attach) may prove when tested in actual use and over time, in spite of its possibly great strength on a static test in a testing laboratory. We will say more about these matters in the next chapter.

II: ENDOPROSTHESES

1) DEFINITION: This term signifies devices which we bury and leave permanently in place in the body, in order to provide or substitute for the mechanical function of some living part lost or damaged or removed because of some injury or disease. Most in current use constitute substitutes for joints and neighboring bony parts. Hip endoprostheses have become quite commonly used, but other analogous devices now also serve or exist in stages of active development in the knee, fingers, wrist, elbow, shoulder and temporomandibular joints, merely as examples. See Figure 22.06.

Some surgeons have also substituted specially fashioned metal parts for the shafts of some long bones and for parts of the mandible. We may expect to see expansion of this practice over the next generation or so, and great improvements both in the devices and in the way in which one employs them.

2) STATE OF THE ART: Judged by the rather harsh criterion of the "Frost Test",* flaws exist in the design or/and usage of all of these devices. While it may often prove better or wiser to accept such flaws rather than avoid using a device enitrely, this should not (and does not) blind us to the need for better understanding of the principles and problems that underly the successes and failures of those devices. Always, progress cannot begin until one frankly faces and accepts the need for it.

And lest someone twist those words to infer meaning that did not lie behind them: They do not imply negligent or incompetent design and/or manufacture of such devices; they

---

* To wit: "If you really understand a system, you can make it behave to suit your own ends 99 out of 100 tries." While this test will reveal whether flaws exist or not, it does not tell us their nature, nor how to find them, nor how to correct them.

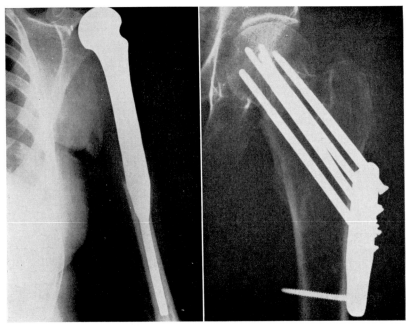

Figure 22.06. *Left:* This lass, aged 17 years at the time of this x-ray, had a highly aggressive giant-cell tumor in her upper humerus which destroyed virtually all of it and was erupting through the biopsy wound at the time of referral to the author. Following an *en bloc* resection the then Austenal Co. (now Howmet) made this endoprosthesis especially for the upper half of her humerus. Living and well 10 years later, good passive shoulder mobility without pain and normal from the elbow down. But poor tension-transfer from living tissue to metal prevents abduction against gravity. Note the lower bone-metal interface; clearly the ideas about its optimum shape voiced later in the text had not materialized when we designed this implant.

    Right: The Wm. Deyerle hip pinning system for internally fixing transcervical hip fractures (photo courtesy of Wm. M. Deyerle, M.D.).

are as good as we can make them with our present limitations in: a) materials, b) in understanding of how the body works, c) in understanding how to devise effective and durable substitutes, d) and how to design effective and durable reconstructive procedures. We do not yet know how to make them better, nor do we even half understand the reason for many of their failures. When we do, then perhaps we can redesign, make and use them in such a way that they do meet the Frost

Test. Our ability to do this now suffers mainly from lack of enough able people to study the varied problems existing in this whole field. The people already working in it prove inadequate in only one consistent respect: too few exist to do the job in a short time. However, their clan grows steadily, and bustles with innovation and ingenuity, and we may expect many great changes and improvements over the next twenty years.

3) PROBLEMS: Failures in these devices fall into five broad categories already referred to:

(a) Fatigue failure, either of the device or of the bone in which it lies implanted, failure manifested by a sudden complete fracture which one can only rarely predict.

(b) Gradual crumbling away of the bony socket before the device and the loads it transfers to the bone, probably (we need direct evidence to confirm this) as a result of a series of microscopic cracks or failures due to too high unit loadings at the bone-metal interface, and/or to locally retarded bone healing, adaptive and remodeling processes which (again) we cannot predict at this time, or to a faulty geometry of the load transfer interface.

(c) Continued pain in the presence of a seemingly excellent fit and technical job of installation, which again one cannot predict and which we often cannot explain satisfactorily.*

(d) Intolerance by the tissue of the material composing the device, some of which still remains unpredictable and which can occur with any and all of the currently marketed alloys and metals, some manufacturer's sales staff's implications to the contrary not withstanding:

(e) And infection, which seems more likely during some of these operations than in many others because of (1) their duration, (2) the amount of dissection and tissue handling

---

* Like most other fields of medicine, orthopaedics abounds with logical explanations. Unfortunately though their logic does not simultaneously assure one of their accuracy.

required in them* (3) the relatively large dead space remaining between the implant and living tissue, which contains a good culture medium—extravasated blood—but with little active biological defense against bacteria, and (4) the inevitable bacterial contamination of tissue that occurs even in modern major surgery. Calling it aseptic or sterile surgery consists of an out-and-out misnomer, of an ideal we aimed at but missed. Indeed, it seems doubtful that we can achieve it in our time at a socially and economically acceptable and reasonable price.

Note that the text said nothing about corrosion. That was because it has become almost unnecessary due to the general knowledge of its existence and importance as a problem, so much so that one cannot easily conceive any contemporary manufacturer using an implant material which had not first been thoroughly tested in this respect. So, rather than beat on a dead horse we pay our respects to those still kicking.

In the next chapter we will take a closer look at some aspects of the general problem of implant failures, partly to improve a clinician's ability to evaluate the new ones we may expect in the coming years, and partly to alert those contemplating construction of new ones to the safeguards they must take into account.

---

* Save in the hand of the truly superior operator (which, believe me, does not mean the same thing as a superior surgeon) .

Chapter 23

Causes of Implant Failures

M<small>ANY REASONS ARISE</small> for failure of a device implanted for one or another reason in the body, and it may help to look briefly at some of them. We will consider separately those of mechanical, biological and iatrogenic origins.

I: MECHANICAL FACTORS

We could subdivide these matters into those related to manufacture, those related to the design of the device, and those related to its use. To repeat, we will assume the general knowledge of metallic corrosion in the body fluids makes it no longer necessary to devote a specific section to it in a chapter such as this; thus, on to other aspects of the problem:

1) M<small>ANUFACTURING</small> P<small>ROBLEMS</small>: Here a large number of things could go wrong. They might include incomplete mixing of the elements forming an alloy, so that it contains some regions rich and others poor in one of its constituent elements or phases (289). This could create differing electromotive potentials on different parts of the device's surface which might lead to galvanic corrosion. In addition, the device may undergo too much cold working during the last phases of manufacture so that strain hardening develops, and along with it the embrittlement and loss of fatigue resistance usually associated with such hardening. Manufacturers often correct this by annealing the device before releasing it for sale. Similarly, some metallic and nonmetallic structural materials exhibit the property of age hardening, meaning that gradually over time, and after they solidify from the melt, diffusional and allotropic changes develop within them which increase both hardness and brittleness (and thus susceptibility to fatigue). This problem does not appear to affect materially the two chief alloy systems cur-

rently in use in making orthopaedic implants, the chrome-cobalt and the 316 stainless series.* In addition to the compositional factors just mentioned, manufacturing procedures can also produce mechanical defects in the device. For example, one form of screw once sold for holding large bone fragments together, was manufactured by a rolling process in which two dies rolling past each other under great pressure spun the stainless steel blank in between them, and impressed therein a helically wound thread. The device looked great on the manufacturers' shelves, but in use many of them developed fatigue fractures prior to completion of bone healing. Microscopic examination of these screws revealed that during the rolling process the metal had flowed so much that in the thread root lay a practically continuous linear fine crack, representing the interface where metal forced to flow down either side of the threads abutted at the roots. Here an excellent basic idea—meaning designing the screw to provide a flexible threaded portion—came to naught because of the method of manufacture. The screws would have held up much better had their threads been cut into blank stock rather than rolled, and the initial trial models used before regular production were so cut—and worked just fine.

Other lessons learned some thirty years ago: One cannot make a complex implant which requires joining two or more pieces of metal together by soldering nor by brazing them. Brazing signifies joining two pieces of metal by flowing a hot melted mass of a bronze or brass-like alloy in between them (289). In part the reasons, of course, constitute the high corrosive susceptibility of solder and brazing metal in saline fluid environments. Welding of steel parts also has not proven an acceptable way to make implants for use in the human body. The heat associated with the welding (which literally melts the metal at the contacting surfaces so they flow and merge into one continuous solid body) in effect adds an additional heat treatment to the steel beyond the

---

* Although both of these systems demonstrate the work hardening property, becoming harder, more brittle and more fatigue sensitive after cold working, for example by bending repeatedly, or as a result of hammering.

weld zone, one which changes its mechanical and chemical properties from the surround sufficiently to permit stress corrosion and even intergranular corrosion to develop in a saline fluid environment. The chrome-cobalt systems do seem to weld satisfactorily (in inert atmospheres) because no such harmful changes in their internal structure follow the attendant heating. In fact the heads of many of the standard lines of hip endoprostheses made of chrome-cobalt alloys usually consist of two hollow halves welded together.

2) PROBLEMS IN DESIGN: Design problems include two categories: those related to the choice of material, and those related to the shape and mechanical relationships of the various parts of the device.

(a) *Materials factors*: We learned more than twenty years ago for example that acrylic plastic and nylon constitute poor choices for in endoprosthetic femoral head. Their wear resistance when moving in contact with normal articular cartilage, proved very poor in service and these devices wore to the point of producing subjective disability in patients after only two or three years of service life. As another example, the polymer going under the trade name of Teflon® originally attracted a great deal of attention by manufacturers because of its very low chemical reactivity and a reasonably low coefficient of friction. For this reason joint surface substitutions, i.e., implants replacing the surfaces of the medial and lateral tibial condyles, became made of it and a good number of them found their way into patients' knees. Most of them had to come out later, because Teflon proves quite susceptible to creep, and in a human knee under compression loads and given time, the stuff flowed like toothpaste under one's thumb. Just that flow led to most of the failures in actual use. Another important cause of failures of such devices relates to the geometry of the bone-implant interface, and we will take it up later. As a third example, back in the early forties when the electrochemical basis of most corrosion of these implants in the body, defined by Doctors Venable and Stuck (275), was either not accepted or clearly understood, a variety of alloys served to construct bone plates and bone screws. The writer has taken out some of these, and discovered thereby how much corrosion a supposedly good vanadium steel or a hardenable stainless steel plate can develop in the human body.

(b) *Problems of implant shape*: These represent matters either of violating ordinary design expertise, i.e., introducing notches or sharp changes in contour which produce stress risers, or making devices too bulky in terms of volume, or failures (excusable or not) to comprehend the manner in which the body will load an implant. As a consequence one can produce a design for a particular purpose which contains within it an unperceived defect that of necessity will cause it to have a high probability of failing following implantation. A variety of such situations have cropped up.

For example, in nailing intracapsular hip fractures some surgeons prefer a sliding nail which allows the fracture to collapse slightly during the initial transient phase of bone resorption which follows most fractures. That collapse (typically some 5mm), thereby maintains good bone contact and promotes early and reliable bone union. Experience has shown that this sliding property does indeed increase significantly the total percentage of unions of such fractures. The Ken and Pugh nails have served satisfactorily in this regard for some years. But one manufacturer, wishing to obtain his part of this market, decided to produce his own such device. It appeared quite satisfactory on the shelf and, in the metallurgical and manufacturing senses, it proved impeccable. However, in use the lengths of the sleeve and the sliding part of the nail proved improperly matched, so that in a large patient with large bones, a failure at their junction in flexure almost had to (and did) occur. You may see in this the wisdom of some old advice which goes about like this: "Be not the first to try new things, nor the last to adopt them after they prove themselves."

As another example, experimental implants of several types have had metal or plastic sleeves that covered a fairly wide area of the periosteal region of the bone within which they lay. That impaired the blood supply to the cortex which as a consequence of that plus cyclic loading, eventually broke in mechanical fatigue, causing bone and appliance to part company as it were.

Still another example: A variety of efforts to find satisfactory total joint replacements have led to the satisfactorily durable Charnley, and Charnley-Mueller metal sliding on plastic, and the Frost metal rolling on metal designs. Also a variety of metal sliding on metal designs have appeared, some of which seem to do well. But in some others of the latter the design choice of metal sliding on metal in an aqueous environment caused the production of much very fine, particulate metallic sludge, representing small particles of the sliding surfaces broken off due to adhesion and abrasion at those surfaces, as described in an earlier chapter in Part I under the discussion of friction. This very fine sludge drastically increased the surface to volume ratio of the metallic debris, and therefore its potential for irritating tissues in contact with it. And in some of these designs, serious irritation and impairment of the biological competence of the apposed bony and solf tissues did occur, requiring the removal of these implants. Of course we could not foresee this, but now that we have learned about it we should try not to redemonstrate it time and time again.

Another example of a shape problem appeared during the evolution of our present day hip endoprosthesis, the Austin-Moore and F. R. Thompson of current manufacture representing the standard, the former appearing in Figure 23.01. As originally evolved and manufactured, the base plates of these prostheses tended to lie at an angle of some 60° inclined from the horizontal. Accordingly, when patients walked on them a fairly sizeable shearing load developed, the femur tending to slide upwards and laterally on the base plate. This shearing load concentrated and transferred across the relatively small bone-metal interface between the upper medial stem of the implant and upper part of the calcar femorale, and led to subjective pain on the part of the user thereof, and to an unusually high percentage of instances of migration of the prosthesis distally down into the femur (181).

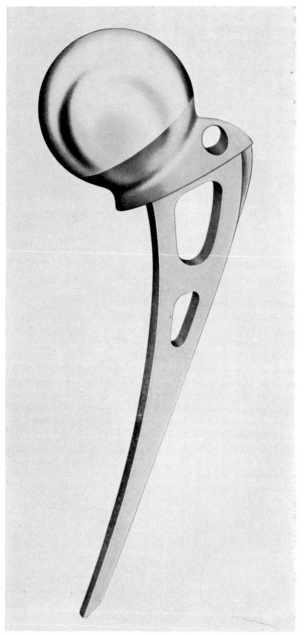

Figure 23.01. A current-production Austin-Moore femoral head-neck replacement endoprosthesis, with approximately a 40° angle of base plate to horizontal instead of the variably steeper inclinations commonly seen in earlier designs.

Some even failed because of an eventual fracture of the bone at the calcar. Over the years as this problem became recognized, the inclination of the base plate was progressively decreased, the current standard representing approximately 40° inclination from the horizontal, and in the femoral component of the Frost total hip system, 25° from the horizontal. Aligning the base plate more normally (i.e., more perpendicularly) to the mechanical compression load resultants usually transferred across such hips, has minimized this shearing load sufficiently that failures from the above mechanism have become uncommon. This situation arose because at the time of their original design nobody had any good idea of the normal mechanical load trajectories across a hip, whether a normal or a painful one, and of some clinical importance, if the latter, then whether overtly or subliminally painful. Indeed, while some of us now think we do have at least a reasonably good idea of those trajectories (if interested, see Volume IV), this still remains debated, not a matter of clear evidence, and probably will so remain until someone produces direct measurements in the living subject with such prostheses in place. Both Carl Hirsch in Sweden and V. Frankel in Cleveland, and their associates, have already begun obtaining such data but for obvious reasons it will take many more studies to remove all doubts and ambiguities about the true loading situation. These studies must somehow resolve a disturbing element, constituting the fact that *when a joint hurts in use, even subliminally, the neurologically determined patterns of muscle contractions actuating it change.* In the hip as a consequence the load resultants align more vertically than they do in a normal hip. With respect to such dynamic load resultants, we might dignify this with a special term. Let us call it the pain-pattern effect.

A final example: Several implants designed in the past thirty years possessed sound mechanical design but fell by the wayside simply because their bulk proved too great for the local anatomical situation. This interfered with motion and function in some cases, or produced such local prominence under the skin in others as to cause pain and/or pressure ulcers which required their removal.

Let us now deal with a few problems related to the use of a device which may prove of sound design and manufacture, but which inherently cannot meet the demands made of it by the patient or his doctor.

(c) *Problems of use*: 1) *Unrealistic expectations of mechanical strength*: One may use a small four or six hole plate to internally fix a fracture of the femur in a large man and then, rather than realizing that this must serve in the same very limited sense as Doctors John Ditmars or Harvey Weiss or J. Poole would use a 6-0 silk suture in a flexor tendon in a hand to serve, allow the patient unrestricted mobility without extra protection by a cast, brace, crutches, or similar devices. Since when one takes the time factor into account such a plate really forms a mechanically frail internal fixation compared to the forces normally generated in that part of the anatomy, it should not surprise anyone when a plate handled postoperatively in this manner bends or breaks, or the screws break or avulse from the bone. The problem here does not lie in the device (which was perfectly satisfactory); the surgeon using it should recognize that as a mechanically feeble form of fixation serving primarily to ensure and maintain an accurate reduction, it requires effective external protection until good bone healing allows living tissues to take over the loads transferred across the part. Having absorbed that, now refer to Figure 23.02.

Equally, when a muscular or obese patient with a fractured femur undergoes internal fixation by intramedullary nailing and then walks on it, the nail accepts large shearing and flexural loads at the level of the fracture. Given a small enough nail or large enough medullary cavity and/or large enough patient, and the nail very likely may not endure those loads long enough for the fracture to heal.

2) *Smoldering infection*: Similarly one should not find it surprising if internal fixation devices used in the presence of smoldering infection lead to subsequently more overt

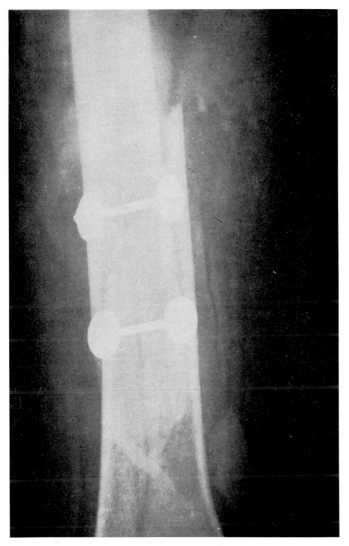

Figure 23.02. Here you see a spiral, pathological fracture of the lower femoral diaphysis in a 70 year old man, due to a metastatic epidermoid carcinoma, originally arising in the lung.

For a variety of medical and situational reasons the author chose to reduce this fracture open, internally fix it with two Webb bolts as shown, have Mss. C. Clinton and R. Smith fit the patient with a suitable brace (including a pelvic band to minimize torque), and ambulate him early with crutches on his good lower limb. Fortunately two bolts were used, for the bone anchorage of the upper one broke 10 days postop. (Common sense in this field suggests: always divide your therapeutic "eggs" up into at least two baskets.) But the lower one held, and with the aid of the brace the patient did ambulate early (i.e., by 3 weeks) and the fracture healed soundly—indeed, enthusiastically—within 10 weeks.

postoperative wound infection and in some cases to rejection of the device.

3) *Endurance*: Nor should it evoke great surprise if a technically good prosthesis or cup arthroplasty fails after serving for running, climbing mountains or playing thirty-six holes of golf every day. Arthroplasties in effect constitute man-made joints, and in the reasonably foreseeable future we probably do not have to worry too much about making these substitutes good enough to allow patients unrestricted function. When we give a patient an artificial joint, an integral part of the procedure usually should constitute teaching him how to minimize the mechanical demands he makes on it throughout its subsequent service life. That offers the device its best opportunity to maintain mobility and to provide freedom from pain for ordinary activities for many years.

4) *Osteoporotic bone*: Equally one should not blame the device if screws pull out when used to secure an osteotomy or fracture in osteoporotic bone (which has very thin cortices). The thin cortices simply mean that a minimum total mechanical interface of bone to the screw threads exists, and therefore minimum holding strength. If one must use screws in such situations, the postoperative plan should provide additional mechanical protection of the part until bone healing has occurred.

5) *Pin diameter problems*: Frequently we may use devices called Steinmann pins or Kirschner wires, either to apply skeletal traction or to transfix fracture fragments in various parts of the body. Small diameter pins present a relatively small projected area to the bone (if diameter is D and length L, then the maximum useful area equals DL) for the transfer of mechanical loads, and given a thin pin and/or large loads and the pin may simply bend or break. Such pins lack flexural stiffness so that while quite satisfactory for fixing the fragments of fractures of the small bones in the hand or foot, they may prove too willowy to do the same job in a radius, humerus, femur or tibia. Given a pin thick enough not to bend but a thin bone cortex, then, again over time, the pin

may appear magically to walk or waltz progressively through the cortical bone in the direction of the traction pull or other load applied to it. Supracondylar traction pins used in elderly patients may migrate a full two centimeters or more in this manner over a period of eight to twelve weeks.* Cure: use pins larger than 3/16 in diameter to increase the total bone-metal interface.

6) *Thermal damage*: When one uses a dull drill to drill holes for bone screws this generates increased heat, due to the friction of the drill point against the bone (here one converts mechanical work or $W = FL$ into its caloric equivalent in heat of 778 ft-lb per B.T.U.; See tables in Part III). This heat can effectively cook and kill a cylinder of bone extending some millimeters distant around the drill hole (180), and can easily reach temperatures in excess of 100° C. The duller the drill and the longer one takes to drill the hole, the greater the diameter of this heat-killed cylinder. When one subsequently inserts a bone screw in it, its immediate mechanical security and strength may prove quite satisfactory but during the subsequent two months or so, as mechanical loads make the screw work micromechanically within its bony bed, the bone in the thread roots gradually weakens by a kind of mechanical fatigue. Lacking any local living mechanisms which can compensate for this loosening effect, the screw may ultimately pull completely out of the bone, destroying the internal fixation. It follows that one should use sharp drills, try to drill the holes quickly, and use increased pressure on the drill point rather than increased revolutions of the drill per minute (i.e., rpm) to achieve this.

---

* A $\frac{1}{8}$ in diameter Steinman pin has a projected area of 1 in² for each 8 in length. In a femoral supracondylar traction set-up only about $\frac{1}{4}$ in of its length may actually lie in contact with bone, which equals about .03 in². Given say 20 lb of weight on the traction bow, then the unit load on that .03 in² bone-metal interface becomes some 700 lb, and it is a constant load, not an intermittent one. Experience shows that the question in this situation does not become: "Will it migrate?" but rather: "How fast will it migrate?".

You suggest then: Drill through the diaphysis to obtain a thicker cortex and thus larger bone-metal interface. While conceding its logic, Dame experience says *no* because with probability $p > .25$, that will lead to a fatigue fracture of the femoral shaft, the pin hole serving as the initiating stress riser.

Such thermally cooked cylinders may later separate out from the living bone as ring sequestrae.

Our faster-driven bone saws provide another source of thermal damage which can delay or actually prevent satisfactory bone healing at an osteotomy site, even in children. It has proven preferable on these biological grounds to cut bone for an osteotomy with an osteotome or a Gigli saw (a hand-driven device), using a large, sharp drill in thick diaphyseal bone to prepare the way for the osteotome. The writer has seen many delayed and nonunions arising from power saw work done on diaphyseal bone.

7) *Proper fitting*: Finally, in using bone plates and screws one should try to drill the screw holes truly concentric with the holes in the plate, which requires a certain amount of mechanical deftness. Drilling such holes eccentrically causes the inserted screws to press and rub quite hard against one side of the plate hole. This concentrates mechanical load between plate and screw on a very small area, and subsequent micromechanical motions of the part will then cause fretting. Given good alloys this need not necessarily lead to fretting corrosion. But in addition, since inserting a screw off center in effect prestresses the screw heads in both flexure and shear, one has an excellent setup for producing a fatigue failure of the screw, usually right below the head. The screw threads should lie across both cortices of the bone in order to obtain the maximum bone metal interface, and also to obtain the best mechanical advantage for the screw to prevent the plate from levering or toggling it within the screw hole. When a screw passes through only one cortex, it has only half of the axial holding power in the threads,* and micromechanical motions of the part can then make the screw toggle within its single hole. This toggling motion, by gradually crushing or crumbling the bone in contact with the threads, can then cause the screw to work loose.

----

* But as to flexure it will have much less than 10% of the strength it has when it extends through both cortices. If that puzzles you, work it out on paper for the case of a femur, using the flexural surface stress equations in Chapter XXI.

II: BIOLOGICAL FACTORS

Device failures related to tissue factors rather than to the mechanical properties of the device would include four types of idiosyncrasies; we will go into this assuming that problems of ordinary galvanic corrosion and chemical reactivity have found solution, and then discuss what kinds of problems remain after solving those two.

1) Tissue Reaction: An occasional patient's tissues will prove quite intolerant to the material of which a particular device is made. It seems to matter not which particular material it is, and none of the currently and widely utilized materials seems really any different in this regard than others. Approximately one patient in five hundred or so will therefore demonstrate an unusual tissue reaction to 316 stainless steel, chrome-cobalt alloy, Teflon, polyethylene and/or methylmethacrylate. While these certainly form problems they do not occur often, and when they do they rarely present problems of great magnitude. At present we lack any accurate way to predict such intolerance.

2) Neoplasia: All observers and students in this field await some evidence that an implant material has stimulated some type of neoplastic response in the host's tissues. The writer does not know of a single instance to date in which that has occurred, and since millions of devices of all types have seen implantation in the human body since 1940, that failure probably tries to tell us something: that such an event will continue to prove exceedingly rare, that it probably will not constitute a causal relationship when it does appear, and that our concern with it may in fact lie far out of proportion to any justification for it.

3) Infection: Another tissue idiosyncrasy which we do see clinically occasionally constitutes an effect of an implant material on the biological competence of the tissue around it, in a manner which impairs the tissue's capacity to combat infection. Consequently delayed infections, as well as infections by organisms which do not ordinarily pro-

duce active infection in healthy people, may occasionally develop after implantation of such mechanical devices.

While seen on occasion, this property too remains an unusual one and probably affects only one in five hundred or so patients who receive an implant. Of all of the materials currently in use, the one that may perhaps prove a little more suspect in this regard than others constitutes polymethyl methacrylate, and this may relate not to the methacrylate itself, but to some of the catalysts and other materials present in its monomer form.

4) ALLERGIC REACTIONS: Finally an implant material should not evoke a response by the host's immunological system. This seems to arise far more often with organic materials than with metals and as a consequence any new artificially made polymers intended for implant use require extensive study in this regard before release for general use. It can form a troublesome problem technically because the immune reaction can trigger off in response to ultramicro quantities of reactants, quantities far below the level which might threaten direct noxious effects upon living tissue.

III: IATROGENIC CAUSES OF OPERATIVE FAILURES

Of course operative procedures on the musculoskeletal system may fail for a very large variety of reasons. We just mentioned some of essentially biomechanical and biological nature, and will now list a few in which we constitute the essential factor in a failure, rather than the design of the implant, its material, its biological peculiarities or its method of manufacture. In reading on, understand clearly the following: no intent exists to criticize orthopaedists who may become entrapped in possibly similar situations. Orthopaedic surgery still constitutes an art rather than a science; we still have only a rudimentary understanding of the biological systems with which we must work, and consequently the bulk of the procedures we perform have a largely empirical basis rather than the solid scientific developmental foundation one expects to find in the engineering, chemical and physical sciences.

Paraphrased, our humanity associates essentially and inherently with fallible perceptiveness, judgement, knowledge and education, so each of us can only try to do his best as he sees it. In that distant day when possibly the lay public may have just reason to expect and demand error-free performance of us, we may perhaps decide to stop practicing medicine rather than risk crucifixion, the reward our antecedents gave to the only other perfect Being listed in our 6000 year history of civilization.

With that in mind, then:

1) DIAGNOSIS: A procedure may fail simply because an incorrect diagnosis served as the basis for a plan of treatment. For example: A woman comes to you asking for a hip (or knee or other) arthroplasty, due to symptoms arising from radiographically evident joint disease. You oblige her. But she is never happy with her new joint because she cannot do what she wants to on it. Too late you discover: She expected a perfectly normally functioning new joint and will not accept anything less. You may have forgotten to make clear in advance that your new joint would have limitations, or she may have had an information-blocking filter in her mind which prevented that information from registering. In either event, such a subjective failure of the procedure and the device lies not in any biomechanical problem but in a more human and less tangible one.

Or, if one substitutes a hip endoprosthesis for an osteoarthritic hip, or for one demonstrating aseptic necrosis of the femoral head, but the patient continues to have his preoperative pain and disability afterwards and ultimately a neurosurgeon cures him of it by removing a herniated lumbar disc, one cannot blame the hip prosthesis for the original procedure's failure to relieve the patient of his disability, nor for any faults he may subsequently find in it. And lest those with limited orthopaedic clinical experience believe that such an error represents a stupid or unforgivable one, hear this: Those with twenty or more years of such experience behind them can attest on that basis that it sometimes can prove impossible to determine where (in the anatomical sense) the disability of some patient arose, because of a variety of reasons we should not discuss here.

As another example, should one elect to do a femoral head replacement arthroplasty for what he assumes forms an osteoarthritic hip, but which in fact forms the early stages of a Charcot hip (due to late lues, diabetes mellitus, multiple sclerosis or a syrinx in the spinal cord), he may expect the procedure to fail, either by dislocation, or by the prosthesis settling into the femur or migrating through the pelvis, or by postoperative wound sepsis.* In point of clinical fact the tissues in the region of a Charcot joint usually demonstrate biological incompetence, in that the normal fatigue-compensating mechanisms react too little and too late, and so do those mechanisms which combat bacterial infection. In my view, these matters reflect a basic regional cellular disorder far more than any simple loss of pain perception, and recent studies on efferent and afferent axon flow of complex organic molecules provide a reasonable and factual basis for assuming that the neurological disease and the biological tissue incompetence bear a causal relationship.

2) PATIENT COOPERATION: A wrong match of a procedure to a particular patient can also lead to an operative failure. For example, under most circumstances one would internally fix an intertrochanteric fracture of the femur in an elderly patient by means of a Jewett nail, or a Smith-Peterson side plate combination, or a Neufeld nail (to mention only a few) and would obtain satisfactory union and a good end result. However, the success of most such procedures requires the patient following the doctor's advice during the postoperative fracture healing time. Part of that advice usually constitutes religiously not bearing weight on the affected limb until

---

* The same impairment in biological competence induced by some artificial materials, one may find arising naturally in body regions affected by Charcot-like neuropathy, which include diabetes mellitus, late lues, peripheral neuropathies of some other kinds, and syrinx. Because of this surgical procedures in such regions prove much more prone to postoperative infection, and if such does develop it may respond so poorly to conventional treatment that an amputation eventually becomes mandatory to save life or eliminate active infection.

fracture healing has occurred, using devices such as crutches or a walker to protect the hip and to facilitate ambulation on one leg. Clearly then, should the patient for whatever reason fail to follow through on that advice, and walk on the operated limb too soon, this may lead either to bending or breakage of the metal, or with about equal frequency to mechanical fatigue-like damage to the bone which anchors, and transfers loads to, the metal. This can cause the bone to crumble, and allow the nail on progressive x-rays apparently to migrate right through the bony substance of the femoral head, penetrate the hip joint and finally enter to some degree the bone of the pelvis above the acetabulum.

But of course the exception always exists; see Figure 23.03.

Be that as it may, such unreliability commonly occurs in patients with mental changes due to advanced age or small vessel disease in the brain, as well as in confirmed alcoholics and drug addicts, and in some patients with psychiatric disorders such as severe depression or manic states. A competent orthopaedic craftsman tries to detect such situations early, and usually attempts to evaluate them before doing that operative procedure so that he can either choose a different device or an entirely different way of handling the problem or by some other means can ensure that the internal fixation will remain protected mechanically after the operation until such time as the bone has healed.

One may also encounter such cooperation difficulties with motorcycle riders, rodeo riders and some rebellious younger men, a clan of wonderful people in all respects except that they have absolutely no regard for the physical safety of their own carcass. The writer well remembers one such individual, both a rodio rider and a motorcycle rider, at the U.S. Veterans Administration Hospital in West Haven, Connecticut. This individual sustained a fracture of the femur at the junction of the middle and lower thirds which underwent an excellent internal fixation with two large Rush pins by Dr. Ned Schutkin. For some season the fracture did not heal; the explanation turned up one day when the patient also turned up with one pin broken at the fracture line and the other bent. It

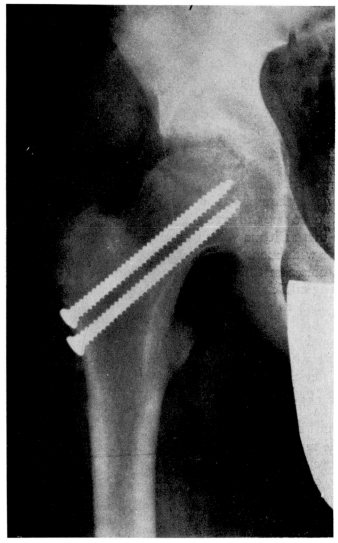

Figure 23.03. This carefree teenager had an epiphyseolisthesis, or slipped capital femoral epiphysis, a condition in which the ball remains in the socket but the neck gradually displaces forwards by a shearing displacement occurring through the epiphyseal plate just below the head. As you see, two Venable screws served to spike it in place, the bone then healed across the plate and the patient (no longer so carefree for he now has a wife, a child and a mortgage) has a functionally normal hip.

Now somewhere in this text, it says that screws in cancellous bone form an inefficient choice of internal fixation, yet here is your author flagrantly seems he began competitive rodeo riding within a week after he left the hospital from the original operation, and the break-bend situation developed when he and his horse parted company the day previous to the second admission (!). Accordingly these devices were removed and a solid Hansen-Street intramedullary nail introduced to fix it. Again a non-union seemed to threaten in spite of the x-ray evidence of abundant callus on either side of the fracture line (meaning it was not a biological failure). Again it turned out that both rodeo and motorcycle riding were in progress, contrary to medical advice. The femur finally healed when I bottled him up in a stout hip spica cast for three months, providing nature a chance to surmount the obstacles hurled at it by an uncaring patient.

3) OPERATIVE PLAN: A failure may occur because the surgeon chose the wrong device for a particular situation.

---

disregarding his own advice, even more than the figure illustrates because the boy was allowed to resume weight bearing only a month after surgery, although it takes some 3–5 months for these slips to heal soundly.

Can you identify the special factors that make these exceptions permissible? They constitute:

One: Children always have more trabecular bone and thicker individual trabeculae than adults (to the tune of $2\times-3\times$) in this part of their skeleton, so the screws do have sound fixation. So sound in fact that you cannot insert them unless you predrill a hole larger than root diameter for them; otherwise the screw driver will simply torque off the screw heads or slots.

Two: Since the epiphyseal plate lies very close to the hip joint, which forms a highly efficient anti-friction device, and since no muscles attach to the ball or the neck, very little shearing drag or flexural loads act on this plate during ordinary activities. The plate accepts loads essentially normal to its plane, and the freely mobile hip above it stress-relieves it from all but compression loads, which simply press the parts together. Thus the two screws really did not have to do much in terms of supplying strength, and in fact the shearing strength provided by this system very greatly exceeds that necessary to make it work with a reliability or probability of $p = .95$.

Lesson: Learn the generalities but always watch for the special circumstances that can modify them in a particular case. You will work more effectively and enjoy it more too.

For example, as mentioned previously the form of mechanical motion usually most deleterious to fracture union constitutes shearing motions of the two fracture surfaces. Should one use an intramedullary nail of a circular cross section and/or of insufficient diameter to completely fill up the marrow cavity of a fractured humerus (or radius or femur or whatever), then if the fracture does not receive some kind of additional mechanical protection from torque during the healing phase, the two fragments can spin around the rod as could two spools threaded on the same spindle. The shearing motion of the cortical surface of one fragment rotating on the other in this manner, can delay union. In fact this represents a not infrequently seen cause of delayed and/or non-unions in orthopaedic practice. This problem does not represent a defect in the design, material or manufacture of the device, but rather a suboptimal use of it.*

Another kind of patient-procedure mismatch: doing a total hip replacement or cup arthroplasty or Moore prosthetic hip replacement operation on a patient who must earn his living by doing hard physical work, such as construction work, plumbing, building, carpentry, stevedoring and the like. With P > .95 such a patient *will not prove able to return to his original job and will require job retraining*. And if you arrange for that retraining first, the deloading of the diseased hip afforded thereby may lead to enough improvement in symptoms *that an operation becomes unnecessary*.

---

* Interestingly in regard to choices of implants and procedures, one finds many different beliefs around the country, many of which probably have little true basis. For example, in some parts of the United States group opinion favors the use of bone plates and screws for internal fixation over all other means, and hold use of an intramedullary device as close to *prima facie* evidence of professional stupidity. Yet, two or three states away exactly the converse may apply. And in our country we frown on treating fractured tibias in traction ("it causes distraction which causes nonunion") but on many parts of the European continent it forms the usual—and most effective—mode of treatment. In point of fact, in most such situations, a group that favors some method to the virtual exclusion of others simply learned to use it properly but never did learn to use properly the techniques they frown on, and blamed their ineptness on the device rather than on their failure or inability to work within its limitations. Not a criticism; just an observation, for *mea culpa* too.

And similarly with shoulder, knee and elbow replacement arthroplasties.

Yet another cause of failure could arise by using an acceptable device in a manner which runs contrary to the biomechanical facts or milieu of the local anatomy. For example, some occasions still arise when a proper solution to a hip problem might constitute using one of the hip endoprostheses which has a perfectly straight stem, somewhat similar to the original Judet and/or Charles Townley's design. However for such a device to function satisfactorily in the hip one must insert it in some valgus so that the head sits or perches fairly upright upon the stump of the neck, creating nearly uniaxial compression loading at the mechanical interface between the two. Should a surgeon insert such a device in too much varus (which you cannot do with Chuck Townley's unless you try—real hard), the postoperative, largely vertical load resultant (arising partly because of inherent motor weakness and partly because of pain which makes the patient protect the hip by inhibiting the muscles that pull midially on the upper femur) will apply very large vertically aligned shearing loads to the implant-bone interface. More often than not these shearing loads will exceed the capacity of the living tissues to accept and adapt to, and they will gradually begin to crumble away before the device—causing it either to work loose in the bone, or making the bone supporting it fracture.

Similarly, certain types of plastic prosthesis made for the interphalangeal joints in the hand, provide by design pure flexural motion at a fairly good level of mechanical endurance and clinicians such as Boyd, Flat, Carroll, Littler, and Swanson make effective use of them. However, the joints in which we implant such devices often actually function so as to apply a very large shearing load across the cross section of these prostheses (38), and when that happens the plastic material of which they are made may prove unable to carry this load and may fracture in shear.

In the same vein, should one choose to internally fix by means of screws, or a screw-plate combination, an osteotomy or a fracture of any bone (such as the humerus, femur, or tibia) which has an unusual amount of osteoporosis, the thin cortex which accompanies that osteoporosis means that relatively little bone/metal interface exists across each screw. As a consequence a local mechanical overload can develop, not of the metal (which in this situation proves far stronger than required) but of the bone. Overloaded beyond its capacity to accept and adapt to, it can then fail mechanically, loosening the screw and the whole internal fixation. Of course one can protect the patient from such a failure by increasing the number of screws to provide a larger total bone/metal contact area or interface, or by using longer plates to provide a greater mechanical advantage for the end screws, and/or by protecting the internal fixation in a mechanical sense during the postoperative healing phase by some practical means such as cast, bed rest, brace and/or the like. This obviously constitutes one of those situations which the surgeon must try to assess accurately in advance, and to compensate for by some means. It does not comprise a situation which the implant designers or manufacturers could reasonably solve for us.

QUESTIONS: CHAPTER 23

1) Given two Steinman pins of ⅛ in O.D. (outside diameter), one threaded and one smooth, which will prove stronger in tension? In flexure? In compression?

2) You must apply supracondylar skeletal traction to the femur of an osteoporotic elderly patient, and have your choice of a 3/32 in. Kirschner wire, a threaded 5/32 in. Steinman pin and a smooth Steinman pin of the same O.D. Which would you select? Why?

3) Your chief tells you not to use screw drivers made of a different metal than the bone screws, because of a danger of corrosion caused by transfer of metal from the screw driver to the screw head (168). Evaluate.

4) a) Given: Intertrochanteric hip fracture well reduced and internally fixed with a Jewett nail, in a hip with

markedly reduced motion due to advanced and preexisting osteoarthritis. Patient sent home on crutches three weeks later; no cast or brace. At four weeks postoperation the nail breaks as the patient gets into a car and the surgeon tells the patient it therefore must have had a manufacturing defect. Evaluate.

b) So the surgeon repeats the operation, and the postoperative advice, and—again!—the nail breaks at four weeks postop. Evaluate.

5) An intramedullary nail requires removal a week after its insertion. May one save it to use in another patient?

6) During an operation to internally fix an osteotomy, it proves necessary to bend or contour a plate with bending irons to make it coapt properly to a curved bone surface. We know that this weakens the plate and some authors have stated for that reason that one should not do it. What do you think?

7) An implant manufacturing combine has undertaken an engineering design study to duplicate in an inanimate total joint replacement, tension loads presumed carried by the tension trabeculae in the:

    a) femoral head and neck
    b) distal femoral condyles
    c) tuber os calcis
    d) humeral head
    e) tibia at the ankle joint.

The engineers expect that in doing so they will more exactly duplicate natural conditions and so better duplicate the function of the living, normal parts.

Evaluate the accuracy of the assumption underlying the project.

Chapter 24

Implant Acceptance Criteria

By IMPLANT, WE mean here any artificial, man-made device intended for implantation within the living body. Table 22.01 listed some of the more commonly used categories of implants currently serving in human bodies, most with acceptable levels of success. We must say a few words about the meaning of acceptable success in this chapter, and some of the considerations involved in assessing it. We will take up three categories of such considerations: biological, materials properties, and design. Before doing so the text must make one quasiphilosophical point, as follows:

No man-conceived design or man-made device will prove perfect. Thus some probability of failure will exist for any and all designs, and separate probabilities of failure will arise in actually making the devices, in actually installing them, and in actually using them. The inverse probabilities (of not failing, i.e., of proving successful) may run all the way from $p = .9999$ (i.e., one failure in 10,000 installations) which is very, very good and not yet attainable in orthopaedic surgical practice, to $p = .0001$, meaning only one in 10,000 such usages will succeed. Increasingly in coming years as we learn to think of such matters as systems, and as our testing expertise improves, we will have to categorize our procedures in such terms. As an illustrative example however, at this writing a success probability of a total hip replacement of $p = .95$, or of a femoral head replacement prosthesis of $p = .90$, represent very high levels of practical and actual achievement. Do not forget then: some probability of failure exists in anything we do, and hangs over our patients like Damocles' sword. It must always be acknowledged, and our decisions must take it into account.

Now for matters of acceptability.

I: BIOLOGICAL CRITERIA FOR IMPLANT MATERIAL ACCEPTABILITY

Whatever material one may use to construct a particular device, whether it serves as a space filler, a suture, as a means for transmitting mechanical loads, as a means for conveying biodynamic information, as a fluid transport system, or as a mechanical articulation substituting for a biological one, it must ideally fulfill the following conditions with respect to the reactions of living tissues to it, particularly those tissues of the musculoskeletal system (109,128).

1) PRIMARY NOXIOUS CELLULAR EFFECT: It should not irritate, poison, or otherwise directly injure the health of the living cells in the tissues in contact with it. If it does irritate them it may evoke a sterile inflammatory response which could lead to its rejection by the body. And such injury could impair local resistance to infection and local healing pro-cesses. *Most such effects arise from chemical reactivity of the implant with the body fluids.* For such a reason the implant material should not prove highly reactive chemically with the body tissues, nor with any of the diverse solutes dissolved in its fluids. One should understand at the outset that no material known remains totally nonreactive in the chemical sense in the human body, so that we must define some minimum level of reactivity below which an implant will prove acceptable, above which it would prove suspect, and much above which it would prove unacceptable. Thus, materials such as iron, brass, aluminum, vanadium steel and the hardenable stainless steels have proven unacceptable for implants buried in body; their level of chemical reactivities cause obvious harm. Correspondingly, materials such as teflon, polyethylene, dacron, nylon, methacrylate, the 316 stainless steels, and the chrome-cobalt and chrome-cobalt-tungsten alloys have proven quite satisfactory in this regard. In this area some manufacturers' agents in promoting their own material have sometimes used specific in vitro chemical tests of the reactivity of their competitors' materials to create the impression that the latter were dangerous, although both of the major alloy systems currently in use have proven rea-

sonably free of such trouble in actual clinical use. Such questionable forms of advertising or salesmanship seem to try to make monetary mountains out of clinical trivia, and reflect adversely upon their users. Keep in mind the following, in reflecting on such problems: Corrosion of mettallic implants has two faces. One represents the possible harmful effects of its solubilized metal atoms on the local cells, and represents a subcategory of the whole class of primary noxious cellular effects. The second constitutes the adverse effects of that loss of metal upon the implant itself, usually in terms of greatly enhanced likelihood of a fatigue failure. Of course both can occur, and with implants of older manufacture (pre-1945) they did. Doctors E. Obletz and P. A. Casagrande introduced me as a resident to clinical examples of this phenomenon in 1950.

Note: Chemical reactivity of an implant material proves a product-function of two independent factors or variables: the inherent chemical reactivity of the material per unit exposed surface area, multiplied by the total surface exposed, in a unit amount of tissue. Thus if we define the chemical reactivity of an implant as A_0, the millimoles of reactive by-products produced in the body per square cm of surface of such material in a year's time as M, and the total surface exposed to a unit volume of those tissues as S, we have this relation:

$$A_0 = MS \hspace{4cm} Equation\ 24.01$$

This relation has already achieved clinical-level significance, in this way. In some total joint designs, metal slides on metal (rolling motion forms another situation entirely). This can produce very fine particles of the metal forming the bearing surfaces (see the chapter dealing with friction in Part I), which accumulate in the tissues and cells in contact with the prosthesis as a sludge. Now when a solid one cm^3 mass of such a metal in the form of a single cube (with a total surface area of 6 cm^2) becomes pulverized to a very fine powder, its total surface area can increase more than 1,000,000 times. *And its chemical effects on tissues will increase in ap-*

proximately similar fashion. Thus the intact cube may not evoke any measurable harmful effects on the embedding tissues but the same amount of material in the form of fine particulate debris may prove a total disaster, evoking irritation, potentiating infection and retarding biological repair and adaptive processes. This phenomenon, another one of the many surface-to-volume ratio effects we find in skeletal physiology, can lead to rejection of a device suffering from such an adverse effect.

2) PRIMARY TISSUE IRRITATIVE EFFECT: Sounds like we repeat ourselves, but we do not. Where the noxious effect deadens a tissue's cellular responses (because it kills cells), the irritative effect primarily exaggerates them. Should the material stimulate directly, or by other indirect means evoke, an excessive repair response or tissue reaction, it may cause the local formation of overly abundant bone, cartilage, and/ or scar production around it. This could create an undesirable bulky mass, one both palpable and visible, depending on its location. Thus a finger, swollen because of such a response to an artificial joint lying between two of its bones, may prove more unsatisfactory to the patient than the original problem it was supposed to alleviate. Such a response may also nullify the ability of the implant to serve its specific purpose. Thus excessive scar and/or bone production around an artificial joint can nearly totally stiffen or ankylose it, defeating at least one of the purposes of the original operation. All of the currently employed alloys have such effects in some patients, although fortunately in a small minority of them. As an entity this effect has not received much recognition yet from materials investigators but it will for clinical experience shows it assuredly occurs.

3) THE NEOPLASTIC EFFECT: The material should not evoke a neoplastic response by tissues, neither locally nor systemically, particularly a malignant one. Needless to say, one would not choose implant materials which could induce cancerous neoplasms in the human body, for reasons too obvious to require further discussion.

4) The Infection-facilitative Effect: It should not enhance the likelihood of developing a local infection. Some materials seem to have the property of reducing the resistance to infection of tissues immediately in contact with them. This can lead to delayed infections, and/or infections by pathogens not ordinarily causing overt infection in otherwise healthy bodies and tissues. Several of the metals, alloys and plastic materials that have served for implant construction in times past (and to some degree even at the present time) have demonstrated this undesirable property. In some of these materials it persists as a permanent effect while in others it seems only temporary and declines with time.

5) Remodeling Effect: The material should not suppress or impair the normal local tissue remodeling mechanisms required to maintain both biological and mechanical competence in bone, cartilage and fibrous tissue structures. As mentioned previously here, and in Volume III too, these mechanisms probably serve to repair mechanical fatigue damage processes in living structural materials while they still remain microscopic and so trivial in extent. As Volume III took some pains to drive home, these effects deal less with cellular biochemistry as conventionally conceived than they do with the problems of mesenchymal cell proliferation, cellular differentiation and the sigma values appropriate for each phase of a sequential process as well as for their summed up value. Consequently an implant which, because of some unexpected chemical or physical property, actually and actively somehow suppresses such remodeling activity in the tissues immediately surrounding it, might subsequently lead to a spontaneous failure, such as a bone fracture or a tendon or ligament rupture, obviously undesirable complications of any implant insertion operation. Lacking any published studies of this effect and property of implant materials at this writing, our chief experience with it and grounds for suspecting it must remain clinical for the present. To study such phenomena effectively and unambiguously, it will prove necessary to use the tetracycline-based system for studying bone modeling and remodeling dynamics de-

veloped in the author's laboratory (90,100,188,193). Fortunately the two alloy systems most commonly used to fashion contemporary metallic implants seem fairly free of such adverse effects, and the same probably holds true of most of the other materials currently used as sutures in present surgical practice.

6) THE CLOTTING EFFECT: When serving as an artificial heart valve, or as a tube to decompress the ventricles of the brain by draining cerebrospinal fluid into some other body compartment (one way of managing hydrocephalus), the implant material should not provoke the production of clots, whether of fibrin primarily or of the platelet-induced type. Orthopaedists have not yet had to cope with such matters but that will probably prove temporary—our specialty diversifies continually into new areas.

7) THE ALLERGENIC EFFECT: We said enough of this in the previous chapter and only list it here for the sake of completeness.

II: MECHANICAL ACCEPTANCE CRITERIA FOR IMPLANT MATERIALS

Setting aside the problems of the chemical and biological reactions that implant materials may evoke in living tissues, and which arise peculiarly by virtue of their living state, we may next consider some of the purely mechanical or physical properties an implant material should possess to make it acceptable for use in the human body. Such criteria would include the following:

1) STRENGTH: The material should possess adequate mechanical strength to serve its purpose. That purpose of course affects one's choice, for obviously totally different strength criteria affect the choice of an implant material serving as a suture with a maximum useful life somewhere under six weeks on the one hand, and on the other the choice of a material to serve as part of an artificial hip joint which will bear sizeable mechanical loads daily for the remaining years of the patient's life. In the former case gradual loss of

strength as the wound heals proves quite acceptable but in the latter case such a process might lead to failure of the device, possibly at a later time in life when age plus the onset of serious medical problems have made it a risky proposition to restore the function of the joint or repair the device by performing another operation.

Table 24.01 lists some of the broad purposes for which we use implants and implant materials.

2) STIFFNESS: The Young's modulus (or in the inverse sense the static compliance) of the material should prove acceptable in the mechanical sense, first for its purpose (including its intended useful service life) and second to the tissue in which it will lie embedded. Again, in designing materials to serve as sutures the material's rigidity rates rather low on the scale of those factors one must take into account in making an optimal choice, simply because of the limited period of time one requires that a suture possess tensile strength.

But when one intends an implant to transfer sizeable mechanical loads from one bone to another for long periods of time, whether across an articulation of any kind or not, the stiffness of the material under dynamic loading conditions *relative to that of the bone under similar conditions* becomes an important matter. This holds true because when one joins by some means two materials of differing stiffness, and then transfers mechanical, and especially changing, loads across them, *the stiffer material becomes the more highly stressed.* However in the case of bone on metal the strength of the latter may so greatly exceed that of the former

TABLE 24.01
PURPOSES OF ORTHOPAEDIC IMPLANTS

Osteosynthesis (temporary)	Load carrying bone replacements (temporary or permanent) (compression and flexure)
Space filler (temporary or permanent)	To alter skeletal growth patterns (temporary)
Total joint replacements (temporary or permanent)	To monitor some physiologic activity (temporary or permanent)
Nerve stimulatory (temporary or permanent)	To transport fluid (temporary or permanent)

(which, remember, is a brittle substance) that the bone actually begins to crumble near the bone-metal interface, but if under such conditions the inanimate part also lacks the necessary endurance in fatigue it then will develop a fatigue failure. It has not yet become customary for designers to give this aspect of implant design much thought, not out of negligence but primarily because the range of choices of biologically acceptable implant materials remains so small that we must accept some penalties, mechanically speaking, to come up with materials acceptable in the biological sense.

3) ENDURANCE IN FATIGUE: Here again one must choose a material appropriate to its purpose and intended service life. Accordingly, a material which fails after 500,000 cycles at its designed stress limits would prove eminently satisfactory for a suture, but disastrous for an arterial graft (cyclically stressed some 100,000 times daily), or an artificial joint, or a partial but load-bearing replacement for a bony diaphysis. On the other hand, a material with indifferent fatigue endurance might prove quite acceptable for making an intramedullary rod or a bone plate which one intends to maintain mechanical alignment and provide fixation only until the bone healing process can make the natural load-carrying tissues able to take over the mechanical function of that portion of the skeleton.

4) DYNAMIC COMPLIANCE: Soon enough we will have to face the problem of trying to match the dynamic stiffness or compliance of an implant material to the tissues embedding it and delivering mechanical loads to it or taking them from it. But we cannot do this effectively with our present range of biologically acceptable materials, and the problem will become more urgent only when newer and better implant materials (and more challenging and taxing designs and usages thereof) become available. A variety of laboratories work on this problem today.

III: DESIGN CRITERIA FOR IMPLANT ACCEPTABILITY

In this area two quite separate problems arise, one relating to the design of the implant itself, the other (and equally important but much less studied) to the interface between it and living tissues.

1) IMPLANT DESIGN CONSIDERATIONS: These consist of achieving shapes, cross sections, and relationships which will allow the implant to perform its assigned function with a high degree of reliability, over a long period of time and yet with a minimum volume of implant material.

Thus, again a 4–0 cotton suture, a poor material from the standpoint of its fatigue properties if used as a tension carrying device upon which life, or some living function, had to depend on for many months or years, nevertheless serves eminently satisfactorily for repairing soft tissue wounds because, within 3 to 4 weeks after suturing, the wounds will have healed well enough that living tissues take over the previous functions of the sutures. The sutures then become an unnecessary and—hopefully and usually—quite inert foreign body embedded in the soft tissues. Accordingly the cross sectional shape of the suture and its surface finish represent trivial matters.

However a patient may need and depend on a hip prosthesis for twenty or more years, so one must choose external shapes of mechanically heavily loaded regions which do not create stress risers that can lead to fatigue failures at some time in the future. For analogous reasons one must also utilize chemical and physical surface-finishing procedures which, by making exposed surfaces smooth and homogeneous, satisfactorily minimize the chance that surface defects (whether physical or chemical in nature) may initiate a future failure in mechanical fatigue. Recall from our earlier discussions of mechanical statics that flexure and torque prove particularly troublesome in causing high surface stresses in structures, and especially when they act in combination. It follows that designs which somehow minimize such loads and combinations should prove better than those which create them. Furthermore one must choose total cross section areas of the implant material so that, given the material's known inherent strength, one reduces unit stress levels within it enough to provide acceptable protection from a fatigue failure.

Finally, in designing implants one must have in mind the manner in which the active human body will apply loads to it. As some of the previous chapters have probably suggested to physicians of my vintage and older, this may differ significantly from what seemed apparent to our own teachers in dissecting room studies of the muscular apparatus that actuates a particular set of joints, or that acts upon a particular bone. To match implant design to body function, we need to arrange or relate the various parts of a device in some way which minimizes surface flexural and torque stresses, and which similarly (but on a much lower priority) minimizes uniaxial loads. In this respect we will need at some time in the fairly near future to construct a lexicon or atlas which outlines the typical magnitudes and spatial orientations of the time-averaged mechanical loads carried by those parts of the skeletal system which we now do, or may in the future attempt to, replace by inanimate implants or endoprostheses. Some of the basic principles required to obtain such atlases appear in the cited references (97,99).

2) BONE-DEVICE INTERFACE: This second and really major problem in biomechanical implant design has received relatively little analytical thought and study to date. It deals with the absolute size, geometry and spatial orientation of the interface between the living and the inanimate structures, and across which mechanical loads will transfer. We can consider these problems from the standpoint of the three principal strains, that is, tension, compression, and shear.

(*a*) *Tension loading design factors*: This design problem poses two separate challenges: providing the necessary durability, and providing an effective tension anchor between living and dead structures. So far we have not yet developed biologically acceptable artificial materials which combine the flexural compliance with the tensile strength and rigidity of collagen, plus living fibrous tissues' resistance to mechanical fatigue in cyclic tension loading. Thus we cannot yet weave ropes out of fine threads of such artificial materials and expect them to provide a useful service life. This does not mean that we cannot find such materials (note that Dacron arterial grafts have proven fairly durable in this respect over periods of 10-plus years, although they carry relatively low loads compared to those applied by major muscles to their tendons). Indeed, materials satisfactory in this respect may already be in production in chemical plants around the world. But we have not gotten around to studying that aspect of their mechanical properties for another, more troublesome and more basic reason, listed next.

For an inanimate prosthetic tendon or ligament to function properly as such in the human body, one needs some means of anchoring each of its ends to the appropriate structures, one end of which will apply a tension load that it has accepted from the other. But at present we have no adhesive capable of performing such a function which simultaneously has the necessary biological and mechanical properties. In order to develop such implants in the future we may have to learn how to make nature do some of our work for us, that is, how to make her interlace such a device with both natural collagen and living cells, and in such a fashion that the mechanical transition from the living to the inanimate becomes gradual, mechanically sound, and durable and self-repairing in fatigue. The description of the natural tension-transfer mechanisms described in an earlier chapter may prove helpful in this regard. This represents an interesting potential area of research in biomechanics which remains virtually untouched at this writing.

(*b*) *Compression*: Here too we face two separate problems: the unit load factor, and the shape factor. With increasing frequency orthopaedists employ devices which transfer compression loads from one bone to another, either across an articulation of some type, or within a single bone, part of which we have replaced with an implant. Failures of such devices, in terms of gradual creeping encroachment of the inanimate into and through the animate, still occur far too frequently for comfort. They probably have two chief causes:

First, excessive unit loading in compression occurs at the mechanical interface between the two.

Second, that interface often has an *improper shape* or contour.

1) *The unit loading factor*: Thus our present Austin-Moore prostheses have a base plate area lying in contact with the calcar femorale that probably lies close to marginal in biomechanical acceptability, because in approximately eighty percent of the patients who accept such a device it appears to function quite well, at least at that location. But in some twenty percent of them a variety of signs appear that the bone side of that interface has gotten into trouble to such an extent that it causes severe pain, or/and it gradually gives way over time before the advancing piston or pile-driver of the metal above it. The unit loading of the bone-metal interface which separates satisfactory from unsatisfactory probably lies somewhere between 10 kg/cm^2 and 100 kg/cm^2*. Certainly my clinical experience indicates that designs which cause the higher unit loadings produce most failures of the creeping encroachment type, and they do so with increasing regularity as the unit loading factor ascends.

One can take two different approaches to reducing the unit loading factor. One, employing some effective combination of mechanical and biological design features, was illustrated in the chapter of joints, in which some of the features of the roller-bearing hip replacement system were described. Another which becomes increasingly popular consists of using a plastic, self-hardening cement as a filler between implant and living bone, a filler which enlarges the total bone-device interface and simultaneously provides nearly total contact at that interface.

2) *The shape of the bone-metal interface*: As to that shape, we might take two clues, one from one of the ways

---

* And it amazes one that no one seems to have tried to determine its approximate value by controlled laboratory experiments.

that nature prefers to do things, and another from some of our past unhappy experiences with certain designs. Both tend to support the intelligence I draw from them.

Basically, the shape of every long bone in the body causes the end loads transferred to it across its articulations to generate a very distinct "necking in" force in the metaphyseal cortex, one which tends to make the cortex constrict upon itself as the end loads develop. This suggests that shapes which deliberately mimic that force at the primary interface between living and inanimate compression-loaded materials, may prove more acceptable to living bone mechanically speaking than perfectly plane interfaces or, even worse, those shapes which have somewhat convex surfaces which generate an exploding or wedging load in the living tissue each time a compression load develops on top of them. This property has not yet received much recognition and has appeared only occasionally in established designs, for example in the base plate of the contemporary Austin-Moore prosthesis, which seems to have evolved largely by trial and error.* Lacking direct experimental tests of course, this property remains a conjecture. However, observation of past device failures makes it quite clear to me that plane and/or convexly curved, intruding interface shapes prove mechanically unacceptable to bone in an unusually high fraction of the instances in which such devices were employed. Accordingly, one should avoid them.

(*c*) *Shear*: By shear at a device-tissue interface we mean as an example the tendency of the base plate of an Austin-Moore prosthesis to move anteriorly or posteriorly on the underlying bone during the normal gait cycle, or for the tibial component of a total knee prosthesis to move similarly on the tibia during the gait cycle. By some means of course one must transfer these shearing forces from the inanimate to the animate, and in such a fashion that the latter does not object, or fail in some way under that onslaught over time.

---

* A perfectly good way to arrive at a serviceable design if one can accept its penalties, such as the slow rate of progress achieved by such means and the human costs of the necessary errors and blind alleys it creates of necessity.

Here we find a fairly reliable clue as to how to do it success-fully, one lying in the way that nature achieved the same purpose in anchoring our children's epiphyseal plates to their metaphyses. If you gelatinize away the cartilage in such plates in an immature animal such as a dog, or even a leg of mutton or a ham hock,* and then examine the apposing

---

* Simply by boiling it for two hours or so.

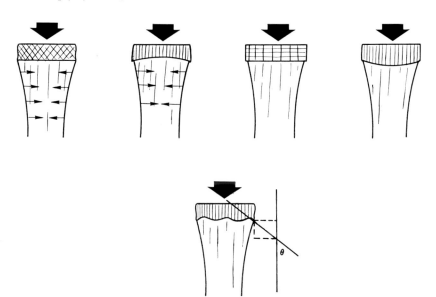

Figure 24.01. *On the left:* You see a "typicalized" bone, which demon-strates an epiphyseal flat portion above (arbitrarily becoming part of the metaphysis after the age at which the epiphyseal plate closes), and the inwaisted metaphyseal-diaphyseal part below. The arrows designate the necking-in force generated by this shape when under uniaxial compression loading.
 Second: For an artificial "epiphysis," such as part of a joint replace-ment design, a concave bone-device interface or surface proves more ac-ceptable to the bone, i.e., bone demonstrates less tendency to crumble ahead of it or to loosen under it in shear, than
 Third: a flat interface, or
 Right: a convex one, the worst type from the standpoint of the biological responses it can evoke.
 Bottom: Nature actually shapes this interface in this manner, and until we have good reason to hold ourselves out as better bioengineers than she, we could do worse than copy her example. Note that the total vertical load across the part exerts a "locking" force in shear, a function of the tangent of the angle of the inclination of the slopes of the hills.

sides of the epiphysis and metaphysis, you will observe that they have hills and valleys, and the hills in one side match exactly the valleys in the other, as shown in Figure 24.01. Since our anatomy arranges matters so that these plates carry large compression loads during normal function, and since our efficient joints cause only approximately one per cent of those loads to translate as drag, creating a lateral shearing load during normal function, you can see that the large compression loads very actively and effectively force the hills of the one structure into the valleys of the other, thereby locking them securely to prevent effectively any shearing displacement. Man could do worse in this instance than to emulate nature and produce contours of similar style for use in similar applications.

CONCLUSION

That does it, *messieurs et mesdames*. After a final quiz, Part III in the remaining pages contains the review matter in nine Appendices, 19 special tables, a Glossary, answers to the questions, a bibliography, an index—and a postscript. I sincerely hope you have found the text informative and that some of it may also prove useful, to you personally, to your residents and most of all to your patients.

QUESTIONS: CHAPTER 24

1) In the accompanying AP x-ray of a child's knee (Figure 24.02) one can see the femoral epiphyseal plate has a hill in its middle, with a mean slope of 14°. Given a 100 kg uniaxial compression load acting across the knee, and so across this epiphyseal plate, how much side thrust must one apply to the epiphysis to unlock this hill and valley arrangement to cause a lateral slip of the epiphysis? You may ignore any inherent shearing strength of the plate and assume it would flow as freely as any liquid.

2) Referring to the same x-ray, account in biomechanical terms for the known fact that children's skeletons prove more difficult to break (i.e., tougher) than adult's from

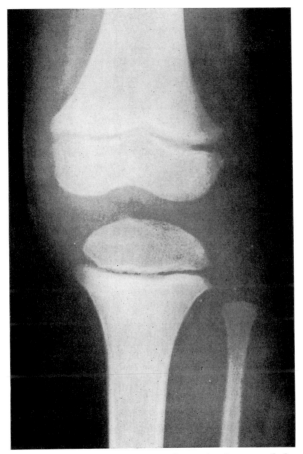

Figure 24.02. X-ray of a child's knee seen from the front, and demonstrating the distal femoral and proximal tibial epiphyses, the clear linear zones representing the unmineralized hyaline cartilage of the epiphyseal plate, and the wide clear zone between the two bones the articular cartilage, rather thick in young children as you can see.

vertically aligned forces, such as might arise by falling erect from a height, or from blunt, slow-moving flexural loads.

Now, for those who like to play "name games" here are a few to tease your colleagues with:

3) Who first claimed that mechanical force played a major role in determining a) bone architecture? b) and chondral architecture?

4) Who first defined the principles of action that actually relate mechanical forces to lamellar bone architecture? Articular architecture? Limb alignment during growth? Total strength of fibrous tissue structures? The time-averaging property of the systems responses involved therein? The concepts of modeling (as distinct from growth), and the modeling barrier?

5) a) Who first described the generation of electrical potentials on the surfaces of strained bone? b) Who discovered piezoelectricity?

6) Who first described the tetracycline bone marking phenomenon?

7) Who first used the tetracycline marking phenomenon to measure an appositional rate? A true bone formation rate (88)? A true bone resorption rate? Values for the BMU population dynamics? To "resolve" cellular, tissue and organ level dynamic phenomena?

8) a) Who first described unmineralized bone, osteoid or organic matrix? b) The scalloping of surfaces by osteoclasts? c) The secondary osteon?

9) Who discovered the electrochemical basis of the corrosion of metallic implants?

10) Who made a workable therapeutic technology or expertise out of a) mould arthroplasty? b) total hip replacement c) femoral head replacement? d) intramedullary nailing?

11) a) Who is responsible for the BMU concept? b) For the sigma concept? c) For recognizing the regional acceleratory effect and the phase lag pool? d) For placing on a quantitative basis the determination of skeletal transients and steady states? e) For the bone "envelope" concept?

12) a) Who initiated most modern studies of the materials properties of bone? b) The concept of the instant center or rotation of joints? c) The concept of the feedback control system? d) Who made the major solutions to the analysis of column instability?

13) a) Who discovered the differential calculus? b) That the sum of the square of its sides equals the square of a right triangle's hypotenuse? c) That a body displaces a mass of fluid equal to its own mass if it floats in it and its own volume if it sinks? d) Who developed common logarithms? e) The slide rule? f) The concept of gravitational attraction? g) Who defined gravitational attraction, mass and weight?

14) Who discovered the alloying of metals? Hardening by heat treatment? Bronze? Brass? The journal? The pulley? The lever? The wheel? The scissors? The knife? Forging? The screw? Pipe? Wire? Columns? Beams? Elasticity? Gyroscopic stabilization? Friction? The concept of number? And of equations?

15) a) Who discovered cobalt? b) Chromium? c) Magnesium? d) Calcium? e) Aluminum? f) Nickle? g) Phosphorus? h) Tantalum? i) Titanium? j) Tungsten?

PART III

APPENDICES

Introduction

LIKE THE GREAT majority of my colleagues, I managed to get through high school, college and medical school in spite of absorbing an absolute minimum of mathematics of all kinds. Then the research bug bit and it became increasingly if alarmingly apparent that some math might serve a useful function. But of course, it had to be learned and/or re-learned by self-study. That effort revealed where some of a physician's hangups in these matters typically lie. And hence in this part of the book some elementary review and explanatory material for those who, like me, probably became exposed to such matters long ago and then promptly forgot them. And, from my generation backwards, it remains possible to practice high quality orthopaedics without using even arithmetic. *But, from your generation forward that can no longer be.* As happened in aviation, mechanical and electrical engineering, physics, chemistry and pharmacology, the slide rule has just begun to become an essential part of our diagnostic and therapeutic action, and within another 20 years residents taking their orthopaedic boards may need to have one (or an electronic, solid-state equivalent) with them in order to answer some of the questions. And that is good, not bad, for it means in the therapeutic sense that we steadily become able to shoot higher and farther, and within tighter cones of dispersion. So for you fellows who go into peripheral vascular collapse (!) when you see $x = Y^2$, or $x = Y + 2Z$, there follows some refresher material intended simply to make some of the math appearing in the first two parts of this book more easily understandable.

Algebra Review

1) PROPORTIONS: One readily understands that 1 is to 2 as 13 is to 26; or 3 is to 4 as 15 is to 20, and so on. We can write these relations as simple proportions (used later to solve some of the trigonometric problems in Appendix 5) as follows:

$$\frac{0.5}{1} = \frac{13}{26}; \frac{3}{4} = \frac{15}{20}$$

But now let us assume that we know the left hand proportion to represent the sine of an angle, meaning the side facing the angle in question, divided by the hypotenuse of a right triangle, given that the hypotenuse has a length of one (of any units of length you choose). The value of the left hand side of the left proportion of course equals $\frac{1}{2}$ or, 0.5, however you prefer to write it for it makes no difference in the result. Assume further that we have another right triangle, representing the alignment of the semitendonosus tendon with the tibia, with a partially flexed knee. The angle between the long axis of the tibia and the tendon equals the same as the one for which the table of sines gave the value of 0.5, namely 30°. Furthermore, we know by measurements that the value of the posteriorly directed component of the semitendonosus muscle's contractile force in this problem consists of 91 kg f.

Problem: Find the muscle's direct-line pull, parallel to its tendon. Simple: we set up a proportion. For *any* angle of 30° in *any* right triangle, no matter how large or small, the trigonometry section shows that the facing side relates to the hypotenuse as $\frac{0.5}{1}$ or $\frac{1}{2}$. So we can write, using x simply to

473

signify the unknown tendon pulling force we wish to determine:

$$\frac{0.5}{1} = \frac{91}{x}$$ (or with perfectly equal validity,

$$\frac{1}{2} = \frac{91}{x}$$

Now we find it as follows:

a) Multiply both sides by x (when you multiply two equals by any same number, their products must also remain equal). Thus we have:

$$\frac{0.5x}{1} = \frac{91x}{x}.$$ On the right, $\frac{x}{x} = 1$, which we need not bother to write. In high school you used to say "they cancel out". This yields $\frac{0.5x}{1} = \frac{91x}{x} = 91$

b) Clearly the number one below the line on the left side also seems redundant so we need not write it either. Thus, upon rewriting it, we have:

$$0.5x = 91$$

c) Now let us get rid of the 0.5 (solving any equation for x means to get x all to itself on one side of the equation by any mathematically legitimate means, so that by doing the necessary arithmetic on the other side we can get our answer) by dividing both sides by 0.5 (dividing two equals by the same number leaves their result still equal) :

$$\frac{0.5x}{0.5} = \frac{91}{0.5};$$ cancel out $\frac{0.5}{0.5}$ (because it equals one

and has become redundant) to obtain x $= \frac{91}{0.5}.$

Now divide 91 by 0.5, and you obtain 182, the value of x. Thus the muscle's stright line contractile force equals 182 kg f, and we found it basically by using proportions.

Note: In this problem the value of *x* depended upon the particular values for the length ratio of the triangle's sides (i.e., the sine of 30°), and upon the 91 kg tension load. Both the sine and the load had particular values independently of any effect the value of *x* has on the solution. Consequently we call *x* the *dependent variable*, and those factors which determine or dictate its particular value the *independent variables*. In plotting or graphing things we conventionally plot dependent variables on the vertical axis or *abcissa*, and the independent ones on the horizontal or *ordinate*.

A couple of more examples:

$$\frac{11}{13} = \frac{x}{19}$$

Procedure: get rid of the 19, by multiplying both side by it, thus:

$$\frac{19 \times 11}{13} = \frac{19x}{9}; \quad \frac{19 \times 11}{13} = x$$

or this example:

$$\frac{3.1 \times 10^{-4}}{13} = \frac{41}{x}$$

Procedure: first we will "move up" the *x*:

$$\frac{X \times 3.1 \times 10^{-4}}{2.71} = \frac{41X}{X}; \quad \text{next cancel out, and then}$$

"move over" the 2.71:

$$\frac{X \times 3.1 \times 10^{-4} \times 2.71}{2.71} = 41 \times 2.71; \quad \text{next cancel}$$

out, and then move 3.1 x 10⁻⁴ over:

$$\frac{X \times 3.1 \times 10^{-4}}{3.1 \times 10^{-4}} = \frac{41 \times 2.71}{3.1 \times 10^{-4}}; \quad \text{so finally:}$$

$$X = \frac{41 \times 2.71}{3.1 \times 10^{-4}}$$

2) EQUATIONS: Now let us deal with a related—and very

common—problem. Consider this relation:

$$2.31 = 123X$$

Now, find X. Simple; we take our cues from the above material on proportions. We need to get X all alone on one side of a relation. So we must get rid of the 123 next to it (but, of course, in a mathematically legitimate way!). So divide both sides through it:

$$\frac{2.31}{123} = \frac{123X}{123}; \text{ cancelling out now yields } \frac{2.31}{123} = X.$$

We can write this in a more general form now, using x, y and z to signify the separate terms (i.e., numbers, values, parameters or whatever):

$$X = y\ z$$

It then follows, and any reader trying to relearn this material for himself should then show to his own satisfaction, that:

$$Y = x/z$$
$$Z = x/y$$

To see that these still remain only simple proportions, write them by reinserting the redundant number one, as follows:

$$\frac{Y}{1} = \frac{X}{Z}, \text{ and } \frac{Z}{1} = \frac{X}{Y}$$

Now consider this relation, and the assignment: find Z:

$$X = Y + 2Z$$

Again we do it by getting Z alone on one side. First then let us get ride of its companion, Y, by subtracting Y from both sides (when you subtract the same number from two equals, the remainders remain equal). So:

$$x - y = y + 2z - y.$$ The plus and minus Y's on the right cancel out to yield $x - y = 2z$. So now divide

both sides by two to move the two over, and leave z alone, and one comes up with $\dfrac{x-y}{2} = z$, or $z = \dfrac{x-y}{2}$. Note another way or form of writing this, one which says exactly the same thing:

$$z - \dfrac{x-y}{2} = 0$$

Now consider this expression, which you must solve for X.

$$a = k\ (x-1)$$

Let us get rid of the k first, thus:

$$\dfrac{a}{k} = \dfrac{k}{k}\ (x-1),\ \text{or:}\ \dfrac{a}{k} = (x-1)\ = x-1;\ \text{now let}$$

us get ride of that minus one, by simply adding plus one to both sides:

$$\dfrac{a}{k} + 1 = X - 1 + 1;\ \text{plus one and minus one}$$

on the right add up to zero so let us not write them, so our expression now reads:

$$\dfrac{a}{k} + 1 = X$$

Simple; and now you are an algebraist.

Probability

In various portions of the text we have used the term probability. When we do so, in effect we make a prediction about the outcome of some future event which has two or more possible eventualities. Flipping a coin forms an excellent example. If one flips it a large number of times, and the geometry of the coin and its distribution of mass lie in truly symmetrical fashion around its center, and if the center of geometry and center of mass coincide so that in effect it does not constitute a "loaded" coin, then one will find the number of heads almost exactly equals the number of tails. And if you take the total number of flips, say 10,000, and divide it into the number of times the coin came up heads, the numerical result will very nearly equal 0.5. While it may depart from that by one or two figures in a third or fourth decimal place, as you increase the number of flips, the uncertainty just referred to moves progressively further and further to the right and the numerical answer comes closer and closer to exactly 0.5. Accordingly we say that each time one flips the coin, the probability that heads will come up equals 0.5. Of course, when you actually flip the coin the next time it may turn up tails but that does not destroy the value of this particular line of argument, because all it did was to predict ahead of time the chance that a given result would ensue. One can demonstrate by a variety of means that that prediction taken only in that sense proves accurate.

Accordingly whenever we say that a fracture will heal under particular circumstances with a probability .5, we imply that in a very large number of fractures in identical circumstances, half of them will develop the predicted result and the remainder some other result.

You can appreciate from the manner in which probability was defined above, that the numerical value of a statement of probability can range somewhere between zero and one, but cannot achieve lesser values than zero—nor greater values than one. This means that if a given event has probability zero of happening, we state in effect that no chance, in even the remotest possible circumstances, exists that it will occur. Similarly to say that an event will occur with probability 1.0, says it constitutes an absolute certainty, with no remotest possible chance of any other outcome.

It follows that the probability of an event occurring of $P = .05$ means that it will occur five times out of a hundred, and will not occur the other 95 times. Or with probability $P = .67$, means that it will occur 67 times out of a hundred and will not occur in the other 33.

Now consider two sequentially related events. Let us say that in order for a fracture to heal the required biological activities must transpire first, and then the technical treatment of the fracture must prove adequate so as not to interfere with the biological factors.

Under a particular circumstance, if the probability that the biological part will succeed equals $P = 0.8$, and that the technical treatment will prove adequate equals $P = 0.6$, what constitutes the probability that the whole fracture healing process (obviously some kind of a summation of both factors) will consummate? One solves problems such as this simply by multiplying the individual probabilities. Thus in the situation 0.8 times 0.6 equals 0.48, equals $P = 0.48$, equals the probability that a given fracture under those circumstances will heal. Equally, that result states that given a hundred such fractures under identical circumstances, and 48 will heal and 52 will not.

In stating such estimates, one of course assumes that no additional and modifying but uncontrolled factors exist. And anyone who works much with biological matters (including men) can hardly fail to acknowledge the existence of innumerable factors over which we not only often have little or no control, but many of which we remain blissfully unaware of.

Clearly, too, from the above, it follows that if one defines the probability of occurrence of a particular event, the probability that it will not occur simply represents the number one minus that probability.

This if for event x *not* to occur P = .01, then it *will* occur with probability $1 - .01 = .99$.

Exponents and Logarithms

1) INTRODUCTION: Very useful mathematical devices derive from some of the properties of exponents, and a brief refresher follows. Thus, when we multiply a number by itself we say we square it, and $2 \times 2 = 4$, $3 \times 3 = 9$ and $4 \times 4 = 16$ can also be written as

$$2^2 = 4; \; 3^2 = 9; \; 4^2 = 16, \text{ and so on.}$$

If we multiply any number by itself three times (as $2 \times 2 \times 2 = 8$), we cube it, or raise it to the third power, written thus:

$$2^3 = 8; \; 3^3 = 27; \; 4^3 = 64, \text{ and so on for even higher}$$
powers. The small upper right-hand number represents the *exponent,* and the behavior and convenience of exponents in some kinds of calculations make then highly useful to the engineer, physicist and chemist. To illustrate let us first describe some of the notational conventions found in technical literature.

First, we could write thus of 2 raised to the eighth power:

$$2^8 = 2.2.2.2 \text{ ——— to 8 times. Or in a more general}$$
form now, using x to signify any read number, and n, and m as its exponents:

$$X^n = x.x.x.x. \text{ ——— to } n \text{ times, where } n \text{ equals an}$$

Equation 1

integer, i.e., a whole number. And where such powers become larger and larger with each raise, the reciprocal of such a number becomes smaller and smaller with each raise. We can write the general expression for the reciprocal as:

$$x^{-n} = \frac{1}{x^n}$$

Equation 2

481

In other words, x^{-n} equals the reciprocal of x^n, a re-reciprocal simply signifying dividing the number in question into the number one. Note too then, that for any value of x you wish to choose:

$$x^0 = 1; \; x^1 = x$$

Or, any number raised to the zeroth power equals unity, and raised to the power of one equals itself.

One writes the square root of a number (i.e., that lesser number which, when squared itself, yields the one in question) as:

$\sqrt{2}$, or $\sqrt{3}$; or $\sqrt{9} = 3$; $\sqrt{4} = 2$, and so on. For the cube root one would write $\sqrt[3]{19}$; or $\sqrt[3]{27} = 3$, and likewise for higher roots, Thus $\sqrt[5]{32} = 2$. Then:

$$x^{\frac{n}{m}} = \sqrt[m]{x^n} = \left(\sqrt[m]{x}\right)^n$$

Note that when n equals one or unity, we have:

$$x^{1/2} = \sqrt{x} \qquad\qquad x^{1/3} = \sqrt[3]{x}$$

$$x^{1/6} = \sqrt[6]{X} \qquad\qquad x^{1/4} = \sqrt[4]{X}$$

and so on. In other words, given a fractional exponent such as the $1/6$ at the lower left, this means nothing more or less than "the 6th root of" whatever number it forms the exponent.

2) LAWS OF EXPONENTS: Four laws or rules govern the behavior of exponents:

(*a*) *Multiplication law*: To multiply a number raised to one power, by the same number raised to another power, simply *add* their exponents and raise the number to that sum. Thus:

$$x^n \cdot x^m = x^{n+m} \qquad\qquad \textit{Equation 3}$$

Thus $2^3 \times 2^5$ equals 2^8.

(*b*) *Division law*: To divide two such numbers simply

subtract their exponents and raise the number to the remainder. Thus:

$$x^n \div x^m = x^{n-m} \qquad \qquad \textit{Equation 4}$$

So $3^5 \div 3^2$ equals 3^3.

Observe that the exponent on the right must consist of n minus m in that order, not the other way around for that would mean dividing the number on the right of the equals by that on the left.

(c) *Power rule*: To raise a power of a number to another power, just multiply the exponents and raise the number of their product. Or:

$$\left(x^n\right)^m = x^{nm} \qquad \qquad \textit{Equation 5}$$

(d) *Root rule*: To find or extract a root of a number raised to a power, divide the exponents by that number:

$$\sqrt[m]{x^n} = x^{\frac{n}{m}} \qquad \qquad \textit{Equation 6}$$

Remember that any particular number represents itself raised to the first power, or $9.365^1 = 9.365$; $3.14159^1 = 3.14159$; or $10013^1 = 10013$. Thus the 6th root of $64 = 64^{1/6}$ (which happens to equal the number 2).

Examples: Find: $X^3 \cdot X^9$; Ans: X^{12}

Find: $X^2 \div X^4$; Ans: $X^{2/4} = X^{1/2} = \sqrt{X}$

Find: $(X^4)^2$; Ans: X^8

3) LOGARITHMS: Take any given number, say N. Then any other number X, has some exponent or power to which if you raise it you will uniquely obtain N. Or in symbols as the *exponential form* or notation:

$$N = X^n$$

In this relation, N represents the particular number we wish to manipulate, n (or the exponent of x) we will now term the logarithm (or equally the *mantissa*), and x the base of the logarithm system. Two such bases serve widely in science. One, the number 10, appears in the tables of common logarithms in Special Table 1 of Part III, and we call it the Briggsian system; another, called the base of natural logarithms or the Naperian system, represents the number 2.71828 and the mathematicians call it *e*. Let us rewrite the above expression into its logarithmic form, which says exactly the same thing but with a different notation. Thus:

$$\text{Log } N_x = n \qquad\qquad \textit{Equation 7}$$

We read that expression as follows: the logarithm of N to the base *x* equals *n*. It means: If you raise *x* to the *n* power you will obtain the number N. Let us compare these two notations briefly to ensure we have the basic idea.

Exponential form	*Logarithmic form*
$3^2 = 9$	$\text{Log}_3 \ 9 \ = 2$
$2^4 = 16$	$\text{Log}_2 \ 16 \ = 4$
$10^3 = 1000$	$\text{Log}_{10} \ 1000 = 3$

Now when we use the base 10, i.e., the Briggsian system, we see the following properties emerge, ones quite convenient in scientific calculations. Thus:

$10^{-4} = .0001$	$\text{Log}_{10} \ .0001 \qquad = -4$
$10^{-3} = .001$	$\text{Log}_{10} \ .001 \qquad = -3$
$10^{-2} = .01$	$\text{Log}_{10} \ .01 \qquad = -2$
$10^{-1} = .1$	$\text{Log}_{10} \ .1 \qquad = -1$
$10^0 = 1$	$\text{Log}_{10} \ 1 \qquad = 0$
$10^1 = 10$	$\text{Log}_{10} \ 10 \qquad = 1$
$10^2 = 100$	$\text{Log}_{10} \ 100 \qquad = 2$
$10^3 = 1000$	$\text{Log}_{10} \ 1000 \qquad = 3$
$10^4 = 10,000$	$\text{Log}_{10} \ 10,000 \qquad = 4$
$10^6 = 1,000,000$	$\text{Log}_{10} \ 1,000,000 = 6$

Now observe a further and very useful property: if we construct a table of the logarithms of all numbers between 1 and 10, we can then use it to find quickly the particular logarithms of all smaller and all larger real numbers. Refer to the Special Table 1 of Common Logarithms, and note that the logarithm of 6.21 (i.e., that exponent or power of 10 which yields the number 6.21) equals .7931. Or in logarithmic form, Log$_{10}$ 6.21 $=$ .7931. Then the logarithm of 62.1 $=$ 1.7931; of 621 $=$ 2.7931; or of 6,210 $=$ 3.7931; or of .621 $=$ -1.7931; or of .0621 $=$ $-$ 2.7931; and so on. If this puzzles you, note that a logarithm of 2.0 means 10^2 $=$ 100; or -3.0 means 10^{-3} $=$ .001, so a logarithm of 2.6931 means 10^2 $\times$ 6.21 $=$ 621.

Now to multiply .621 $\times$ 163,000 by the longhand method would take a bit of time. But with logarithms one simply looks up the logs of each, adds them *and finds in the table the number (N) corresponding to their sum.* Depending upon the accuracy needed one can use tables accurate to anywhere from three figures (i.e., three place tables) to over eight (eight-place tables). When one does a great deal of trigonometric computation, he can buy tables providing the logarithms of the trigonometric functions too, which facilitates such work.

The slide rule: Since one simply adds and subtracts exponents of the number 10 to multiply and divide the numbers they represent, one could array on a linear scale the numbers actually corresponding to those exponents of 10, and then by sliding one scale on another perform the analogous and very simple functions of mechanically adding and subtracting the scale lengths corresponding to the exponents, and read off the scale the real numbers written there which they correspond to. Hence the slide rule, invented by an artillery officer named Mannheim. The leaflets accompanying a new slide rule explain their functions in all required detail so we need not attempt to do so here.

Angular Measure

Conventionally we express angles in degrees, but for some purposes *radian measure* (also called circular measure) has considerable convenience. One radian of angular measure equals that angle subtended by the radius of a circle as it sweeps over a length of the circle's perimeter *equal to the length of the circle's radius*. Thus, and since the perimeter of a circle equals 2 π r, and *r*, its radius, equals that length of its perimeter enclosed by an angle of one radian,

$$180° = \pi \text{ radians}; \quad 360° = 2\pi \text{ radians}.$$

$$1° = \frac{\pi}{180} = \frac{1}{57.3} \text{ radians}; \quad 57.3° = 1 \text{ radian}.$$

And any angle equals (where c equals that part of the circumference of the circle actually embraced by the angle, otherwise known as the length of arc) :

$$\text{Angle in radians} = \frac{c}{r} \qquad\qquad \textit{Equation 8}$$

Another unit encountered sometimes constitutes the *mil,* representing the angle subtended by one meter at a distance of a kilometer, i.e., 1000 meters. *Note:* You will find 360°, 2π radians and 6,400 mils of angular measure in a full circle. See Figure 1.

EXAMPLES:

1) A man's forearm extends at the elbow at a rate of 100 radians/second. Given that the distance between the elbow's axis of rotation and the baseball he holds in his hand equals one foot, find the speed given the baseball by this isolated part of the man's body.

Answer: The radius here equals one foot, so the speed of

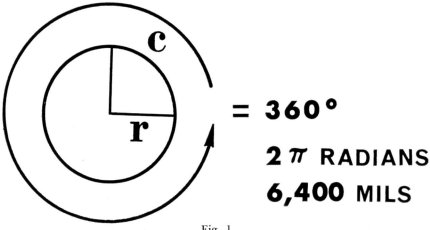

= **360°**

2 π RADIANS

6,400 MILS

Fig. 1

the hand in feet per second relative to the elbow joint equals

$$S = r \text{ radian/sec}$$

or

$$S = 1 \times 100/\text{sec}; \quad s = 100 \text{ ft/sec}$$

2) Now compute *s* for a different situation, one in which a two-foot radius exists.

Answer: $s = 2 \times 100/\text{sec} = 200 \text{ ft/sec}$

3) An object known to have a length of two meters subtends an angle, θ, of one mil from an observation point. Find the object's distance.

$$Answer: \text{ mils at observation point} = \frac{\text{length of object}}{(\text{true range} \div 1000)}$$

Rearranging this, we have: $\text{true range} = \dfrac{\text{length} \times 1000}{\text{mils observed}},$

or

$$\frac{2 \times 1000}{1}$$

So the object lies 2000 meters distant.

Note that the 2 meter length here equals, not a true *arc* of a circle but a *chord*. But for such small angles (below 5° or 6°) the difference betweeen the arc and chord remains so small that one can ignore it for most purposes. Note another sometimes useful property of small angles: The numerical values of their sines and tangents, and their radian measure, correspond so closely one may interchange them at will for most needs. If you wonder why, set each function up on paper for angles of 0.5°, 1°, 2° and 4°, and you will discover it for yourself.

4) An angle, θ has a value of 1.37 radians. Express it in degrees.

Answer: 1 radian $= 57.3°$. Consequently θ (in degrees) $=$ radians $\times$ 57.3 $= 1.37 \times 57.3 = 78.6°$.

5) An angle, θ has a value of 21.4°. Express it in circular measure.

Answer: θ (in degrees) $=$ radians $\times$ 57.3.

Rearranging to solve for radians:

$$\frac{\theta}{57.3} = \text{radians};\qquad \frac{21.4}{57.3} = .374 \text{ radians.}$$

Trigonometry Review

Trigonometric functions in essence relate the angles of triangles to the lengths of their sides. The following exposition will use the degree as a measure of an angle, 360° representing a complete traverse of a point on a circle around its center. And we will follow the further convention of using two axes or lines which intersect at right angles, and which serve as a means for providing coordinates (i.e., as reference lines) which can locate uniquely any point, or any line, in the plane defined by them. These have become known as *Cartesian coordinates.*

1) SINE, COSINE, TANGENT: The three direct trigonometric functions consist of the *sine, cosine* and *tangent,* and in Figure 2 they represent (relative to the angle θ in the right triangle shown therein) the vertical distance AB divided by the hypotenuse, the horizontal OB divided by the hypotenuse; and AB divided by OB, respectively. One may also define the reciprocals* of the above functions, as follows.

$$\text{cosecant } \theta = \frac{1}{\text{Sin } \theta} \quad \text{and:} \quad \tan \theta = \frac{\text{Sin } \theta}{\cos \theta}$$

$$\text{secant } \theta = \frac{1}{\text{Cos } \theta} \quad \text{so:} \quad \cot \theta = \frac{\text{Cos } \theta}{\text{Sin } \theta}$$

$$\text{cotangent } \theta = \frac{1}{\text{Tan } \theta}$$

---

* A reciprocal, to repeat, signifies a simple function of, or operation upon, some number quantity. For example, some parameter has a value of 2.5 units; then its reciprocal equals $\frac{1}{2.5}$. The reciprocal of (as examples now) 5 equals 1/5; of 11 equals 1/11; of 123.6 equals 1/123.6; of 3^2 equals $1/3^2$; of 3.2 log × equals $\frac{1}{3.2 \log x}$, and so on.

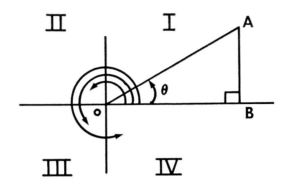

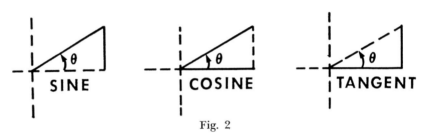

Fig. 2

Obviously the angle θ in Figure 2 represents an arbitrary choice; and the circular lines partly surrounding the origin (i.e., point of intersection where all values on the coordinate axes equal zero) of the coordinate axes simply signify that one may have any variety of larger angles, some of which can wind up to the left of the vertical axis or abcissa, and others below the horizontal axis or ordinate, so that negative values should arise for some of the trigonometric functions. And they do; the following table illustrates those quadrants which have positive and those negative values for particular trigonometric functions. Note that the Roman numbered quadrants correspond to those labeled in the drawing in Figure 2.

Note too that an angle of 1100° represents three complete 360 rotations of a point (such as A) around the origin (0) of a Cartesian coordinate graph, or the center of a circle; plus 20° more left over (i.e., 360° × 3 = 1080°; 1100° − 1080° = 20°). So it follows that the trigonometric functions

Table 1 (a)

Quadrant	I	II	III	IV
Sine, cosec	+	+	—	—
Cos, Sec	+	—	—	+
Tan, cot	+	—	+	—

of an 1100° angle constitute exactly those of any residual left after substracting all possible multiples of 360°.

2) PYTHAGOREAN RELATIONS: Pythagoras noted that for a right triangle (i.e., a triangle in which one of the internal angles equalled exactly 90°) the length of the hypotenuse (the side facing the right angle) squared equalled the sum of the squares of the other two sides. Or if we use lower case letters, *a, b* and *c,* to signify the length of each of its sides, *a* representing the hypotenuse:

$$a^2 = b^2 + c^2$$

or

$$a = \sqrt{b^2 + c^2} \qquad\qquad Equation\ 9$$

From that relation one can deduce, and you can work out for yourself if your curiosity bump so impells you (but we will merely state here) , the comparable trigonometric Pythagorean relations. Thus:

$$Cos^2\theta + Sin^2\theta = 1 \qquad\qquad Equation\ 10$$
$$Sec^2\theta - Tan^2\theta = 1 \qquad\qquad Equation\ 11$$
$$Cosec^2\theta - Cot^2\theta = 1 \qquad\qquad Equation\ 12$$

3) COFUNCTIONS: Recall that the sum of all three angles within a triangle equals 180°, and in any right triangle, given one of the other internal angles (such as θ in Figure 2) , the other one (here, angle OAB) must equal 90° minus θ, and one calls it the complement of θ. Note in that figure that it also equals the angle between the vertical axis and the hypotenuse. Thus one can readily show that (where 90° minus θ = the complement of θ) :

$$Sin\ \theta = cos\ (90 - \theta) \qquad\qquad Equation\ 13$$

And, so, Cos $(90 - \theta)$ equals the cofunction of Sin θ. In fact this idea generalizes to this statement: any trigonometric function of any multiple of $90° \pm \theta$ equals that of θ, and of an odd multiple of $90°$ equals that of its cofunction of θ (one changes the sign in some of those but we need not get into that here).

4) FUNCTIONS OF SPECIAL ANGLES:

The 30-60-90 triangle shown in Figure 3, top left: We may list these:

$$\text{Sin } 30° = \frac{1}{2} = \cos 60°$$

$$\text{Cos } 30° = \frac{\sqrt{3}}{2} = \sin 60°$$

$$\text{Tan } 30° = \frac{1}{\sqrt{3}} = \cot 60°$$

Note one meaning of the above: If the length of the hypotenuse equals unity, then the side facing the $30°$ angle has a length of $1/2$, and that facing the $60°$ angle a length of $\frac{\sqrt{3}}{2}$.

Thus given any other real length for one of the sides of such a triangle one can find the other from these relations by means of proportions.

Now for the 45-45-90 triangle in Figure 3, we can write

$$\text{Sin } 45° = 1/\sqrt{2} = \cos 45°$$
$$\text{Cosec } 45° = \sqrt{2} = \sec 45°$$
$$\text{Tan } 45° = 1 = \cot. 45°$$

And for the angle of zero degrees, we may write:

$$\text{Sin } 0° = 0 = \tan 0°$$
$$\text{Cos } 0° = 1 = \sec 0°$$
$$\text{Cosec } 0° = \infty = \cot 0°$$

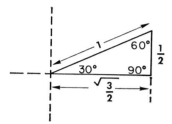

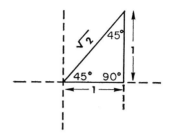

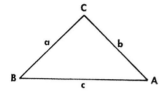

Fig. 3

These relations also apply to 180° angles and all multiples of 180° except for some sign changes we will not deal with.

For 90° angles we can write these functions, which apply also (but with some sign changes) to all odd multiples of 90°, such as 270°, 450°, etc.

$$\text{Sin } 90° = 1 = \text{cosec } 90°$$
$$\text{Cos } 90° = 0 = \text{cot } 90°$$
$$\text{Sec } 90° = \infty = \text{tan } 90°$$

5) GENERAL RELATIONS: Now four more general trigonometric relations, and then on to other matters. Thus, the sine addition formula (they do not add as ordinary numbers do) :

$$\text{Sin } (\theta + B) = \text{Sin } \theta \text{ Cos } B = \text{Cos } \theta \text{ Sin } B$$
Equation 14

and the cosine addition formula

$$\text{Sin } (\theta - B) = \text{Sin } \theta \text{ Cos } B - \text{Cos } \theta \text{ Sin } B$$
Equation 15

and for the cosine subtraction formula:

$$\text{Cos } (\theta - B) = \cos \theta \cos B + \sin \theta \sin B$$
Equation 16

$$\text{Sin } 2\theta = 2 \sin \theta \cos \theta$$
Equation 17

$$\text{Cos } 2\theta = \cos^2\theta - \sin^2\theta$$

Equation 18

Inverse trigonometric function notation: This can really confuse a beginner trying to feel his way in this jungle, and I describe it here simply because some authors seem to delight in the confusion it can create. Observe then that saying:

Writing the sine of an angle $\theta = 0.5$, means exactly the same things as writing:

$$\theta = \text{arc sin } 0.5,$$

or, equally, writing

$$\theta = \sin^{-1} 0.5$$

Likewise, saying that the tangent of an angle equals 0.1 means exactly the same as:

$$\theta = \text{arc tan } 0.1$$

or,

$$\theta = \tan^{-1} \ 0.1$$

The -1 above the sin, cos or tan expressions does not signify a power or exponent in the above system of notation*; it merely signifies that one employs the inverse trigonometric notation, a particular way of writing the information in which, rather than specifying an angle in degrees, you specify it as the numerical value of one of its trigonometric funcitons.

The Law of Sines: Given any two angles within any triangle, and one can then express all of its sides as ratios, so that given a measured value for one side one can then find the actual values of the others. This can serve as a useful relation in many vector problems. The lower left drawing in Figure 3 applies here.

Thus if we know angles A and C, we can always find B thus:

$$180° - A - C = B$$

---

* Note that all notational systems represent purely and strictly arbitrary choices and, presumably, possess convenience and simplicity as their justification for existence.

The lengths of the sides relate to these angles as follows, the colon notation reading "is to", the equals sign "as"

$$a:b:c = \sin A: \sin B: \sin C \qquad Equation\ 19$$

Or in words: side *a* is to side *b* is to side *c,* as sin A is to sin B is to sin C.

The law of cosines: For the same figure, this relation holds true:

$$a^2 = b^2 + c^2 - 2b\ c\ \cos A \qquad Equation\ 20$$

The law of tangents: For the same figure, this relation holds true:

$$\frac{a+b}{a-b} = \frac{\mathrm{Tan}\ \dfrac{A+B}{2}}{\mathrm{Tan}\ \dfrac{A-B}{2}} \qquad Equation\ 21$$

Examples: Let us now solve several problems to illustrate the use of these relations. Refer to the same drawing as we work through them.

Assume we know *c*, C and B. Find the remaining terms. $\dfrac{c}{b} = \dfrac{\sin C}{\sin B}$, or $b = C\dfrac{\sin B}{\sin C}$, so we find *b*. A equals the other two angles subtracted from 180; or A = 180° − (B + C). And we can find *a* as

$$\frac{a}{b} = \frac{\sin A}{\sin B}, \quad a = b\ \frac{\sin A}{\sin B}$$

Assume we know *a, b* and A. Then:

$$\frac{b}{a} = \frac{\sin A}{\sin B}, \quad \text{and}\ \sin B = \frac{b}{a}\ \sin A.$$

Knowing both B and A, we can find C, so finding *c* becomes a matter of

$$c = b\ \frac{\sin C}{\sin B}$$

Given b, c and A, find the remaining terms. Here we use the law of tangents. First, note that we invert that law as previously written, and that $B + C = 180° − A$; dividing through by 2 on both sides we get $\dfrac{B+C}{2} = 90° − \dfrac{A}{2}$, so tan $(\dfrac{B+C}{2}) = \tan (90° − \dfrac{A}{2})$.

Now if (in inverted form) :

$$\frac{\tan (\dfrac{B-C}{2})}{\tan (\dfrac{B+C}{2})} = \frac{b-c}{b+c}, \text{ then multiplying through by}$$

the denominator we have:

$$\tan (\frac{B-C}{2}) = \frac{b-c}{b+c} \cdot \tan (\frac{B+C}{2})$$

Substituting the identity $\tan (\dfrac{B+C}{2}) = \dfrac{b-c}{b+c} \cdot \tan (90 − \dfrac{A}{2})$ on the right we have: $\tan (\dfrac{B-C}{2}) = \dfrac{b-c}{b+c} \cdot \tan (90° − \dfrac{A}{2})$

We have values for all the right hand terms and so can obtain one for the left by doing the necessary arithmetic. By inserting its value into the law of tangents formula as written just above, and solving for the denominator we can obtain its value, and by the difference can find B, and then C. The law of sines will then provide a.

Given a, b and c, find A, B and C. Use the law of cosines here, thus:

$$a^2 = b^2+c^2 − 2bc \cos A, \text{ and solve for } \cos A,$$

which yields

$$\text{Cos } A = \frac{b^2 + c^2 - a^2}{2\,b\,c}$$

The law of sines will then yield Sin B and Sin C.

6) SOLUTIONS OF RIGHT TRIANGLES: For working out force resultants and for breaking loads down into their components within a structure one must either use the parallelogram rules, or the more exact trigonometric procedures. We will describe the more commonly needed of the latter next.

Thus in the accompanying Figure 4 which describes a right triangle, assume that AB at the top left represents a

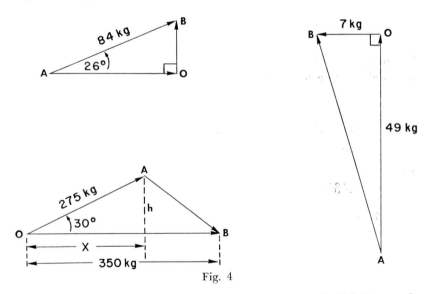

Fig. 4

muscle contractile force of 84 kg, acting at angle BAO equals 26°, relative to the longitudinal axis of that tibia, an axis defined by the line AO. Find the magnitudes of the load components AO and BO, and the angle ABO.

Vector Component AO: Ratio of AO divided by the hypotenuse represents the cosine of the angle, BAO, or

$$\text{cosBAO} = \frac{AO}{AB}$$

Solve for AO as described in Appendix 1, to obtain

(CosBAO) AB = AO,

insert the respective numerical values:

Cos 26° × 84 = AO
.899 × 84 = 75.5 kg

We already know its line of action as 26° relative to the primary load vector, AB.

Vector component OB:

Our basic trig tells us that

$$\text{Sin BAO} = \frac{\text{BO}}{\text{AB}}$$

Solving for BO, we have (using brackets simply to avoid any confusion over what multiplies by what):

(Sin BAO) AB = BO

and inserting the proper values we have:

Sin 26° × 84 = BO

or

.438 × 84 = 36.8 kg

As to its line of action, the sum of the angles in any triangle equals 180°, and in this one we know two of them to consist of 26° and 90°. Thus 180° − (26° + 90°) = angle ABO = 64°

Resultant: Now in the right hand part of Figure 4, we start with the following information, inferred perhaps from strain-gauge measurements of femoral neck strains under a particular set of loading conditions. We have one load component OB of 7 kg force, plus another of 49 kg acting at right angles to it. Find the resultant AB, and the angles BAO and OBA. As for the angle BAO, its tangent consists of:

$$\text{Tan BAO} = \frac{\text{BO}}{\text{AO}}, \text{ or tan BAO} = \frac{7}{49} = \frac{1}{7}$$

tan BAO = .143; or tan⁻¹ BAO = .143

The table of trigonometric functions shows this, the line of action of AB relative to AO, to correspond to an angle of 8° 10′. The other angle, OBA, therefore must equal 180° − (90° + 8° 10′) = 81° 50′.

As for the magnitude of AB, it forms the hypotenuse of this triangle, and this relation obtains:

$$\cos \text{ OAB} = \frac{AO}{AB}$$

Solving for AB, we have:

$$AB = \frac{AO}{\text{Cos OAB}};$$ inserting the appropriate numbers

yields: $$AB = \frac{49}{\cos \ 8° \ 10′} = \frac{49}{.989}$$

Note: These do not form the only ways of providing these answers; interested readers will find others by playing around with the problems.

7) SOLUTION OF NONRIGHT TRIANGLES: In the lower left drawing in Figure 4 two loads act on a part of the human knee, represented by OA = 275 kg (a known factor), and AB = ? (an unknown which x will signify). They produce a reaction on the tibia actually measured by some means of 350 kg, and the angle between the known load and the known reaction equals 30°. Find the load AB, both as to its magnitude and its direction.

Answer: Begin by dropping a line h from the apex A, perpendicular to CB, and solving the left hand triangle. We need to find both h and x. Note that the sine of 30° equals $\frac{h}{275}$, so (multiplying both sides by 275 and cancelling where indicated) h equals sine 30° × 275, or:

$$h = 275 \times \sin 30° = 137$$

A similar procedure will now provide x: cos 30° $= x/275$, so:

$$x = 275 \times \cos 30° = 238 \text{ kg}$$

Now for the right hand triangle the remainder of line OB must equal 350 − 238 = 112 kg. We already know h to equal 137. Inspecting the diagram shows that h/350-x equals the tangent of the angle OBA. So we can find angle OBA as its tangent, thus:

$$\tan \text{ ABO} = \frac{137}{112} = 1.22; \text{ or if you like being mys-}$$

terious, write it thus:

$$\tan^{-1} \text{ ABO} = 1.22, \text{ or arc tan ABO} = 1.22.$$

Looking this up in the table of trigonometric functions tells us that ABO equals 50.5°, and that defines the line of action of force AB towards force OB. With respect to OA, the line of action of force AB equals angle OAh plus hAB, or 99.5° (using the property that the sum of the angles in each triangle must equal 180°). To find the magnitude of the load AB, use the relation:

$$\sec \text{ ABO} = \frac{AB}{350\text{-x}}, \text{ so AB} = \sec \text{ ABO } (350\text{-x}) . \text{ In-}$$

serting the numbers then yields AB $= \sec 50.5° \times 112 = 1.57 \times 112 = 176$ kg.

Note: The only trigonometric demands the text will make of you, you can handle with simple sines, cosines and tangents.

Electrical Fundamentals

Because bone, tendon and cartilage develop electrical voltages when strained, and because these voltages may prove related, whether directly or indirectly, to the "signals" we presume these materials deliver to their cells, signals which participate in a feedback system that adapts their bulk mechanical properites to the mechanical demands made of them by our bodies, we will review briefly here a few matters of electrical physics which help to understand some of the research going on in this whole field. Many who read this may expect some day to see such research produce a new body of clinically useful expertise.

We may define electricity as the field which deals with the properties of large numbers of freely movable electrons. When those electrons nevertheless do not move, the properties of the collection represent the field of electrostatics. When they do move we deal with electrical currents, or current electricity (62).

1) ELECTROSTATICS: Electrons have a unit negative electrical charge, opposite to the positive electrical charge of the atomic nucleus. And as to the interactions between such charges:

Bodies with like charge repel each other, those with unlike charge attract. And as a matter of fact these repulsions and attractions conform to this equation:

$$F = \frac{QQ'}{k \; r^2} \qquad\qquad\text{\textit{Equation 22}}$$

where F equals the force in dynes, Q and Q′ signify two electrical charges (i.e., groups of positive and/or negative charges) stated in e.s.u. system units (electrostatic system) of statcoulombs, and *r* the distance between them in cm.

One statcoulomb equals that amount of electrical charge which at 1 cm distance from another one exerts a force of 1 dyne on it (repulsive if the charges have the same sign, attractive if otherwise). In this equation, k signifies the dielectric constant of the medium between the two charges, and in vacuum it equals unity, i.e., the number one. Clearly, for such attractions or repulsions to occur at a distance some kind of invisible force field must emanate from each charge. It has been named the electric field. The electric field demonstrates a gradient of potential, i.e., a rate of change per unit distance. We may define the unit of such change in e.s.u. units thus: It requires one erg to move one statcoulomb from zero potential to one statvolt potential.

A good analogy here: Water pressure, which analogizes the volt (in any system of electrical units). A volt thus resembles a kind of electrical pressure. The ordinary volt (of zinc-carbon 1.5 volt battery context) equals a much smaller unit of potential: That in which one joule of work (10^7 ergs) moves one ordinary coulomb of charge (3×10^9 statcoulombs) from zero to one ordinary volt potential. Thus one ordinary volt equals one three hundredths of a volt e.s.u.

Capacitance: Just as an air tank of some fixed volume may hold widely differing amounts of air according to the pressure at which one fills it, so various materials and physical arrangements may hold varying amounts of electric charge depending upon the potential (i.e., voltage) one uses to "fill" it or charge it. A device intended to hold electric charge has become known as a condenser or capacitor, and the measure of the capacity for electric charge constitutes the farad. In e.s.u. units then:

One statfarad of capacitance will change its potential by one statvolt when a change in its charge of one statcoulomb occurs.

And the charge Q, relates to capacitance C, and electrical potential V, as follows:

$$Q = CV \qquad\qquad Equation\ 23$$

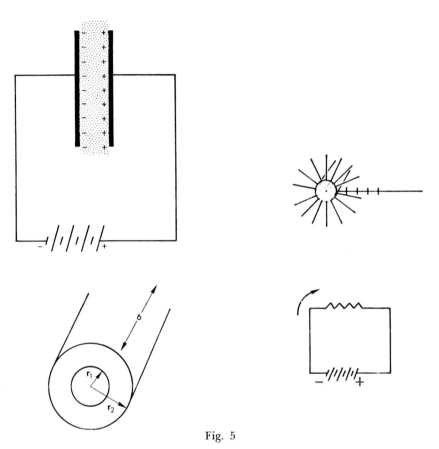

Fig. 5

Consider a capacitor consisting of two plates with a voltage of one e.s.u. volt impressed across it as shown in Figure 5. The size of two plates (which here form conductors, such as aluminum foil) has been chosen so that it holds one statcoulomb, and so has a capacitance of one statfarad *when the medium between the plates constitutes a good vacuum.* Now fill the space between the plates with very pure water. Immediately another 79 statcoulombs of charge flow from the battery to the capacitor. In other words, the medium separating the capacitor plates affects the capacity of the capacitor. The ability of various forms of electrically insulating matter to do this forms a property called the dielectric constant, mentioned earlier. Table 1 lists some dielectric con-

TABLE 1 (b)
DIELECTRIC CONSTANT OF MATERIALS (k)

Material	k	Material	k
Vacuum	1.000	Glass	6
Air	1.0006	Sulfur	3.8
Mica	6.5	Water	80
Paraffin	2.1	Titanates	1000 $\pm$
Paper	2.0	Wood	2.5–3.5
Methylmethacrylate	3.0	Polyethylene	2.3
Cell membrane: 1000 MHz	10–20X		
Cell membrane: 1000 1Hz $\approx$ 1,000,000			

* per cm^2 of membrane.

stants for your information. Observe the dependence of cell membrane capacitance upon frequency: it rises steeply as the frequency at which one conducts the test declines. Parenthetically, the cell membrane has a capitance of 1 μF (one microfarad) /cm^2 at 37°C temperature, and a resistance on the order of 100 ohms/cm^2. To continue now, if A represents the area of these plates, d their separation (both expressed in cm^2 or cm respectively) and k the dielectric constant of the intervening medium, then the following relation expresses the capitance of such a capacitor in e.s.u. units:

$$C = \frac{k\ A}{4\ \pi\ d} \qquad\qquad Equation\ 24$$

Note: The capacitance (as well as the strength of the electric field of Equation 24 in terms such as voltage differ-ence per cm) increases as the separation decreases, and as the area and dielectric constant increase. Also, one can alter the geometry of the plates for special purposes, and one of possible interest in skeletal physiology deals with the essen-tially cylindrical capacitor in which electrically conducting media on either side of a cylinder of dielectric material form a condenser. If L equals the length of such a cylinder (here the length of a bone), r_1 the radius of its inner surface and r_2 that of the outer, and k the dielectric constant, units given in cm and statfarads, the capacitance of such a con-denser becomes:

$$C = \frac{kL}{2\ \log_e\ r_1/r_2} \qquad\qquad Equation\ 25$$

2) ORDINARY ELECTRICAL UNITS: The practical units familiar to all of us, as the 12-volt car battery, the ampere and the microfarad of radio and TV usage, relate to the analogous e.s.u. units as follows:

1 volt = 1/300 statvolt; one statvolt = 300 volts.
1 coulomb = 3 × 10⁹ statcoulomb; one statcoulomb
= 3 × 10⁻⁹ = 3 billionths of a coulomb
1 farad = 9 × 10¹¹ statfarads; one statfarad = 9 ×
10⁻¹¹ = 9 hundredths of one billionth of a farad

Remember this property of two electrically charged cylindrical surfaces separated by an insulator (which, by definition must then have some dielectric constant) : The intensity of the electrical field surrounding it in a vacuum falls off according to the radius of the distance from the surface, and in multiples of that radius. That is, at 2 radii the field strength equals ½ that lying on the surface; at three radii it equals ⅓ and so on. But when a dielectric with a constant k of 10 intervenes, the field strength at 2 radii falls to $\frac{1}{2 \times 10} = \frac{1}{20}$; and with a dielectric constant of 50, at 3 radii the field strength falls to $\frac{1}{3 \times 50} = \frac{1}{150}$ that at the surface, i.e., at unit radius. Thus, given the right dielectric, then the electrical field strengths can fall off quite rapidly as one moves away from that surface.

Note: We have defined one set of electrical units derived from electrostatic phenomena and abbreviated e.s.u. units; and a second system of ordinary units which will face orthopaedists in most of the literature they will probably read. A third one, derived from studies of magnetism and current flow, also exists and includes the abampere, abvolt, abfarad but we need not go into that further here. In these ordinary units then, this relation holds:

1 coulomb = the amount of charge (i.e., number of electrons) in 1 ampere flowing for 1 second.

And we can now define the joule, a unit of work, as 1 Joule = the work done in moving 1 coulomb of charge along a voltage difference or gradient of 1 volt. Henceforth we will use ordinary electrical units.

Resistance: An electrical charge does not flow effortlessly down (or up) a voltage gradient; it experiences a resistance, and we name the *ohm* as the unit of electrical resistance. It relates to the voltage potential V, and the current flowing in amperes I, as follows, known as Ohm's Law:

$$R = \frac{V}{I}; \text{ or } V = R \text{ I}; \text{ or } I = V/R$$

Equation 26

and in words: one ohm allows only 1 ampere to flow down a voltage gradient of one volt.

Often when one needs to work with small fractions of a volt or an ampere, one uses millivolts and milliamperes (i.e., thousandths of one unit) or microvolts and microamperes (millionths of one unit).

Let us next examine the manner in which an electrical current field decays with distance from a cylindrical source supplying charge to a surrounding conducting medium. If on each square millimeter of the cylinder's surface 1/1000 coulomb of charge flows outwards per second (i.e., one milliampere per mm^2 current density), then at two radii from the center of the cylinder (and thus one from its surface) the current flux equals ½ milliampere, at 5 radii it equals 1/5 milliampere, and at 12 radii it equals 1/12 milliampere.

Thus we have a basic difference in the manner in which the electric field and a current field can decay in the cylindrical situation described: The former may decay very rapidly with distance but the latter cannot. It follows that possible biological effects of the former, the electric field, may remain confined to regions close to the surfaces of charged cylinders but the effects of the latter must decay linearly with distance from the surface and reach half their surface value at one radius distant from it (two radii out from the cylinder's center).

Now one further property of electrical current flow: The total current flow through a circuit equals the voltage divided by the total resistance (Ohm's Law again), but at least two resistances exist in series in any circuit: that external resistance of the circuit, signified by the resistor at the lower right of Figure 5, and that internal resistance of the source, here the battery. Thus:

$$I = \frac{V}{R_e + R_1} \qquad\qquad Equation\ 27$$

Assume one measures an electron current flow of .01 milliampere per mm^2 of a bone surface straining concavely in combined flexure and compression. Given that the resistance of the body fluids between the bone surface emitting it and the electrode collecting that current lies below one ohn, while that of the bone equals some 5,000 ohms, the internal voltage required to drive this system becomes:

$$
\begin{aligned}
V &= (R_e + R_1) \\
&= .0001\ (5,000 + .01) \\
&= .50\ volts
\end{aligned}
$$

Note that this voltage potential arises across the whole thickness of the cortex, and to detect it one would have to have electrodes placed directly on each cortical surface (no one has done this *in vivo* at this writing).

Piezoelectricity

We describe this physical property of some crystalline states of matter primarily because bone and tendon have demonstrated at least analogous properties, and those properties promise to relate in some meaningful way to the transducing mechanisms which allow skeletal systems to adapt their architecture (by properly chosen and patterned cellular responses arising on their surfaces or envelopes) to the major time averaged mechanical demands made of them. We credit Jean and Pierre Curie with discovering in 1880 that when a quartz crystal becomes mechanically strained in compression along a particular direction with respect to its optic axis, an electric charge arises across the two compressed surfaces, one side becoming electrically negative relative to the other. Upon destraining the crystal, the charge difference then disappears, and one can cycle it back and forth in this manner indefinitely.

Correspondingly, when one impresses a varying voltage across the crystal by means of two copper or aluminum plates in contact with it, the crystal will alternately contract and expand physically and parallel to the electric field gradient. In fact this reverse process serves to provide crystal oscillators of very stable frequency for a variety of purposes in the electronics industry. The thickness of the crystal (given the density of its material) determines its mechanical resonant vibration frequency, and one can increase it by grinding it thinner. When this resonant mechanical vibration frequency matches that of a varying electric field across it, one can lock the electronic oscillator to it to maintain equally stable electrical oscillation. A variety of other crystals have shown the piezoelectric property and we may expect more will turn up in the future.

The surface charge developed by a piezoelectric material

does not represent a current source; rather it represents a temporary movement of positive and negative charges around the centers of some of the crystal lattice positions, and so it produces *an essentially pure electric field,* one which displays primarily the properties of electrostatics rather than of current electricity. Thus any effects such a phenomenon might exert upon cells should prove maximal at the surface of the piezoelectric material (in our biomechanical concerns, bone and fibrous tissues, and possibly cartilage and teeth too) and would display considerable shielding effects by the outlying layers of cell membranes because of the respectable capacitance of those membranes and the series-decay effect produced by multiple layers of such membranes. Note that those membranes not only can shield effectively cells twenty or more microns distant from a charged surface; equally they can shield that surface from an experimenter's attempt to impose an external electric field on it, and thus to make the biological system dance to his drum rather than to its own.

Because of the physical nature of this effect one cannot measure it accurately with a device such as an ammeter, for the latter measures current flow, not voltage, and a good piezoelectric substance will "leak" only trivial amounts, in the range of microamperes per cm^2 of surface. To measure the effect accurately one should employ a device such as an operational amplifier, which measures voltages not by drawing current from the voltage source but by generating an equal but *opposing* voltage so that *net current flow becomes trivial.* One then measures that latter voltage by electronic means. The electronics engineer says of such voltage measuring devices that they have very high input impendance, usually greater than 10 megohms (i.e., 10×10^6 ohms). This pratical property of piezoelectric phenomena just begins to receive recognition by investigators studying such properties in skeletal tissues and one cannot say at present how far it may take us when properly pursued and developed. But one thing has become clear to date: the simplistic amperometric approach taken by most investigators so far cannot tap whatever biological depths this field may contain.

Remember then in reading about or pondering on studies of the biological piezoelectric phenomena: They represent *reversible electric charge separations* which produce electric fields (105) ; they do not represent in essence amperometric or current-flow phenomena. Consequently capacitive effects of cell membranes should prove important in their biological effects and in determining the geographic distributions of those effects relative to the structures and surfaces on which the charge separations arise. Because these charge separations involve very small coulomb movements, membrane and electrode polarization phenomena in the measuring electrodes should prove quite troublesome and important technical problems.

Finally, keep this in mind too: The actual chemical or physical effect which orders the skeletal cells around for architectural purposes may constitute something else than the charge separations we discussed above, and those separations could prove indirect secondary effects of that more important one.

Free Body Diagrams

While the main text made no use of or reference to this method of analyzing the forces and reactions in structures, it has begun to appear in orthopaedic board exams, so we will describe it briefly here in order that a resident may understand what it represents.

In essence a free body diagram sketches or abstracts some part of a mechanical system whose stresses one wishes to understand (55,70,71). One then represents each force and/or stress acting upon or within it as an arrow, its orientation signifying that of the force, its length, the magnitude of that force, and its arrow head the sense of that force's action. Similar arrows designate all other forces acting on the system, and they also designate all of the reactions (90,111). A reaction consists of a secondary force acting on a structure—or body—as some consequence of another active primary force also acting on it and which resists the acceleratory effect of that active, primary force. If the forces and reactions on a body do not all cancel out, then it experiences acceleration and so it does not exist in static equilibrium. But if all forces—including moments—do cancel out then it does exist in static equilibrium (210). Thus for the equilibrium state we may write, using the upper case Greek letter sigma—Σ—to signify "the sum of":

$$\Sigma F_x = 0; \quad \Sigma F_y = 0; \quad \Sigma M = 0 \qquad Equation\ 28$$

meaning, respectively, that the sum of all force components acting in the x or horizontal direction equal zero; likewise for all components acting in the y or vertical direction; and likewise for all of the moments (i.e., torques). We can complicate things further if we wish by adding the third dimension of space, which requires additional terms. But we do not wish.

Thus, in the accompanying Figure 6 of a beam carrying a vertical load P, and lying on two end supports, we see that the weight of the beam W plus the load P, must equal the sum of the two reactions R_1 and R_2 in magnitude, but they must act in that sense which causes all the forces and torques to cancel out. Or in symbols:

$$P + W - R_1 - R_2 = 0$$

or, if you prefer the usual high-school physics format:

$$P + W = R_1 + R_2$$

Now let us examine a very thin section of the beam taken somewhere to the left of the point of application of the load, shown below. On its right side a vertical shearing force acts downwards, applied by the part of the beam lying off to its right; observe that that part of the beam attempts to drop under the influence of P on top of it. This shearing load generates a shearing strain, and a stress that resists any further shearing strain. On the left side of the free body lies an oppositely directed (i.e., upwards) shearing force or load, applied by that part of the beam to its left, which presses upwards on it. Obviously the load represented by that force generates another and matching vertical shearing stress in the left face of the free body.

These two shearing forces, equal in magnitude but opposite in direction and separated by the length of the free body, when averaged and added up over the length of the whole beam, constitute its flexure and form a couple, and as we noted in Part I such a couple must tend to rotate the free body, here in a clockwise direction around its center of mass (216). While that couple assuredly exists, yet in a beam under the static equilibrium condition shown no such rotation occurs. Then forces of exactly equal magnitude but opposite in direction or sense must arise in the beam which cancel it. These represent the flexural moments shown by the short arrows which form another couple, consisting of compression forces in the beam's top fibers, and tension in the bottom ones, both lying parallel to the beam's upper and

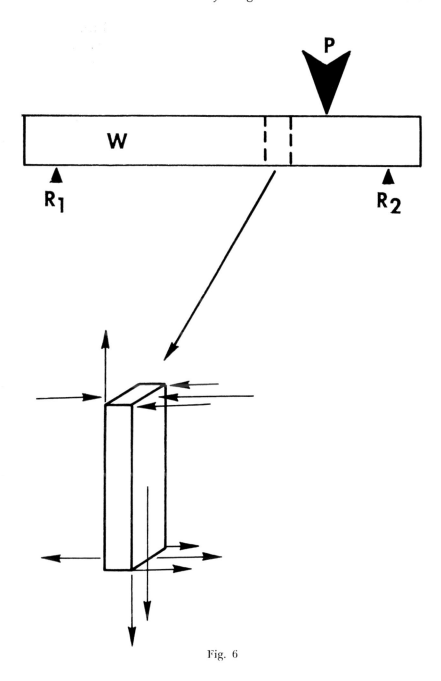

Fig. 6

lower surface fibers. With these forces all added in, the free body diagram has become essentially complete. It lacks only sufficient excess in magnitude of the upwards acting shear vector to offset the downwards acting mass of the free body section itself. In most exploratory analyses one omits consideration of that mass, or defers it.

Beam and Column Flexure

1) BEAMS: If we know both the unit stress within a material and its Young's modulus, we can calculate the strain as the former divided by the latter, or:

$$\epsilon = \sigma/E \qquad\qquad \textit{Equation 29}$$

In an elastic beam loaded in flexure, the strain of its surface fibers also must equal their distance from the neutral plane Y, divided by the radius of curvature of the beam under flexural deformation. Signify that radius by r; then:

$$\frac{\sigma}{E} = \frac{y}{r} \qquad\qquad \textit{Equation 30}$$

Then these relations hold true, where M signifies the flexural moments at a given section of a beam and I the rectangular moment of inertia:

$$r = \frac{E\,I}{M} \qquad\qquad \textit{Equation 31}$$

$$\sigma = \frac{E\,Y}{r} \qquad\qquad \textit{Equation 32}$$

2) COLUMNS: In one important regard, strain behavior in columns loaded near the failure point differs from that in beams. Beam flexure varies in direct proportion to the flexural load, so that doubling the load doubles the deflection, or decreasing the one to one-third decreases the other in equal proportion. Thus one has visible evidence of an approaching or impending beam failure.

But given a column with both ends free to rotate (an excellent analogy with our bones, most of which have low-friction joints at either end), and carrying a uniaxial compression load, little seems to happen as the load increases progressively except for some compression strain (equal to σ/E), until at a critical point the column suddenly buckles (i.e., bends sideways) and fractures in flexure. This critical load or Euler load, named after the European mathematician who described it, occurs when a trivial eccentricity adds a flexural strain to the uniaxial compression strain, leading to or precipitating a positive feedback relation between the strain and the loads. The resulting failure occurs suddenly, unexpectedly and tends to be catastrophic in nature. Euler provided several ways of calculating the value of this critical load; the one of direct interest here constitutes the following relation, where P_{cr} signifies the critical load, E the Young's modulus in compression, I the rectangular moment of inertia, and L the column length:

$$P_{cr} = \frac{\pi^2 \ E \ I}{L^2} \qquad\qquad Equation\ 33$$

When the column ends lie fixed in cement, earth or steel in such a way as to resist flexural deformation of the column at its ends, its effective strength increases and one must use a different relation to find P_{cr}.

The critical unit stress at the moment of failure, σ_{cr}, equals (where A equals the cross sectional area of the column):

$$\sigma_{cr} = \frac{P_{cr}}{A}$$

For those who want to practice with the math, the beam flexure formulas and the logarithm tables, try this one.

Given: At midshaft a femur of length 39 cm has a cortical thickness of 5.0 mm and a total cortical cross section area of 3.0 cm². Calculate its rectangular and polar moments of inertia at that midshaft level, and its maximum surface stress in compression at that level for a bending load of 10 kg applied at a point 10 cm from its upper end. Then, given a breaking stress in tension of 11 kg/mm² find the flexural load applied to it at midshaft that will break the femur. You may assume a perfectly circular cross sectional geometry in your analysis (answer #16, Chapter 24).

Common Logarithms

These three-place tables provide logarithms of numbers from one to ten, to values in the second decimal point. To use them, look up the first two digits of the number you are working with in the left hand column, and the third in the corresponding row. The number found at the intersect constitutes the logarithm, or the exponent of ten that yields the number you are working with.

For any number between one and ten, the table provides its logarithm directly. For numbers between 10 and 100, put the number one to the left of the decimal of the logarithm; between 100–1000 the number 2; 1000–10,000 the number 3, and so on.

Exs:	Find log 2.31	Answ:	.3636
	Find log 0.0231		−2.3636
	Find log 62.7		1.7973
	Find log 627.0		2.7973
	Find log 627,000		5.7973

Problem: Multiply 11.2 by 16.7
Answ: $Log_{10} 11.2 = 1.0492$
$Log_{10} 16.7 = 1.2227$
(now add them);
Log_{10} product = 2.2719; product = 187

Problem: Divide 163 by 2.72
Answ: $Log_{10} 163 = 2.2122$
$Log_{10} 2.72 = .4346$ (now subtract them);
Log_{10} of answer 1.7776; answer = 59.9

Orthopaedic Biomechanics

SPECIAL TABLE 1

COMMON LOGARITHMS OF NUMBERS

N	0	1	2	3	4	5	6	7	8	9
1.00	.0000	.0004	.0009	.0013	.0017	.0022	.0026	.0030	.0035	.0039
.01	0043	0048	0052	0056	0060	0065	0069	0073	0077	0082
.02	0086	0090	0095	0099	0103	0107	0111	0116	0120	0124
.03	0128	0133	0137	0141	0145	0149	0154	0158	0162	0166
.04	0170	0175	0179	0183	0187	0191	0194	0199	0204	0208
1.05	.0212	.0216	.0220	.0224	.0228	.0233	.0237	.0241	.0245	.0249
.06	0253	0257	0261	0265	0269	0273	0278	0282	0286	0290
.07	0294	0298	0302	0306	0310	0314	0318	0322	0326	0330
.08	0334	0338	0342	0346	0350	0354	0358	0362	0366	0370
.09	0374	0378	0382	0386	0390	0394	0398	0402	0406	0410
1.0	.0000	.0043	.0086	.0128	.0170	.0212	.0253	.0294	.0334	.0374
.1	0414	0453	0492	0531	0569	0607	0645	0682	0719	0755
.2	0792	0828	0864	0899	0934	0969	1004	1038	1072	1106
.3	1139	1173	1206	1239	1271	1303	1335	1367	1399	1430
.4	1461	1492	1523	1553	1584	1614	1644	1673	1703	1732
1.5	.1761	.1790	.1818	.1847	.1875	.1903	.1931	.1959	.1987	.2014
.6	2041	2068	2095	2122	2148	2175	2201	2227	2253	2279
.7	2304	2330	2355	2380	2405	2430	2455	2480	2504	2529
.8	2553	2577	2601	2625	2648	2672	2695	2718	2742	2765
.9	2788	2810	2833	2856	2878	2900	2923	2945	2967	2989
2.0	.3010	.3032	.3054	.3075	.3096	.3118	.3139	.3160	.3181	.3201
.1	3222	3243	3263	3284	3304	3324	3345	3365	3385	3404
.2	3424	3444	3464	3483	3502	3522	3541	3560	3579	3598
.3	3617	3636	3655	3674	3692	3711	3729	3747	3766	3784
.4	3802	3820	3838	3856	3874	3892	3909	3927	3945	3962
2.5	.3979	.3997	.4014	.4031	.4048	.4065	.4082	.4099	.4116	.4133
.6	4150	4166	4183	4200	4216	4232	4249	4265	4281	4298
.7	4314	4330	4346	4362	4378	4393	4409	4425	4440	4456
.8	4472	4487	4502	4518	4533	4548	4564	4579	4594	4609
.9	4624	4639	4654	4669	4683	4698	4713	4728	4742	4757
3.0	.4771	.4786	.4800	.4814	.4829	.4843	.4857	.4871	.4886	.4900
.1	4914	4928	4942	4955	4969	4983	4997	5011	5024	5038
.2	5051	5065	5079	5092	5105	5119	5132	5145	5159	5172
.3	5185	5198	5211	5224	5237	5250	5263	5276	5289	5302
.4	5315	5328	5340	5353	5366	5378	5391	5403	5416	5428
3.5	.5441	.5453	.5465	.5478	.5490	.5502	.5514	.5527	.5539	.5551
.6	5563	5575	5587	5599	5611	5623	5635	5647	5658	5670
.7	5682	5694	5705	5717	5729	5740	5752	5763	5775	5786
.8	5798	5809	5821	5832	5843	5855	5866	5877	5888	5899
.9	5911	5922	5933	5944	5955	5966	5977	5988	5999	6010
4.0	.6021	.6031	.6042	.6053	.6064	.6075	.6085	.6096	.6107	.6117
.1	6128	6138	6149	6160	6170	6180	6191	6201	6212	6222
.2	6232	6243	6253	6263	6274	6284	6294	6304	6314	6325
.3	6335	6345	6355	6365	6375	6385	6395	6405	6415	6425
.4	6435	6444	6454	6464	6474	6484	6493	6503	6513	6522
4.5	.6532	.6542	.6551	.6561	.6571	.6580	.6590	.6599	.6609	.6618
.6	6628	6637	6646	6656	6665	6675	6684	6693	6702	6712
.7	6721	6730	6739	6749	6758	6767	6776	6785	6794	6803
.8	6812	6821	6830	6839	6848	6857	6866	6875	6884	6893
.9	6902	6911	6920	6928	6937	6946	6955	6964	6972	6981

SPECIAL TABLE 1 (*Continued*)

N	0	1	2	3	4	5	6	7	8	9
5.0	.6990	.6998	.7007	.7016	.7024	.7033	.7042	.7050	.7059	.7067
.1	7076	7084	7093	7101	7110	7118	7126	7135	7143	7152
.2	7160	7168	7177	7185	7193	7202	7210	7218	7226	7235
.3	7243	7251	7259	7267	7275	7284	7292	7300	7308	7316
.4	7324	7332	7340	7348	7356	7364	7372	7380	7388	7396
5.5	.7404	.7412	.7419	.7427	.7435	.7443	.7451	.7459	.7466	.7474
.6	7482	7490	7497	7505	7513	7520	7528	7536	7543	7551
.7	7559	7566	7574	7582	7589	7597	7604	7612	7619	7627
.8	7634	7642	7649	7657	7664	7672	7679	7686	7694	7701
.9	7709	7716	7723	7731	7738	7745	7752	7760	7767	7774
6.0	.7782	.7789	.7796	.7803	.7810	.7818	.7825	.7832	.7839	.7846
.1	7853	7860	7868	7875	7882	7889	7896	7903	7910	7917
.2	7924	7931	7938	7945	7952	7959	7966	7973	7980	7987
.3	7993	8000	8007	8014	8021	8028	8035	8041	8048	8055
.4	8062	8069	8075	8082	8089	8096	8102	8109	8116	8122
6.5	.8129	.8136	.8142	.8149	.8156	.8162	.8169	.8176	.8182	.8189
.6	8195	8202	8209	8215	8222	8228	8235	8241	8248	8254
.7	8261	8267	8274	8280	7287	8293	8299	8306	8312	8319
.8	8325	8331	8338	8344	8351	8357	8363	8370	8376	8382
.9	8388	8395	8401	8407	8414	8420	8426	8432	8439	8445
7.0	.8451	.8457	.8463	.8470	.8476	.8482	.8488	.8494	.8500	.8506
.1	8513	8519	8525	8531	8537	8543	8549	8555	8561	8567
.2	8573	8579	8585	8591	8597	8603	8609	8615	8621	8627
.3	8633	8639	8645	8651	8657	8663	8669	8675	8681	8686
.4	8692	8698	8704	8710	8716	8722	8727	8733	8739	8745
7.5	.8751	.8756	.8762	.8768	.8774	.8779	.8785	.8791	.8797	.8802
.6	8808	8814	8820	8825	8831	8837	8842	8848	8854	8859
.7	8865	8871	8876	8882	8887	8893	8899	8904	8910	8915
.8	8921	8927	8932	8938	8943	8949	8954	8960	8965	8971
.9	8976	8982	8987	8993	8998	9004	9009	9015	9020	9025
8.0	.9031	.9036	.9042	.9047	.9053	.9058	.9063	.9069	.9074	.9079
.1	9085	9090	9096	9101	9106	9112	9117	9122	9128	9133
.2	9138	9143	9149	9154	9159	9165	9170	9175	9180	9186
.3	9191	9196	9201	9206	9212	9217	9222	9227	9232	9238
.4	9243	9248	9253	9258	9263	9269	9274	9279	9284	9289
8.5	.9294	9.299	.9304	.9309	.9315	.9320	.9325	.9330	.9335	.9340
.6	9345	9350	9355	9360	9365	9370	9375	9380	9385	9390
.7	9395	9400	9405	9410	9415	9420	9425	9430	9435	9440
.8	9445	9450	9455	9460	9465	9469	9474	9479	9484	9489
.9	9494	9499	9504	9509	9513	9518	9523	9528	9533	9538
9.0	.9542	.9547	.9552	.9557	.9562	.9566	.9571	.9576	.9581	.9586
.1	9590	9595	9600	9605	9609	9614	9619	9624	9628	9633
.2	9638	9643	9647	9652	9657	9661	9666	9671	9675	9680
.3	9685	9689	9694	9699	9703	9708	9713	9717	9722	9727
.4	9731	9736	9741	9745	9750	9754	9759	9763	9768	9773
9.5	.9777	.9782	.9786	.9791	.9795	.9800	.9805	.9809	.9814	.9818
.6	9823	9827	9832	9836	9841	9845	9850	9854	9859	9863
.7	9868	9872	9877	9881	9886	9890	9894	9899	9903	9908
.8	9912	9917	9921	9926	9930	9934	9939	9943	9948	9952
.9	9956	9961	9965	9969	9974	9978	9983	9987	9991	9996

Natural Trigonometric Functions

To use, look up the angle (in degrees and 10 minute intervals) along the left column for angles under 45°, and along the right hand column for those over. When using the left column (A), read the name of the trigonometric functions off the top row, but when using the right column (i.e., 45–90°), read the functions off the bottom row.

Note that for trigonometric purposes the sine of 110° equals the sine of (110°–90°) or 20°; the cosine of 183° equals the sine of 183–90) =93°, and (93°–90°) = −3° (see the Quadrant Table, Appendix 5).

SPECIAL TABLE 2

NATURAL VALUES OF TRIGONOMETRIC FUNCTIONS

A	sin A	cos A	tan A	cot A	sec A	cosec A	
0°	.00000	1.0000	.00000		1.0000		90°
	.00291	1.0000	.00291	343.77	1.0000	343.78	
	.00582	1.0000	.00582	171.88	1.0000	171.89	
	.00873	1.0000	.00873	114.59	1.0000	114.59	
	.01164	.9999	.01164	85.940	1.0001	85.946	
	.01454	.9999	.01455	68.750	1.0001	68.757	
1°	.01745	.9998	.01746	57.290	1.0002	57.299	89°
	.02036	.9998	.02036	49.104	1.0002	49.114	
	.02327	.9997	.02328	42.964	1.0003	42.976	
	.02618	.9997	.02619	38.188	1.0003	38.202	
	.02908	.9996	.02910	34.368	1.0004	34.382	
	.03199	.9995	.03201	31.242	1.0005	31.258	
2°	.03490	.9994	.03492	28.6363	1.0006	28.654	88°
	.03781	.9993	.03783	26.4316	1.0007	26.451	
	.04071	.9992	.04075	24.5418	1.0008	24.562	
	.04362	.9990	.04366	22.9038	1.0010	22.926	
	.04653	.9989	.04658	21.4704	1.0011	21.494	
	.04943	.9988	.04949	20.2056	1.0012	20.230	
3°	.05234	.9986	.05241	19.0811	1.0014	19.107	87°
	.05524	.9985	.05533	18.0750	1.0015	18.103	
	.05814	.9983	.05824	17.1693	1.0017	17.198	
	.06105	.9981	.06116	16.3499	1.0019	16.380	
	.06395	.9980	.06408	15.6048	1.0021	15.637	
	.06685	.9978	.06700	14.9244	1.0022	14.958	
4°	.06976	.9976	.06993	14.3007	1.0024	14.336	86°
	.07266	.9974	.07285	13.7267	1.0027	13.763	
	.07556	.9971	.07578	13.1969	1.0029	13.235	
	.07846	.9969	.07870	12.7062	1.0031	12.746	
	.08136	.9967	.08163	12.2505	1.0033	12.291	
	.08426	.9964	.08456	11.8262	1.0036	11.808	
5°	.08716	.9962	.08749	11.4301	1.0038	11.474	85°
	.09005	.9959	.09042	11.0594	1.0041	11.105	
	.09295	.9957	.09335	10.7119	1.0044	10.758	
	.09585	.9954	.09629	10.3854	1.0046	10.433	
	.09874	.9951	.09923	10.0780	1.0049	10.128	
	.10164	.9948	.10216	9.7882	1.0052	9.839	
	cos A	sin A	cot A	tan A	cosec A	sec A	A

SPECIAL TABLE 2 *(Continued)*

A	sin A	cos A	tan A	cot A	sec A	cosec A	
6°	.10453	.9945	.10510	9.5144	1.0055	9.5668	84°
	.10742	.9942	.10805	9.2553	1.0058	9.3092	
	.11031	.9939	.11099	9.0098	1.0061	9.0652	
	.11320	.9936	.11394	8.7769	1.0065	8.8337	
	.11609	.9932	.11688	8.5555	1.0068	8.6138	
	.11898	.9929	.11983	8.3450	1.0072	8.4647	
7°	.12187	.9925	.12278	8.1443	1.0075	8.2055	83°
	.12476	.9922	.12574	7.9530	1.0079	8.0157	
	.12764	.9918	.12869	7.7704	1.0083	7.8344	
	.13053	.9914	.13165	7.5958	1.0086	7.6613	
	.1305	.9914	.1317	7.5958	1.0086	7.6613	
	.1334	.9911	.1346	7.4287	1.0090	7.4957	
	.1363	.9907	.1376	7.2687	1.0094	7.3372	
8°	.1392	.9903	.1405	7.1154	1.0098	7.1853	82°
	.1421	.9899	.1453	6.9682	1.0102	7.0396	
	.1449	.9894	.1465	6.8269	1.0107	6.8998	
	.1478	.9890	.1495	6.6912	1.0111	6.7655	
	.1507	.9886	.1524	6.5606	1.0116	6.6363	
	.1536	.9881	.1554	6.4348	1.0120	6.5121	
9°	.1564	.9877	.1584	6.3138	1.0125	6.3925	81°
	.1593	.9872	.1614	6.1970	1.0129	6.2772	
	.1622	.9868	.1644	6.0844	1.0134	6.1661	
	.1650	.9863	.1673	5.9758	1.0139	6.0589	
	.1679	.9858	.1703	5.8708	1.0144	5.9554	
	.1708	.9853	.1733	5.7694	1.0149	5.8554	
10°	.1736	.9848	.1763	5.6713	1.0154	5.7588	80°
	.1765	.9843	.1793	5.5764	1.0160	5.6653	
	.1794	.9838	.1823	5.4845	1.0165	5.5749	
	.1822	.9833	.1853	5.3955	1.0170	5.4874	
	.1851	.9827	.1883	5.3093	1.0176	5.4026	
	.1880	.9822	.1914	5.2257	1.0182	5.3205	
11°	.1908	.9816	.1944	5.1446	1.0187	5.2408	79°
	.1937	.9811	.1974	5.0658	1.0193	5.1636	
	.1965	.9805	.2004	4.9894	1.0199	5.0886	
	.1994	.9799	.2035	4.9152	1.0205	5.0159	
	.2022	.9793	.2065	4.8430	1.0211	4.9452	
	.2051	.9787	.2095	4.7729	1.0217	4.8765	
12°	.2079	.9781	.2126	4.7046	1.0223	4.8097	78°
	.2108	.9775	.2156	4.6382	1.0230	4.7448	
	.2136	.9769	.2186	4.5736	1.0236	4.6817	
	.2164	.9763	.2217	4.5107	1.0243	4.6202	
	.2193	.9757	.2247	4.4494	1.0249	4.5604	
	.2221	.9750	.2278	4.3897	1.0256	4.5022	
	cos A	sin A	cot A	tan A	cosec A	sec A	A

SPECIAL TABLE 2 *(Continued)*

A	sin A	cos A	tan A	cot A	sec A	cosec A	
13°	.2250	.9744	.2309	4.3315	1.0263	4.4454	77°
	.2278	.9737	.2339	4.2747	1.0270	4.3901	
	.2306	.9730	.2370	4.2193	1.0277	4.3362	
	.2334	.9724	.2401	4.1653	1.0284	4.2837	
	.2363	.9717	.2432	4.1126	1.0291	4.2324	
	.2391	.9710	.2462	4.0611	1.0299	4.1824	
14°	.2419	.9703	.2493	4.0108	1.0306	4.1336	76°
	.2447	.9696	.2524	3.9617	1.0314	4.0859	
	.2476	.9689	.2555	3.9136	1.0321	4.0394	
	.2504	.9681	.2586	3.8667	1.0329	3.9939	
	.2532	.9674	.2617	3.8208	1.0337	3.9495	
	.2560	.9667	.2648	3.7760	1.0345	3.9061	
15°	.2588	.6959	.2679	3.7321	1.0353	3.8637	75°
	.2616	.9652	.2711	3.6891	1.0361	3.8222	
	.2644	.9644	.2742	3.6470	1.0369	3.7817	
	.2672	.9636	.2773	3.6059	1.0377	3.7420	
	.2700	.9628	.2805	3.5656	1.0386	3.7032	
	.2728	.9621	.2836	3.5261	1.0394	3.6652	
16°	.2756	.9613	.2807	3.4874	1.0403	3.6280	74°
	.2784	.9605	.2899	3.4495	1.0412	3.5915	
	.2812	.9596	.2931	3.4124	1.0421	3.5559	
	.2840	.9588	.2962	3.3759	1.0430	3.5209	
	.2868	.9580	.2994	3.3402	1.0439	3.4867	
	.2896	.9672	.3026	3.3052	1.0448	3.4532	
17°	.2924	.9563	.3057	3.2709	1.0457	3.4203	73°
	.2952	.9555	.3089	3.2371	1.0466	3.3881	
	.2979	.9546	.3121	3.2041	1.0476	3.3565	
	.3007	.9537	.3153	3.1716	1.0485	3.3255	
	.3035	.9528	.3185	3.1397	1.0495	3.2951	
	.3062	.9520	.3217	3.1084	1.0505	3.2653	
18°	.3090	.9511	.3249	3.0777	1.0515	3.2361	72°
	.3118	.9502	.3281	3.0475	1.0525	3.2074	
	.3145	.9492	.3314	3.0178	1.0535	3.1792	
	.3173	.9483	.3346	2.9887	1.0545	3.1516	
	.3201	.9474	.3378	2.9600	1.0555	3.1244	
	.3228	.9465	.3411	2.9319	1.0566	3.0977	
19°	.3256	.9455	.3443	2.9042	1.0576	3.0716	71°
	.3283	.9446	.3476	2.8770	1.0587	3.0458	
	.3311	.9436	.3508	2.8502	1.0598	3.0206	
	.3338	.9426	.3541	2.8239	1.0609	2.9957	
	.3365	.9417	.3574	2.7980	1.0620	2.9714	
	.3393	.9407	.3607	2.7725	1.0631	2.9474	
	cos A	sin A	cot A	tan A	cosec A	sec A	A

SPECIAL TABLE 2 *(Continued)*

A	sin A	cos A	tan A	cot A	sec A	cosec A	
20°	.3420	.9397	.3640	2.7475	1.0642	2.9238	70°
	.3448	.9387	.3673	2.7228	1.0653	2.9006	
	.3475	.9377	.3706	2.6985	1.0665	2.8779	
	.3502	.9367	.3739	2.6747	1.0676	2.8555	
	.3529	.9356	.3772	2.6511	1.0688	2.8334	
	.3557	.9346	.3805	2.6279	1.0700	2.8118	
21°	.3584	.9336	.3839	2.6051	1.0712	2.7904	69°
	.3611	.9325	.3872	2.5826	1.0724	2.7695	
	.3638	.9315	.3906	2.5605	1.0736	2.7488	
	.3665	.9304	.3939	2.5386	1.0748	2.7285	
	.3692	.9293	.3973	2.5172	1.0760	2.7085	
	.3719	.9283	.4006	2.4960	1.0773	2.6888	
22°	.3746	.9272	.4040	2.4751	1.0785	2.6695	68°
	.3773	.9261	.4074	2.4545	1.0798	2.6504	
	.3800	.9250	.4108	2.4342	1.0811	2.6316	
	.3827	.9239	.4142	2.4142	1.0824	2.6131	
	.3854	.9228	.4176	2.3945	1.0837	2.5949	
	.3881	.9216	.4210	2.3750	1.0850	2.5770	
23°	.3907	.9205	.4245	2.3559	1.0864	2.5593	67°
	.3934	.9194	.4279	2.3369	1.0877	2.5419	
	.3961	.9182	.4314	2.3183	1.0891	2.5247	
	.3987	.9171	.4348	2.2998	1.0904	2.5078	
	.4014	.9159	.4383	2.2817	1.0918	2.4912	
	.4041	.9147	.4417	2.2637	1.0932	2.4748	
24°	.4067	.9135	.4452	2.2460	1.0946	2.586	66°
	.4094	.9124	.4487	2.2286	1.0961	2.4426	
	.4120	.9112	.4522	2.2113	1.0975	2.4269	
	.4147	.9100	.4557	2.1943	1.0990	2.4114	
	.4173	.9088	.4592	2.1775	1.1004	2.3961	
	.4200	.9075	.4628	2.1609	1.1019	2.3811	
25°	.4226	.9063	.4663	2.1445	1.1034	2.3662	65°
	.4253	.9051	.4699	2.1283	1.1049	2.3515	
	.4279	.9038	.4734	2.1123	1.1064	2.3371	
	.4305	.9026	.4770	2.0965	1.1079	2.3228	
	.4331	.9013	.4806	2.0809	1.1095	2.3088	
	.4358	.9001	.4841	2.0655	1.1110	2.2949	
26°	.4384	.8988	.4877	2.0503	1.1126	2.2812	64°
	.4410	.8975	.4913	2.0353	1.1142	2.2677	
	.4430	.8962	.4950	2.0204	1.1158	2.2543	
	.4462	.8949	.4986	2.0057	1.1174	2.2412	
	.4488	.8936	.5022	1.9912	1.1190	2.2282	
	.4514	.8923	.5059	1.9768	1.1207	2.2154	
	cos A	sin A	cot A	tan A	cosec A	sec A	A

Natural Trigonometric Functions

SPECIAL TABLE 2 *(Continued)*

A	sin A	cos A	tan A	cot A	sec A	cosec A	
27°	.4540	.8910	.5095	1.9626	1.1223	2.2027	63°
	.4566	.8897	.5132	1.9486	1.1240	2.1902	
	.4592	.8884	.5169	1.9347	1.1257	2.1779	
	.4617	.8870	.5206	1.9210	1.1274	2.1657	
	.4643	.8857	.5243	1.9074	1.1291	2.1537	
	.4669	.8843	.5280	1.8940	1.1308	2.1418	
28°	.4695	.8829	.5317	1.8807	1.1326	2.1301	62°
	.4720	.8816	.5354	1.8676	1.1343	2.1185	
	.4746	.8802	.5392	1.8546	1.1361	2.1070	
	.4772	.8788	.5430	1.8418	1.1379	2.0957	
	.4797	.8774	.5467	1.8291	1.1397	2.0846	
	.4823	.8760	.5505	1.8165	1.1415	2.0736	
29°	.4848	.8746	.5543	1.8040	1.1434	2.0627	61°
	.4874	.8732	.5581	1.7917	1.1452	2.0519	
	.4899	.8718	.5619	1.7796	1.1471	2.0413	
	.4924	.8704	.5658	1.7675	1.1490	2.0308	
	.4950	.8689	.5696	1.7556	1.1509	2.0204	
	.4975	.8675	.5735	1.7437	1.1528	2.0101	
30°	.5000	.8660	.5774	1.7321	1.1547	2.0000	60°
	.5025	.8646	.5812	1.7205	1.1567	1.9900	
	.5050	.8631	.5851	1.7090	1.1586	1.9801	
	.5075	.8616	.5890	1.6977	1.1606	1.9703	
	.5100	.8601	.5930	1.6864	1.1626	1.9606	
	.5125	.8587	.5969	1.6753	1.1646	1.9511	
31°	.5150	.8572	.6009	1.6643	1.1666	1.9416	59°
	.5175	.8557	.6048	1.6534	1.1687	1.9323	
	.5200	.8542	.6088	1.6426	1.1708	1.9230	
	.5225	.8526	.6128	1.6319	1.1728	1.9139	
	.5250	.8511	.6168	1.6212	1.1749	1.9049	
	.5275	.8496	.6208	1.6107	1.1770	1.8959	
32°	.5299	.8480	.6249	1.6003	1.1792	1.8871	58°
	.5324	.8465	.6289	1.5900	1.1813	1.8783	
	.5348	.8450	.6330	1.5798	1.1835	1.8699	
	.5373	.8434	.6371	1.5697	1.1857	1.8612	
	.5398	.8418	.6412	1.5597	1.1879	1.8527	
	.5422	.8403	.6453	1.5497	1.1901	1.8444	
33°	.5446	.8387	.6494	1.5399	1.1924	1.8361	57°
	.5471	.8371	.6536	1.5301	1.1946	1.8279	
	.5495	.8355	.6577	1.5204	1.1969	1.8198	
	.5519	.8339	.6619	1.5108	1.1992	1.8118	
	.5544	.8323	.6661	1.5013	1.2015	1.8039	
	.5568	.8307	.6703	1.4919	1.2039	1.7960	
	cos A	sin A	cot A	tan A	cosec A	sec A	A

SPECIAL TABLE 2 *(Continued)*

A	sin A	cos A	tan A	cot A	sec A	cosec A	
34°	.5592	.8290	.6745	1.4826	1.2062	1.7883	56°
	.5616	.8274	.6787	1.4733	1.2086	1.7806	
	.5640	.8258	.6830	1.4641	1.2110	1.7730	
	.5664	.8241	.6873	1.4550	1.2134	1.7655	
	.5688	.8225	.6916	1.4460	1.2158	1.7581	
	.5712	.8208	.6959	1.4370	1.2183	1.7507	
35°	.5736	.8192	.7002	1.4281	1.2208	1.7435	55°
	.5760	.8175	.7046	1.4193	1.2233	1.7362	
	.5783	.8158	.7089	1.4106	1.2258	1.7291	
	.5807	.8141	.7133	1.4019	1.2283	1.7221	
	.5831	.8124	.7177	1.3934	1.2309	1.7151	
	.5854	.8107	.7221	1.3848	1.2335	1.7082	
36°	.5878	.8090	.7265	1.3764	1.2361	1.7013	54°
	.5901	.8073	.7310	1.3680	1.2387	1.6945	
	.5925	.8056	.7355	1.3597	1.2413	1.6878	
	.5948	.8039	.7400	1.3514	1.2440	1.6812	
	.5972	.8021	.7445	1.3432	1.2467	1.6746	
	.5995	.8004	.7490	1.3351	1.2494	1.6681	
37°	.6018	.7986	.7536	1.3270	1.2521	1.6616	53°
	.6041	.7969	.7536	1.3190	1.2549	1.6553	
	.6065	.7951	.7627	1.3111	1.2577	1.6489	
	.6088	.7934	.7673	1.3032	1.2605	1.6427	
	.6111	.7916	.7720	1.2954	1.2633	1.6365	
	.6134	.7898	.7766	1.2876	1.2662	1.6304	
38°	.6157	.7880	.7813	1.2799	1.2690	1.6243	52°
	.6180	.7862	.7860	1.2723	1.2719	1.6183	
	.6202	.7844	.7907	1.2647	1.2748	1.6123	
	.6225	.7826	.7954	1.2572	1.2779	1.6064	
	.6248	.7808	.8002	1.2497	1.2808	1.6005	
	.6271	.7790	.8050	1.2423	1.2837	1.5948	
39°	.6293	.7771	.8098	1.2349	1.2868	1.5890	51°
	.6316	.7753	.8146	1.2276	1.2898	1.5833	
	.6338	.7735	.8195	1.2203	1.2929	1.5777	
	.6361	.7716	.8243	1.2131	1.2960	1.5721	
	.6383	.7698	.8392	1.2059	1.2991	1.5666	
	.6406	.7679	.8342	1.1988	1.3022	1.5611	
	cos A	sin A	cot A	tan A	cosec A	sec A	A

SPECIAL TABLE 2 *(Continued)*

A	sin A	cos A	tan A	cot A	sec A	cosec A	
40°	.6428	.7660	.8391	1.1918	1.3054	1.5557	50°
	.6450	.7642	.8441	1.1847	1.3086	1.5504	
	.6472	.7623	.8491	1.1778	1.3118	1.5450	
	.6494	.7604	.8541	1.1708	1.3151	1.5398	
	.6517	.7585	.8591	1.1640	1.3184	1.5346	
	.6539	.7566	.8642	1.1571	1.3217	1.5294	
41°	.6561	.7547	.8693	1.1504	1.3250	1.5243	49°
	.6583	.7528	.8744	1.1436	1.3384	1.5192	
	.6604	.7509	.8796	1.1369	1.3318	1.5142	
	.6626	.7490	.8847	1.1303	1.3352	1.5092	
	.6648	.7470	.8899	1.1237	1.3386	1.5042	
	.6670	.7451	.8952	1.1171	1.3421	1.4993	
42°	.6691	.7431	.9004	1.1106	1.3456	1.4945	48°
	.6713	.7412	.9057	1.1041	1.3492	1.4897	
	.6734	.7392	.9110	1.0977	1.3527	1.4849	
	.6756	.7373	.9163	1.0913	1.3563	1.4802	
	.6777	.7353	.9217	1.0850	1.3600	1.4755	
	.6799	.7333	.9271	1.0786	1.3636	1.4709	
43°	.6820	.7314	.9325	1.0724	1.3673	1.4663	47°
	.6841	.7294	.9380	1.0661	1.3711	1.4617	
	.6862	.7274	.9435	1.0599	1.3748	1.4572	
	.6884	.7254	.9490	1.0538	1.3786	1.4527	
	.6905	.7234	.9545	1.0477	1.3824	1.4483	
	.6926	.7214	.9601	1.0416	1.3863	1.4439	
44°	.6947	.7193	.9657	1.0355	1.3902	1.4396	46°
	.6967	.7173	.9713	1.0295	1.3941	1.4352	
	.6988	.7153	.9770	1.0235	1.3980	1.4310	
	.7009	.7133	.9827	1.0176	1.4020	1.4267	
	.7030	.7112	.9884	1.0117	1.4061	1.4225	
	.7050	.7092	.9942	1.0058	1.4101	1.4184	
45°	.7071	.7071	1.0000	1.0000	1.4142	1.4142	45°
	cos A	sin A	cot A	tan A	cosec A	sec A	A

Conversion Factors

To convert a given length in one system of units to the same length in any other system units, or likewise with any other physical parameters of concern to this text, use the conversion factors given in these tables. We include the following for convenience:

SPECIAL TABLE 3
LENGTHS

To Obtain ↓ / Multiply Number Of → by	Centimeters	Feet	Inches	Kilometers	Nautical miles	Meters	Mils	Miles	Millimeters	Yards
Centimeters	1	30.48	2.540	10^5	1.853	100	2.540×10^{-3}	1.609×10^5	0.1	91.44
Feet	3.281×10^{-2}	1	8.333×10^{-2}	3281	6080.27	3.281	8.333×10^{-5}	5280	3.281×10^{-3}	3
Inches	0.3937	12	1	3.937×10^4	7.296×10^4	39.37	0.001	6.336×10^4	3.937×10^{-2}	36
Kilometers	10^{-5}	3.048×10^{-4}	2.540×10^{-5}	1	1.853	0.001	2.540×10^{-8}	1.609	10^{-6}	9.144×10^{-4}
Nautical miles		1.645×10^{-4}		0.5396	1	5.396×10^{-4}		0.8684		4.934×10^{-4}
Meters	0.01	0.3048	2.540×10^{-2}	1000	1853	1		1609	0.001	0.9144
Mils	393.7	1.2×10^4	1000	3.937×10^7		3.937×10^4	1		39.37	3.6×10^4
Miles	6.214×10^{-6}	1.894×10^{-4}	1.578×10^{-5}	0.6214	1.1516	6.214×10^{-4}		1	6.214×10^{-7}	5.682×10^{-4}
Millimeters	10	304.8	25.40	10^6		1000	2.540×10^{-2}		1	914.4
Yards	1.094×10^{-2}	0.3333	2.778×10^{-2}	1094	2027	1.094	2.778×10^{-5}	1760	1.094×10^{-3}	1

SPECIAL TABLE 4
FORCE

Multiply Number Of by / To Obtain	Dynes	Grams	Joules per cm	Joules per meter	Kilograms	Pounds	Poundals
Dynes	1	980.7	10^7	10^5	9.807×10^5	4.448×10^5	1.383×10^4
Grams	1.020×10^{-2}	1	1.020×10^4	102.0	1000	453.6	14.10
Joules per cm	10^{-7}	9.807×10^{-5}	1	.01	9.807×10^{-2}	4.448×10^{-2}	1.383×10^{-2}
Newtons or joules per meter	10^{-5}	9.807×10^{-2}	100	1	9.807	4.448	0.1383
Kilograms	1.020×10^{-6}	0.001	10.20	0.1020	1	0.4536	1.410×10^{-2}
Pounds	2.248×10^{-6}	2.205×10^{-3}	22.48	0.2248	2.205	1	3.108×10^{-2}
Poundals	7.233×10^{-5}	7.093×10^{-2}	723.3	7.233	70.93	32.17	1

Conversion factors between absolute and gravitational units apply only under standard acceleration due to gravity conditions.

MASS

To Obtain \ Multiply Number Of by →	Grains	Grams	Kilograms	Milligrams	Ounces	Pounds	Tons (long)	Tons (metric)	Tons (short)
Grains	1	15.43	1.543×10^4	1.543×10^{-2}	437.5	7000			
Grams	6.481×10^{-2}	1	1000	0.001	28.35	453.6	1.016×10^6	10^6	9.072×10^5
Kilograms	6.481×10^{-5}	0.001	1	10^{-6}	2.835×10^{-2}	0.4536	1016	1000	907.2
Milligrams	64.81	1000	10^6	1	2.835×10^4	4.536×10^5	1.016×10^9	10^9	9.072×10^8
Ounces	2.286×10^{-3}	3.527×10^{-2}	35.27	3.527×10^{-6}	1	16	3.584×10^4	3.527×10^4	3.2×10^4
Pounds	1.429×10^{-4}	2.205×10^{-3}	2.205	2.205×10^{-6}	6.250×10^{-2}	1	2240	2205	2000
Tons (long)		9.842×10^{-7}	9.842×10^{-4}	9.842×10^{-10}	2.790×10^{-5}	4.464×10^{-4}	1	0.9842	0.8929
Tons (metric)		10^{-6}	0.001	10^{-9}	2.835×10^{-5}	4.536×10^{-4}	1.016	1	0.9072
Tons (short)		1.102×10^{-6}	1.102×10^{-3}	1.102×10^{-9}	3.125×10^{-5}	0.0005	1.120	1.102	1

SPECIAL TABLE 6
TIME

To Obtain ↓ / Multiply Number Of by →	Days	Hours	Minutes	Months (average)	Seconds	Weeks
Days	1	4.167×10^{-2}	6.944×10^{-4}	30.42	1.157×10^{-5}	7
Hours	24	1	1.667×10^{-2}	730.0	2.778×10^{-4}	168
Minutes	1440	60	1	4.380×10^{4}	1.667×10^{-2}	1.008×10^{4}
Months (average)	3.288×10^{-2}	1.370×10^{-3}	2.283×10^{-5}	1	3.806×10^{-7}	0.2302
Seconds	8.64×10^{4}	3600	60	2.628×10^{6}	1	6.048×10^{5}
Weeks	0.1429	5.952×10^{-3}	9.921×10^{-5}	4.344	1.654×10^{-6}	1

SPECIAL TABLE 7
WORK

To Obtain / Multiply Number Of by	Dyne-centimeters	Gram-centimeters	Kilogram-meters	Pound-feet	Newton-meter
Dyne-centimeters	1	980.7	9.807×10^7	1.356×10^7	10^7
Gram-centimeters	1.020×10^{-2}	1	10^5	1.383×10^4	1.020×10^4
Kilogram-meters	1.020×10^{-8}	10^{-5}	1	0.1383	0.1020
Pound-feet	7.376×10^{-8}	7.233×10^{-5}	7.233	1	0.7376
Newton-meter	10^{-7}	9.807×10^{-4}	9.807	1.305	1

SPECIAL TABLE 8
SPEED

To Obtain \ Multiply Number Of by →	Centimeters per Second	Feet per minute	Feet per second	Kilometers per hour	Kilometers per minute	Knots	Meters per minute	Meters per second	Miles per second	Miles per minute
Centimeters per second	1	0.5080	30.48	27.78	1667	51 48	1.667	100	44.70	2682
Feet per minute	1.969	1	60	54.68	3281	101.3	3.281	196.8	88	5280
Feet per second	3.281×10^{-2}	1.667×10^{-2}	1	0.9113	54.68	1.689	5.468×10^{-2}	3.281	1.467	88
Kilometers per hour	0.036	1.829×10^{-2}	1.097	1	60	1.853	0.06	3.6	1.609	96.54
Kilometers per minute	0.0006	3.048×10^{-4}	1.829×10^{-2}	1.667×10^{-2}	1	3.088×10^{-2}	0.001	0.06	2.682×10^{-2}	1.609
Knots*	1.943×10^{-2}	9.868×10^{-2}	0.5921	0.5396	32.38	1	3.238×10^{-2}	1.943	0.8684	52.10
Meters per minute	0.6	0.3048	18.29	16.67	1000	30.88	1	60	26.82	1609
Meters per second	0.01	5.080×10^{-2}	0.3048	0.2778	16.67	0.5148	1.667×10^{-2}	1	0.4770	26.82
Miles per hour	2.37×10^{-2}	1.136×10^{-2}	0.6818	0.6214	37.28	1.152	3.728×10^{-2}	2.237	1	60
Miles per minute	2.778	1.892								

SPECIAL TABLE 9
CALORIMETRIC ENERGY

Multiply Number Of — by →

To Obtain	British thermal units	Centimeter-grams	Ergs or centimeter dynes	Foot-pounds	Horsepower-hours	Joules or watt-seconds	Kilogram-calories	Kilowatt-hours	Meter-kilograms	Watt-hours
British thermal units	1	9.297×10^{-8}	9.480×10^{-11}	1.285×10^{-2}	2545	9.480×10^{-4}	3.969	3413	9.297×10^{-3}	3.413
Centimeter-grams	1.076×10^{7}	1	1.020×10^{-3}	1.383×10^{4}	2.737×10^{10}	1.020×10^{4}	4.269×10^{7}	3.671×10^{10}	10^{5}	3.671×10^{7}
Ergs or centimeter-dynes	1.055×10^{10}	980.7	1	1.356×10^{7}	2.684×10^{13}	10^{7}	4.186×10^{10}	3.6×10^{13}	9.807×10^{7}	3.6×10^{10}
Foot-pounds	778.3	7.233×10^{-5}	7.367×10^{-8}	1	1.98×10^{6}	0.7376	3087	2.655×10^{6}	7.233	2655
Horsepower-hours	3.929×10^{-4}	3.654×10^{-11}	3.722×10^{-14}	5.050×10^{-7}	1	3.722×10^{-7}	1.559×10^{-3}	1.341	3.653×10^{-6}	1.341×10^{-3}
Joules or watt-seconds	1054.8	9.807×10^{-5}	10^{-7}	1.356	2.684×10^{6}	1	4186	3.6×10^{6}	9.807	3600
Kilogram-calories	0.2520	2.343×10^{-8}	2.389×10^{-11}	3.239×10^{-4}	6413.	2.389×10^{-4}	1	860.0	2.343×10^{-3}	0.8600
Kilowatt-hours	2.930×10^{-4}	2.724×10^{-11}	2.778×10^{-14}	3.766×10^{-7}	0.7457	2.778×10^{-7}	1.163×10^{-3}	1	2.724×10^{-6}	0.001
Meter-kilograms	107.6	10^{-5}	1.020×10^{-8}	0.1383	2.737×10^{5}	0.1020	426.9	3.671×10^{5}	1	367.1
Watt-hours	0.2930	2.724×10^{-8}	2.778×10^{-11}	3.766×10^{-4}	745.7	2.778×10^{-4}	1.163	1000	2.724×10^{-3}	1

SPECIAL TABLE 10
PRESSURE

Multiply Number Of → by / To Obtain ↓	Atmospheres	Baryes or dynes per square centimeter	Centimeters of mercury at 0°C	Inches of mercury at 0°C	Inches of water at 4°C	Kilograms per square meter	Pounds per square foot	Pounds per square inch	Tons (short) for square foot	Newtons per square meter
Atmospheres	1	9.869×10^{-7}	1.316×10^{-2}	3.342×10^{-2}	2.458×10^{-3}	9.678×10^{-5}	4.725×10^{-4}	6.804×10^{-2}	0.9450	9.869×10^{-6}
Baryes or dynes per square centimeter	1.013×10^{6}	1	1.333×10^{4}	3.386×10^{4}	2.491×10^{2}	98.07	478.8	6.895×10^{4}	9.567×10^{5}	10
Centimeters of mercury at 0°C	76.00	7.501×10^{-5}	1	2.540	0.1868	7.356×10^{-3}	3.591×10^{-2}	5.171	71.83	7.501×10^{-4}
Inches of mercury at 0°C	29.92	2.953×10^{-5}	0.3937	1	7.355×10^{-2}	2.896×10^{-3}	1.414×10^{-2}	2.036	28.28	2.953×10^{-4}
Inches of water at 4°C	406.8	4.015×10^{-4}	5.354	13.60	1	3.937×10^{-2}	0.1922	27.68	384.5	4.015×10^{-3}
Kilograms per square meter	1.033×10^{4}	1.020×10^{-2}	136.0	345.3	25.40	1	4.882	703.1	9765	0.1020
Pounds per square foot	2117	2.089×10^{-3}	27.85	70.73	5.204	0.2048	1	144	2000	2.089×10^{-2}
Pounds per square inch	14.70	1.450×10^{-5}	0.1934	0.4912	3.613×10^{-2}	1.422×10^{-3}	6.944×10^{-3}	1	13.89	1.450×10^{-4}
Tons (short) per square foot	1.058	1.044×10^{-6}	1.392×10^{-2}	3.536×10^{-2}	2.601×10^{-3}	1.024×10^{-4}	0.0005	0.072	1	1.044×10^{-5}
Newtons per square	1.013	10^{-1}	1.333	3.386	2.491	9.807	47.88	6.895	9.576	1

SPECIAL TABLE 11
SPECIFIC GRAVITY

Multiply Number Of by	Grams per cubic Centimeter	Kilograms per cubic meter	Pounds per cubic foot	Pounds per cubic foot
To Obtain				
Grams per cubic centimeter	1	0.001	1.602×10^{-2}	27.68
Kilograms per cubic meter	1000	1	16.02	2.768×10^4
Pounds per cubic foot	62.43	6.243×10^{-2}	1	1728
Pounds per cubic inch	3.613×10^{-2}	3.613×10^{-5}	5.787×10^{-4}	1
Pounds per mil foot*	3.405×10^{-2}	3.405×10^{-10}	5.456×10^{-9}	9.425×10^{-6}

*Unit of volume is a volume one foot long and one circular mill in cross-section area.

To Obtain ↓ / Multiply Number Of → by	Acres	Circular mils	Square centimeters	Square feet	Square inches	Square kilometers	Square meters	Square miles	Square millimeters	Square yards
Acres	1			2.296×10^{-5}		247.1	2.471×10^{-4}	640		2.066×10^{-4}
Circular mils		1	1.973×10^{5}	1.833×10^{8}	1.273×10^{6}		1.973×10^{9}		1973	
Square centimeters		5.067×10^{-6}	1	929.0	6.452	10^{10}	10^{4}	2.590×10^{10}	0.01	8361
Square feet	4.356×10^{4}		1.076×10^{-3}	1	6.944×10^{-3}	1.076×10^{7}	10.76	2.788×10^{7}	1.076×10^{-5}	9
Square inches	6,272,640	7.854×10^{-7}	0.1550	144	1	1.550×10^{9}	1550	4.015×10^{9}	1.550×10^{-3}	1296
Square kilometers	4.047×10^{-3}		10^{-10}	9.290×10^{-8}	6.452×10^{-10}	1	10^{-6}	2.590	10^{-12}	8.361×10^{-7}
Square meters	4047		0.0001	9.290×10^{-2}	6.452×10^{-4}	10^{6}	1	2.590×10^{6}	10^{-6}	0.8361
Square miles	1.562×10^{-3}		3.861×10^{-11}	3.587×10^{-8}		0.3861	3.861×10^{-7}	1	3.861×10^{-13}	3.228×10^{-7}
Square millimeters		5.067×10^{-4}	100	9.290×10^{4}	645.2	10^{12}	10^{6}		1	8.361×10^{5}
Square yards	4840		1.196	0.1111	7.716	1.196	1.196	3.098	1.196	1

VOLUME

Multiply Number Of → by

To Obtain ↓	Bushels (dry)	Cubic centimeters	Cubic feet	Cubic inches	Cubic meters	Cubic yards	Gallons (liquid)	Liters	Pints (liquid)	Quarts (liquid)
Bushels (dry)	1		0.8036	4.651×10^{-4}	28.38			2.838×10^{-2}		
Cubic centimeters	3.524×10^{4}	1	2.832×10^{4}	16.39	10^{6}	7.646×10^{5}	3785	1000	473.2	946.4
Cubic feet	1.2445	3.531×10^{-5}	1	5.787×10^{-4}	35.31	27	0.1337	3.531×10^{-2}	1.671×10^{-2}	3.342×10^{-2}
Cubic inches	2150.4	6.102×10^{-2}	1728	1	6.102×10^{4}	46.656	231	61.02	28.87	57.75
Cubic meters	3.524×10^{-2}	10^{-6}	2.832×10^{-2}	1.639×10^{-5}	1	0.7646	3.785×10^{-3}	0.001	4.732×10^{-4}	9.464×10^{-4}
Cubic yards		1.308×10^{-6}	3.704×10^{-2}	2.143×10^{-5}	1.308	1	4.951×10^{-3}	1.308×10^{-3}	6.189×10^{-4}	1.238×10^{-3}
Gallons (liquid)		2.642×10^{-4}	7.481	4.329×10^{-3}	264.2	202.0	1	0.2642	0.125	0.25
Liters	35.24	0.001	28.32	1.639×10^{-2}	1000	764.6	3.785	1	0.4732	0.9464
Pints (Liquid)		2.113×10^{-3}	59.84	3.463×10^{-2}	2113	1616	8	2.113	1	2
Quarts (Liquid)		1.057×10^{-3}	29.92	1.732×10^{-2}	1057	807.9	4	1.057	0.5	1

SPECIAL TABLE 14
ANGULAR MEASURE

To Obtain → / Multiply Number Of by	Degrees	Minutes	Quadrants	Radians	Revolutions (Circumferences)	Seconds
Degrees	1	1.667×10^{-2}	90	57.30	360	2.778×10^{-4}
Minutes	60	1	5400	3438	2.16×10^{4}	1.667×10^{-2}
Quadrants	1.111×10^{-2}	1.852×10^{-4}	1	0.6366	4	3.087×10^{-6}
Radians	1.745×10^{-2}	2.909×10^{-4}	1.571	1	6.283	4.848×10^{-6}
Revolutions (Circumferences)	2.778×10^{-2}	4.630×10^{-5}	0.25	0.1591	1	7.716×10^{-7}
Seconds	3600	60	3.24×10^{5}	2.063×10^{5}	1.296×10^{6}	1

HARDNESS TABLE

Brinell, mm. diam. indentation	Vickers diamond Pyramid	Rockwell A 60kg	Rockwell C 150kg	D 100kg	Approx. Tensile Strength p.s.i., thousands
2.25	840	84.1	65.3	74.8	
2.35	737	82.2	61.7	72.0	
2.60	591	78.4	54.7	66.7	300
2.80	508	75.6	49.6	62.7	252
2.95	455	93.4	45.7	59.7	219
3.15	383	70.1	39.1	54.6	177
3.35	350	68.1	35.5	51.9	159
3.55	309	65.7	30.9	48.3	141
3.80	269	63.0	25.4	44.2	123
4.0	241	60.8	20.5	40.5	111
4.25	213	—	13.8	—	98

Note: hardness of fresh wet bone equals $\approx$ 40 Rockwell H, 25 Brinell and 25 Vickers.

SPECIAL TABLE 16
GREEK ALPHABET

A α alpha	I ι iota	P ρ rho
B β beta	K κ kappa	Σ σ sigma
Γ γ gamma	Λ λ lambda	T ς tau
Δ δ delta	M μ mu	Υ υ upsilon
E ε epsilon	N ν nu	Φ φ phi
Z ζ zeta	Ξ ξ xi	X χ chi
H η eta	O o omicron	Ψ ψ psi
Θ θ theta	Π π pi	Ω ω omega

SPECIAL TABLE 17

Cross sectional Figure	Moment inertia (I_o)	Radius of gyration (r_o)	Polar moment inertia (J_o)
Rectangular, width b and total height y	$\dfrac{1}{12} b\, y^3$	$\dfrac{y}{12}$	$\dfrac{1}{12}$ by $(b^2 + y^2)$
Circular, outer diameter D	$\dfrac{1}{64} \pi\, D^4$	$D/4$	$\dfrac{1}{32} \pi\, D^4$
Tubular, inner diameter d, outer diameter D	$\dfrac{1}{64} \pi\, (D^4 - d^4)$	$\dfrac{D^2 + d^2}{4}$	$\dfrac{1}{32} \pi\, (D^4 - d^4)$
Triangular, of width b and height y	$\dfrac{1}{36} b\, y^3$	$\dfrac{y}{18}$	$\dfrac{1}{48}$ by $(\dfrac{4}{3} y^2 + b^2)$

(Valid only if neutral axis/plane lies in the center of the cross section.)

SPECIAL TABLE 18
SYSTEMS OF UNITS

Quantity	c g s	M K S	M T S	Technical	English
length	centimeter (cm)	meter (m)	meter (m)	meter (m)	foot (ft)
time	second (sec)	second (sec)	second (sec)	second (sec)	second (sec)
mass	gram (g)	kilogram (kg)	ton (1000 kg)	9.81 kg mass	pound (lb)
force	dyne	Newton (10^5 dynes)	Sthene (10^8 dynes)	kilogram force (kg f)	pound force (lb f)
power	erg/sec	watt	Kilowatt	9.8 watt	horsepower (hp)
energy	erg	Joule (10^7 ergs)	kilojoule	kg f/m	B.T.U.; ft-lb

SPECIAL TABLE 19
MORE CONVERSION FACTORS

1 acre	= 4,3560 ft²	1 B.t.u./sec	= 1.05 × 10¹⁰	
	= 4840 yd²		ergs/sec	
	= 160 rods²		= 1.41 h p	
	= .0016 mi²		= 1.05 kilowatts	
1 ampere	= .1 abampere	1 bushel	= 8 gallons	
	= 1 coulomb/sec		= 36.4 liters	
	= 3.0 × 10⁹	1 calorie (gm)	= .0039 B.t.u.	
	statamperes		= 4.18 × 10⁷ ergs	
1 Ångstrom	= 1 × 10⁻⁸ cm		= 3.08 ft-lb	
	= 3.9 × 10⁻⁹ in		= 42665 gm-cm	
	= .0001 microns		= 4.184 Joules	
	= .1 millimicrons	1 cm	= 10⁸ Ångstroms	
1 atmosphere	= 1.01 bar		= .033 ft	
	= 76 cm Hg		= 10,000 microns	
	= 1033 cm H₂O		= 10 mm	
	= 1033 gm/cm²	1 dram (fluid)	= 3.69 cc	
	= 14.7 lb/in²		= .0225 in³	
	= 760 torrs		= 60 minims	
1 B.t.u.	= 252 gm cal.		= .125 oz	
	= 1.05 × 10¹⁰ ergs	1 dyne	= .0157 grains	
	= 778 ft-lb		= .0010 gm	
	= 1054 Joules		= 1 × 10⁻⁵ Newtons	
	= 107 kg — m		= 2.25 × 10⁻⁶ lb	
	= 1054 watt-sec	1 electron volt	= 1.6 × 10⁻¹² ergs	
1 erg	= 2.39 × 10⁻⁸ cal	1 hectare	= 2.47 acres	
	= 1 dyne-cm		= 10,000 m²	
	= 6.2 × 10¹¹		= .0039 mi²	
	electron volts	1 horsepower	= 42.4 B.t.u./min.	
	= 7.4 × 10⁻⁸ ft-lb	(mechanical)	= 10,678 cal/min	
	= .0010 gm-cm		= 33,000 ft-lb/min	
	= 1 × 10⁻⁷ Joules		= 550 ft-lb/sec	
1 fathom	= 6 feet		= 745 Joules/sec	
	= 2 yards		= .745 kilowatt	
1 foot	= 30.5 cm		= 745 watts	
1 ft-lb	= .0013 B.t.u.		= .076 hp (boiler)	
	= .324 cal (gm)		= 1.0 hp (metric)	
	= 13825 gm-cm		= 1.0 hp (electric)	
	= .138 kg-m	1 inch	= 2.54 × 10⁸	
1 gallon (U.S.)	= .031 barrels		Ångstrom	
	= .107 bushels		= 2.54 cm	
	= .155 ft³ <		= 6.02 Picas	
	= 268.8 in³		(printers)	
	= 4.4 liters		= 72.3 points	
1 grain	= .324 carats		(printers)	
	= 63.5 dynes	1 Joule	= .0095 B.t.u.	
	= 64.7 mg		= .239 cal (gm)	
1 gm	= carats		= 1 × 10⁷ ergs	
	= 980.6 dynes		= .737 ft-lb	
	= 15.4 grains		= 10,197 gm-cm	
	= .032 oz (troy)		= 1.00 watt-sec	

SPECIAL TABLE 19 (Continued)

1 kg	= 9.8 × 10⁻⁵ dynes	1 Joule/sec	= .0013 hp
	= 32.1 oz (troy)		= 1.00 watts
	= 643 pennyweights		= .737 ft-lb/sec
	= 2.20 lb (advp)	1 micron	= 10,000 Ångstroms
	= .068 slugs		= .001 mm
1 kilowatt	= 3414 B.t.u./hr		= 3.9 × 10⁻⁵ in
	= 239 cal/sec	1 mile	= 9.72 cables
	= 44.254 ft-lb/in	(statute)	= 1.70 fathoms
	= 1.34 hp		= 5280 ft
	= 1000 Joules/sec		= 1.609 km
1 knot	= 1 mph		= .868 mi (naut, Brit)
	= 1.85 km/hr		= 320 yd
	= 1.69 ft/sec		= 1760 yd
	= 51.4 cm/sec	1 milliliter	= 1 cm³
1 league	= 18.240 ft		= .061 in³
	= 5.5 km		= 16.2 minims
	= 3.45 mi		= .034 oz
	= 3038 fathoms	1 Newton	= 10,000 dynes
1 liter	= 61.0 in³		= .225 lb
	= .227 gallons	1 Newton-meter	= 1 × 10⁷ dyne/cm
	= 1.05 quarts		= 10,200 gm/cm
	= 1000 cc		= .102 kg-m
1 meter	= 100 cm		= .737 lb-ft
	= 1546 fathoms	1 peck (U.S.)	= .077 barrels
	= 3.28 ft		= .25 bushels
	= 1.09 yd		= 2.33 gallons
1 lb (advp)	= 7000 grains		= 8 quarts
	= 453.6 gm	1 pennyweight	= 24 grains
	= .453 kg		= 1.55 gm
	= 15 oz (advp)	1 ton (short)	= 907 kg
	= 14 oz (troy)		= 2000 lb (advp)
	= 291.6 pennyweight		= 2430 lb (troy)
	= .031 slugs		= .893 tons (long)
1 Reyn	= 6.89 × 10⁶		= .907 tons (metric)
	centipoises	1 watt	= 3.41 B.t.u./hr
1 revolution	= 360 degrees		= 14.3 cal/min
	= 4 gradrants		= 1 Joule/sec
	= 6.28 radians		= .0013 hp
1 rod	= 16.5 ft		= .001 kilowatt
	= 5.03 m		
	= 5.5 yd		
1 scruple	= 20 grains		
	= 1.29 gm		
1 slug	= 14.6 kg		
	= 32.2 lb		
1 span	= 9 inches		
1 square mile	= 640 acres		
	= 259 hectares		
	= 2.59 km²		

SPECIAL TABLE 20
MILLIMETERS-TO-INCHES CONVERSION

Inches	Millimeters	Inches	Millimeters	Inches	Millimeters	Inches	Millimeters	Inches	Millimeters	Inches	Millimeters	Inches	Millimeters
1/64	0.3969	51/64	20.2406	2 3/32	53.1814	3 9/16	90.4877	5 1/32	127.794	6 7/8	174.625	9 1/2	241.300
1/32	0.7937	13/16	20.6375	2 1/8	53.9751	3 19/32	91.2814	5 1/16	128.588	6 15/16	176.213	9 9/16	242.888
3/64	1.1906	53/64	21.0344	2 5/32	54.7688	3 5/8	92.0752	5 3/32	129.382	7	177.800	9 5/8	244.475
1/16	1.5875	27/32	21.4312	2 3/16	55.5626	3 21/32	92.8689	5 1/8	130.175	7 1/16	179.388	9 11/16	246.063
5/64	1.9844	55/64	21.8281	2 7/32	56.3564	3 11/16	93.6627	5 5/32	130.969	7 1/8	180.975	9 3/4	247.650
3/32	2.3812	7/8	22.2250	2 1/4	57.1501	3 23/32	94.4564	5 3/16	131.763	7 3/16	182.563	9 13/16	249.238
7/64	2.7781	57/64	22.6219	2 9/32	57.9439	3 3/4	95.2502	5 7/32	132.557	7 1/4	184.150	9 7/8	250.825
1/8	3.1750	29/32	23.0187	2 5/16	58.7376	3 25/32	96.0439	5 1/4	133.350	7 5/16	185.738	9 15/16	252.413
9/64	3.5719	59/64	23.4156	2 11/32	59.5314	3 13/16	96.8377	5 9/32	134.141	7 3/8	187.325	10	254.001
5/32	3.9687	15/16	23.8125	2 3/8	60.3251	3 27/32	97.6314	5 5/16	134.938	7 7/16	188.913	10 1/16	255.588
11/64	4.3656	61/64	24.2094	2 13/32	61.1189	3 7/8	98.4252	5 11/32	135.732	7 1/2	190.500	10 1/8	257.176
3/16	4.7625	31/32	24.6062	2 7/16	61.9126	3 29/32	99.2189	5 3/8	136.525	7 9/16	192.088	10 3/16	258.763
13/64	5.1594	63/64	25.0031	2 15/32	62.7064	3 15/16	100.013	5 13/32	137.319	7 5/8	193.675	10 1/4	260.351
7/32	5.5562	1	25.4001	2 1/2	63.5001	3 31/32	100.806	5 7/16	138.113	7 11/16	195.263	10 5/16	261.938
15/64	5.9531	1 1/32	26.1938	2 17/32	64.2939	4	101.600	5 15/32	138.907	7 3/4	196.850	10 3/8	263.526
1/4	6.3500	1 1/16	26.9876	2 9/16	65.0876	4 1/32	102.394	5 1/2	139.700	7 13/16	198.438	10 7/16	265.113
17/64	6.7469	1 3/32	27.7813	2 19/32	65.8814	4 1/16	103.188	5 17/32	140.494	7 7/8	200.025	10 1/2	266.700
9/32	7.1437	1 1/8	28.5751	2 5/8	66.6751	4 3/32	103.981	5 9/16	141.288	7 15/16	201.613	10 9/16	268.288
19/64	7.5406	1 5/32	29.3688	2 21/32	67.4689	4 1/8	104.775	5 19/32	142.082	8	203.200	10 5/8	269.876
5/16	7.9375	1 3/16	30.1626	2 11/16	68.2626	4 5/32	105.569	5 5/8	142.875	8 1/16	204.788	10 11/16	271.463
21/64	8.3344	1 7/32	30.9563	2 23/32	69.0564	4 3/16	106.363	5 21/32	143.669	8 1/8	206.375	10 3/4	273.051
11/32	8.7312	1 1/4	31.7501	2 3/4	69.8501	4 7/32	107.156	5 11/16	144.463	8 3/16	207.963	10 13/16	274.638
23/64	9.1281	1 9/32	32.5438	2 25/32	70.6439	4 1/4	107.950	5 23/32	145.257	8 1/4	209.550	10 7/8	276.226
3/8	9.5250	1 5/16	33.3376	2 13/16	71.4376	4 9/32	108.744	5 3/4	146.050	8 5/16	211.138	10 15/16	277.813
25/64	9.9219	1 11/32	34.1313	2 27/32	72.2314	4 5/16	109.538	5 25/32	146.844	8 3/8	212.725	11	279.401
13/32	10.3187	1 3/8	34.9251	2 7/8	73.0251	4 11/32	110.331	5 13/16	147.638	8 7/16	214.313	11 1/16	280.988
27/64	10.7156	1 13/32	35.7188	2 29/32	73.8189	4 3/8	111.125	5 27/32	148.432	8 1/2	215.900	11 1/8	282.576
7/16	11.1125	1 7/16	36.5126	2 15/16	74.6126	4 13/32	111.919	5 7/8	149.225	8 9/16	217.488	11 3/16	284.163
29/64	11.5094	1 15/32	37.3063	2 31/32	75.4064	4 7/16	112.713	5 29/32	150.019	8 5/8	219.075	11 1/4	285.751
15/32	11.9062	1 1/2	38.1001	3	76.2002	4 15/32	113.506	5 15/16	150.813	8 11/16	220.663	11 5/16	287.338
31/64	12.3031	1 17/32	38.8938	3 1/32	76.9939	4 1/2	114.300	5 31/32	151.607	8 3/4	222.250	11 3/8	288.926
1/2	12.7000	1 9/16	39.6876	3 1/16	77.7877	4 17/32	115.094	6	152.400	8 13/16	223.838	11 7/16	290.513
33/64	13.0969	1 19/32	40.4813	3 3/32	78.5814	4 9/16	115.888	6 1/16	153.988	8 7/8	225.425	11 1/2	292.101
17/32	13.4937	1 5/8	41.2751	3 1/8	79.3752	4 19/32	116.681	6 1/8	155.575	8 15/16	227.013	11 9/16	293.688
35/64	13.8906	1 21/32	42.0688	3 5/32	80.1689	4 5/8	117.475	6 3/16	157.163	9	228.600	11 5/8	295.276
9/16	14.2875	1 11/16	42.8626	3 3/16	80.9627	4 21/32	118.269	6 1/4	158.750	9 1/16	230.188	11 11/16	296.863
37/64	14.6844	1 23/32	43.6563	3 7/32	81.7564	4 11/16	119.063	6 5/16	160.338	9 1/8	231.775	11 3/4	298.451
19/32	15.0812	1 3/4	44.4501	3 1/4	82.5502	4 23/32	119.856	6 3/8	161.925	9 3/16	233.363	11 13/16	300.038
39/64	15.4781	1 25/32	45.2438	3 9/32	83.3439	4 3/4	120.650	6 7/16	163.513	9 1/4	234.950	11 7/8	301.626
5/8	15.8750	1 13/16	46.0376	3 5/16	84.1377	4 25/32	121.444	6 1/2	165.100	9 5/16	236.538	11 15/16	303.213
41/64	16.2719	1 27/32	46.8313	3 11/32	84.9314	4 13/16	122.238	6 9/16	166.688	9 3/8	238.125	12	304.801
21/32	16.6687	1 7/8	47.6251	3 3/8	85.7252	4 27/32	123.031	6 5/8	168.275	9 7/16	239.713		
43/64	17.0656	1 29/32	48.4188	3 13/32	86.5189	4 7/8	123.825	6 11/16	169.863				
11/16	17.4625	1 15/16	49.2126	3 7/16	87.3127	4 29/32	124.619	6 3/4	171.450				
45/64	17.8594	1 31/32	50.0063	3 15/32	88.1064	4 15/16	125.413	6 13/16	173.038				
23/32	18.2562	2	50.8001	3 1/2	88.9002	4 31/32	126.206						
47/64	18.6531	2 1/32	51.5939	3 17/32	89.6939	5	127.000						
3/4	19.0500	2 1/16	52.3876										
49/64	19.4469												
25/32	19.8437												

Answers to Questions

PART I

CHAPTER 1:

1) a) That which can accelerate matter. b) A force applied to a structure. c) A quantity of mechanical work or its equivalent. d) The rate at which one does mechanical work or its equivalent.

2) a and b: Yes, by expending it in a short enough span of time (i.e., to reach a level of power dissipation great enough) to generate stresses that exceed the strength of those materials.

3) Stresses (three principal ones) : friction; viscosity; loads; electrical voltage; coulomb forces; gravity.

4) a) 50 lb; b) 33.3 lb; c) zero; d) zero; e) zero.

5) Load; stress; friction; weight (but not mass) ; the volt; torque; dynamic flexure; hydrostatic pressure; magnetism.

6) a, c, d, e: scalar; vectorial: b, f, g.

CHAPTER 2:

1) See the text.

2) a) It forms a compression load, not a stress nor a strain *in this context.* b) A load on the walls of the chamber.

3) a) .01 mm; b) 100 kg; c) 100 kg; d) compression; e) .01 mm; f) compression; g) .0014.

4) Break the solid bulk of the column up into numerous columns of equal length but very much smaller diameter. When you do this a one cm height of the column can now shorten in compression much more without breaking. If this intrigues you, refer to the column formulas and the beam deflection formulas in Appendix 9, Part III, and see if you can work it out for yourself. Keep in mind as the clincher

546

on the reality of this effect the solid glass rod and the glass rope, each of equal cross section as far as the amount of glass contained in a one cm. length goes.

CHAPTER 3:

1) a) Returns to original shape and dimensions after deforming. b) Returns as mechanical work all of that put into deforming it. c) Stress remains proportional to strain. d) Absorbs a lot of energy before breaking. e) Absorbs little energy before breaking.

2) They would form a straight line.

3) It lost resilience but most probably remained elastic.

4) By expending it very slowly in the first instance and very rapidly in the second.

5) a) Mass times velocity. b) The transfer of momentum from one body to another, usually over a very short period of time. c) Force times the distance over which it acts. d) The resistance of the intermolecular bonds of a material to deformation under an applied load. e) Kinetic energy.

6) Let us try English units. Since 7 mm equals about 0.26 in., and 850 fps equals 850×12 inches/sec, or 10,000 ips, if we ignore the deceleration of the slug in the bone then the momentum transfer occurred over $\dfrac{0.26}{10,600}$ seconds or .000024 seconds, or 2.4×10^{-5} second.

The Special Tables—Part III—allow you to find that 800 mg equals roughly .07 lb. Since momentum equals mv, $850 \times .07$ equals 5.9 lb-ft. (Note: The usual formula for muzzle kinetic energy equals $\frac{1}{2} mv^2$, and yields a much larger number). We assumed the bullet transferred $\frac{2}{3}$ of that to the metatarsal. And $5.9 \times .66$ equals 3.9 lb-ft.

CHAPTER 4:

1) a) Resistance of a fluid to shearing strain or flow. b) That resistance given as dyne-sec/cm². c) Motion of atoms or molecules of one substance between those of another.

2) a) Pressure transmits equally through all parts of a fluid. b) Given equal volumes of fluid flowing past in unit time, the transverse pressure in slowly moving regions exceeds that in quickly moving ones. c) The study of fluids at rest in the mechanical sense.

3) Shearing stress.

4) Shearing strain.

5) Unit pressure equals $700/20$ kg/cm^2, or 35 kg/cm^2. By Pascal's principle that amounts to 35 kg/cm or about 3×10^8 dynes, far above the fluid's some 8×10^1 dynes/cm surface tension. No way!

CHAPTER 5:

1) a) A regular arrangement of atoms or molecules. b) A lattice large enough to have long range order. c) The weak attraction of one part of a molecule with a local excess of positive charge, for the negative region of another molecule. d) A linear defect in a crystal lattice.

2) Not true; the metal existed in the crystalline state ever since the time it froze out of the melt at the steel plant where the original ingot was poured.

3) a) A spontaneous change in the structure of the crystalline lattice, dependent usually upon temperature. b) Part of a single crystal surrounded by others of like or dissimilar kind.

4) By annealing it.

5) Dislocation systems arising in physical and chemical imperfections in the crystals which form the bulk, markedly weaken it in shear.

CHAPTER 6:

1) a) A constant-ratio mixture of atoms that forms out of the melt during cooling, and which has constant physical, thermal and mechanical properties. b) A mixture of two or more metallic elements.

2) Yes—this constitutes cold working when done at room

temperature and it can cause work hardening or strain hardening.

3) a) Ferric carbide, Fe_3C. b) An allotropic form of iron and carbon in which the carbon atoms have been "frozen" in the interstitial positions without forming significant amounts of cementite.

4) After rapidly cooling or quenching from the austenitic temperature to produce martensite, one reheats partially to allow some transformation of the martensite to ferrite and cementite. At the expense of loss of hardness, this greatly increases the toughness and resistance to fatigue.

5) It causes a surface film of chromium oxide to form by combining with ambient oxygen. The film proves highly resistant to corrosion and has the self-healing property if mechanically broken.

6) No, the heat generated in the steel by the rapidly moving abrasive wheel, heat reflected by the showers of bright, glowing sparks produced by the grinding, in effect overtempers the steel, that is it dehardens it so it will not hold its new cutting edge. One must sharpen such tools by hand on an abrasive stone, a process which does not generate heat quickly enough to alter the hardness of the steel.

7) The very hard martensite contains strains in its lattice. This strain of course represents strain energy, or if you prefer, prestress. It therefore becomes much easier for the corrosive solutes in cells and the body fluids to react chemically with these prestressed bonds, leading to a kind of stress corrosion which dulls the knife edge more quickly than mechanical abrasion would dull it in cutting dry, seasoned wood for example.

8) The hardened bolts supply much greater strength, rigidity and toughness in an equal volume of metal than annealed bolts.

9) The hacksaw teeth generate so much heat in cutting the alloy that they rapidly reach their tempering temperature, the martensite then converts to ferrite, and as a result the teeth become softer than the chrome-cobalt alloy, where-

upon the latter simply burnishes the carbon steel blade. But the alloy blade contains elements such as vanadium, nickle and/or molybdenum which stabilize the martensite even at high temperatures, so the teeth retain enough hardness to continue cutting the nail.

10) To avoid heating to the point that the metal in the blade edge overtempers or loses its hardness. That hardness supplies the resistance to wear by abrasion which we signify when we say of a knife: "It holds its edge well."

11) a) Because they have, and/or readily develop when strained, numerous dislocation systems. b) Shear.

CHAPTER 7:

1) a) One which lacks the crystalline state, i.e., lacks long range order in its atomic arrangements. b) That range of temperature (not sharply defined at either end) over which a polymer acts like a rubber due to disruption, caused by thermal motions of its molecules and atoms. c) van der Waal's bonds.

2) a) The basic molecule serving as the building block for a polymer. b) Long chains (whether of one, two or three dimensional structure) made up of mers joined to each other in repeating arrays.

3) a) Strain and then fix a polymer between two clamps or other restraints; the force it exerts on those restraints then gradually decreases with time. b) A polymer which exhibits elastic behavior (often meaning resilient behavior more than elastic) .

CHAPTER 8:

1) Because their highly prestressed lattices require little extra tension or shear to reach the failure point, but have a considerable capacity for absorbing compression loads.

2) In effect it markedly lowers the mechanical power one must put into the system to build up that total quantity of strain energy which will break it. The fracturing energy

probably remains approximately a constant for a given material, and the step-by-step mode of putting that energy into the system prolongs the time allowed for doing it (i.e., reduces the power needed to do it).

3) Solid (meaning rigid to all three principal stresses and strains) but lacking long range order of its atomic and ionic constituents, and so a supercooled liquid.

CHAPTER 9:

1) a) A porous ceramic then infiltrated with molten metal to form a tough matrix filling the pores. b) A bulk material containing two or more mechanically separate phases. c) A composite material in which fibers of a strong material carry most of the load, while the embedding matrix distributes it evenly to each fiber.

2) The biological structural materials represent members of this class, and include the various types of bone and cartilage, plus dentine, cementum, enamel, and all fibrous tissue structures.

3) A crack in any one fiber generates increased local strain but the matrix yields readily to it, protecting neighboring fibers from its effects.

CHAPTER 10:

1) The latter, while rigid in pure tension and/or compression, lacks rigidity in shear.

2) a) No. b) Yes. c) No.

3) a) Yes. b) Yes.

4) a) False. b) True. c) False. d) False. e) False.

5) Fracture or failure of a part which nevertheless has never been loaded beyond its safe design limits, usually under cyclically changing loads.

CHAPTER 11:

1) Uniaxial tension and compression; shear; flexure, and torque.

2) A couple of tension-compression stresses which opposes the rotary force or torque of another couple of shearing stresses (see freebody diagrams, Appendix 8).

3) a) How effectively a given cross sectional shape withstands a flexural load. b) How effectively a given cross sectional shape withstands a torque, or tendency to rotation around its longitudinal axis.

4) a) False. b) False.

5) If a solid: flexure. If a gas or liquid: meaningless.

6) Improved endurance in all types of fatigue; greater strain tolerance than characteristic of the fiber material in solid, bulk form (i.e., greater compliance); greater toughness; piezoelectric response to strain without fragility corresponding to solid bulk material.

7) Given the adhesive strength of the matrix to each unit area of fiber, the total fiber surface must provide a total shearing strength matching the total uniaxial load on the fiber. This reduces then to the fiber surface-to-volume ratio, the particular optimum one becoming a function of the matrix-fiber adhesion strength in shear.

8) No.

9) a) Contract all of the muscles arising from the medial humeral condyle; their tension load across the medial elbow neutralizes the distracting effect of the torque. And that is exactly what happens; try it.

b) The muscles spanning both the shoulder and elbow joints contract, and progressively harder as the torque you apply rises. They add a uniaxial compression load on the bone which neutralizes enough of the torque-engendered tension to prevent a fracture. These muscles include especially the biceps, brachialis and coracobrachialis; try it.

c) The muscles arising from the medial epicondyle and inserting at and distal to the wrist apply an eccentric tension load, which cancels out the flexural tension stresses in the forearm bones, chain-brace fashion. Work it out on paper. And do you begin to sense some rather brilliant engineering here?

d) The control system (in the CNS) must cause them to happen, and its lack of error in doing so implies precise and sensitive receptors for dangerous levels of strain in the affected structures, coupled with exact computation of the needed muscle forces according to highly efficient, predetermined biomechanical "game rules", all integrated into a system of essential simplicity (for in essence only the very simple can provide the very reliable).

CHAPTER 12:

1) To allow one part to move upon another.
2) To minimize wear of the bearing surfaces.
3) Review the text (!).
4) a) True. b) True. c) False. d) True. e) True.

PART II

CHAPTER 13:

1) Fibrous and lamellar bone, hyaline and fibrocartilage; fibrous tissue; elastic cartilage and tissue; dentine and enamel; cementum.

2) Add internal structural order to a simple tissue; combine any two tissues; or both.

3) a) False. b) True. c) False (see Volume IV). d) False.

4) Growth; modeling; remodeling; repair; defense; maturation; homeostasis.

5) Mesenchymal cell activation and proliferation; differentiation of cells into functionally specialized lines; performance of those special functions by the cell populations elaborated by proliferative-differentiative activity (see Vols. II, III).

6) Same answers as in answer no. 4 just above.

7) Collagen *fibers*; mucopolysaccharide *matrix*; inorganic *mineral; water.*

8) a) Yes. b) No. c) Yes. d) Yes.

9) a) Solve this by assuming you divide 1 mm³ into enough regularly stacked sub-cubes to yield 18,000 corner intersections. By working the geometry of this out on paper you can see that a cube with n units on a side will have essentially n^3 corner intersections in it if n equals a number larger than 10 (we will ignore certain matters that become increasingly important as n takes values less than 10).

Thus we need the cube root of 18,000. If you look up the logarithm of 18,000 (i.e., 5.0 + log of 1.800) and divide it by three, then find the number corresponding to that logarithm, you obtain the result 26. In other words, if you break one cubic mm up into the proper number of smaller cubes all of the same size, then when $\dfrac{1}{26}$ of a millimeter separates one cubic face from the next nearest parallel one, you will have 18,000 corners at each of which an osteocyte lies. Hence mean osteocyte separation equals 1/26 mm or .038 mm, or 38 microns.

b) This must then equal 38 microns plus some minor fraction because they do not travel in straight lines (they actually spiral through the bone).

c) Assuming 70 canaliculae/osteocyte, each 38 microns or .038 mm long and we have 70 × 18,000 × .038 mm of canaliculae per mm³ of bone, or 4,200 mm length in a cubic mm of bone. To get the cylindrical surface area use S = II DL; S = 3.14 × .0045 × 4800.

S = 68 mm²/mm³. And per liter: $10^3 \times 10^3$ or 10^6 mm³ exist in 1000 cc, so S = .68 × 10^8 mm²/liter. If this surface plays a role in the microdamage detection system, enough of it exists to ensure not overlooking anything, at least on the basis of the availability of the "monitor".

d) Per one mm length, a single canaliculus would have a surface area S of .0045 × π × 1 mm, or .014 mm². Its volume equals 1/4 π .045² or .0005 mm³. So the S/V ratio of .014 mm² ÷ .0005 mm³ equals roughly 28.

CHAPTER 14:

1) Creation of new skeletal tissue; growth of the skeleton; architectural adaptations to mechanically imposed demands; repair; biological bearing manufacture.

2) Three: collagen *fibers;* mucopolysaccharide *matrix; water.*

3) a) No. b) No. c) No. d) No. e) No.

4) Growth proceeds slower in tension than compression; it has a biphasic response to compression; a physiologic range of loading exists, on either side of which lies a pathological range (see Volume II).

CHAPTER 15:

1) Collagen *fibers;* mucopolysaccharide *matrix; water.*

2) See the text.

3) a) To provide rigidity and strength in tension loading alone. b) To provide rigidity but good static compliance to all three principal mechanical loads and strains. c) To provide anisotropic rigidity and low static compliance to all three principal strains.

4) No. Their strength depends upon several things: a) the total amount of collagen in the cross section, which can vary inversely as the amount of mucopolysaccharide embedding matrix present, to vary the total strength without changing the cross section area. b) Changes in collagen cross linking and in mean polymer length made of the tropocollagen mer molecules can also vary total strength without changing cross section area.

5) Old, because cross linking (which binds different fibrils together side to side, thereby bonding across the ends of separate polymer molecules lined up end to end) increases as a function of (i.e., with increasing) time.

6) Testing its flexural compliance (or, if you prefer, its flexural stiffness). Cross linking directly limits shear parallel to the grain, just as in beams as described in Part I.

7) a) It implies that strain-sensitive nerve endings exist in both tendon and bone, and that normally they prevent a person from applying forces to the bony and fibrous tissue parts of the skeleton sufficient in magnitude to endanger their structural integrity. b) It should greatly enhance the chance of complete ruptures during the game. c) One would favor those procedures and techniques which tend to preserve any innervation originally present in the fibrous tissue structure to serve as the new—or reconstructed—ligament. Thus repair of the original should prove better than a replacement, and a replacement whose innervation remains intact should excel over any free (and thus infarcted) graft.

CHAPTER 16:

1) a) One in which shearing stress increases proportionally to flow speed. b) Resistance does not increase as fast as flow.

2) See the text.

3) Same answer to all: synovial fluid.

4) a) No. b) Yes. c) Yes. d) No. e) No. g) No.

CHAPTER 17:

1) a) Its volume. b) Its maximum cross section area. c) The resting length of its belly.

2) a) Shortens against a constant load or resistance. b) Contracts against an immovable resistance.

3) See the text.

4) The central nervous system, according to patterns determined inherently therein.

5) The anatomy, or spatial disposition and alignment, of the muscle relative to the structures it attaches to.

CHAPTER 18:

1) Maximal at the articular surface, minimal at midshaft, graded nearly continuously between.

2) By varying the total cross section one can vary total

strength; by subdividing it into more and more numerous but progressively thinner fibers or beams one can increase its compliance over a wide range.

3) a) To permit motion of one rigid part on another. b) To minimize wear. c) To promote durability and reliability of function.

4) By making their backing compliant enough to yield readily in advance of loading eccentricities tending to destroy it.

5) Flexible but load carrying pads enhancing adaptational compliance to loading eccentricities.

6) Four: the wedge-flow effect; negative pressure effect; the anatomical pump; the Bernouilli contour effect.

7) Structural features which reduce wear to some minimum value or level, combined with biodynamic ones which repair what damage does occur while it remains trivial in extent, thereby preventing cumulative wear.

8) The particular and sometimes seemingly weird combinations of such motions in the living joint do not serve directly the primal function of the joint. Rather they serve to protect living bearing surfaces with very particular properties and needs from regional overloads. The inanimate artificial bearing surfaces pose us no such demands, so the effort represents mostly waste in terms of time, talent, complexity (which augments unreliability) and, ultimately, expense to the recipient, the patient. A minor lesson appears here, highlighted by the observation that youthful and inexperienced doctors tend to find more complex solutions to problems than their older colleagues who tend to proceed more directly—and simply—through a problem towards its solution. Time and the experience it brings does that to us. Thus residents and students puzzle over how swiftly and effortlessly somebody like D. Bosworth or D. Lucas or R. A. Robinson, or C. Thompson seemingly can solve clinical problems. But it was not effortless or swift—do not forget those 20–30 earlier years they invested in finding out what *not* to do. They may not show but they are there.

9) By coapting essentially completely to both bone and implant, it greatly enlarges the bone-implant interface area, thereby reducing unit loads below that upper limit which living bone cannot tolerate and/or adapt to. And in the process it produces much more uniform loading of that interface which also promulgates mechanical acceptance.

10) When an inanimate device of different compliance than bone has an interface with bone across which mechanical loads transfer, *it will always become loose* in its bony bed in actual use, and several arthrographic studies have now confirmed this for the case of cemented-in total hips. Yet in spite of that these systems continue to give satisfactory service. b) No real need exists anyway to try to affix these implants rigidly and permanently to bone. We can accept some micromechanical motion and concentrate instead upon other matters such as improving the implant materials, geometry and biological acceptability. c) Geometry of bone-implant interface; the ideal unit loading factor on that interface; durability of the intact system.

11) a) They wear mostly by abrasion, producing a sludge of very fine metal particles which, because of surface-to-volume ratio effects, can irritate the adjacent soft tissues.

b) Cause one metal part to roll on the other; or design the device in some manner that hydrodynamic flotation occurs during active motion.

CHAPTER 19:

1) Trivial case:

2) All surfaces move towards the concavity arising during dynamic flexural strains. b) It constitutes a time averaging system which ignores the momentary and/or transient exception. c) Covering bone surface with cartilage, teeth or implant, or devitalizing it.

3) Anatomical curves generate cantilever-arrangement flexural moments which cancel static-arrangement dynamic ones of muscular origin.

4) False.

5) As a brittle material bone should—and does—fracture before it deforms plastically under torque or flexure. And the very limited tolerance of the skin to constant pressure makes it impossible to apply torques of such magnitude for any length of time—serious pressure sores would quickly result.

6) a) Nope. The high tops serve no more esoteric function than keeping the shoes from falling off of small feet liberally padded with baby fat. b) Prescribe high top shoes. While they do no good, they do no harm either. And if you do not she will take the child to someone who will, but who may in addition do something else that does prove harmful.

7) a) No (and clinical experience substantiates this). While logical, this treatment remains ineffective, probably because it does not apply a large enough force for a long enough time to move the growth rate of the relevant parts of the growing chondral planes over onto the descending limb of the growth/force-response curve.

b) Surgical derotational osteotomy (but rarely necessary for this deformity); or apply external devices which turn the feet out more than 45°, and keep them on day and night until correction has developed. Devices might include Dennis-Browne or Fillauer splints, casts, or properly designed ambulatory braces. Or identify the overactive muscles causing the deformity and temporarily weaken them (not standard practice with this deformity in neurologically normal children, but it rapidly becomes so in spastic children).

c) You will probably make the pes planus worse, and must decide at what point the trade becomes uneconomical or harmful. Note that for the most part these two deformities pose cosmetic problems primarily, not functional ones, and so often represent more problems of parental overconcern than of children's orthopaedics. Good clinicians such as A. Haddad, Worcester or R. Shimo, Tokyo or T. Tajima, Kagoshima, take this so much for granted in their daily decision making process that they remain unaware that they have made a judgement based upon an assignment or priorities that would prove difficult for a student to grasp.

d) The diapers worn by the younger child cause him or her to hold both hips externally rotated by about 40° to make room for the diaper between the thighs. Thus the splint holds the feet in only 20° beyond neutral relative to the whole lower limb and the hip, and generates a logical but ineffective corrective force. But in the older toilet trained and walking child the lower limbs now usually point directly forward, so that 60° represents considerable external rotation of the foot relative to the hip. This provides both a logical and an effective corrective force.

8) a) Implanting the electrodes constituted a local bone tissue injury which of necessity would lead to local repair and the production of woven bone. Electrolytic products at the positive electrode impaired that repair, but did not at the negative one. Thus the experiment produced no information about bone modeling which, note, occurs naturally on totally undamaged surfaces and can lead to direct apposition of new circumferential lamellar bone. Lest these words be misunderstood, understand they do not deny that such microcurrents may actually potentiate bone healing; they only say that if so, experiments such as this do not demonstrate it unambiguously.

b) The only way one can evaluate such a problem: Begin with a model in which you have somehow caused biological incompetence of fracture healing. Since this occurs only very rarely in common laboratory animals and no real effort was made to produce it in them, the experiment provided no information about this either.

c) The only way one can evaluate this problem: Produce a technical failure first, and then try to make it heal. Since this was not done, no information of known relevance to this matter was obtained.

d) See Appendix 7, *Piezoelectric Effect*. The experiment did not begin with a very good grasp of the physical realities of the situation chosen to study.

e) Nothing, for it did not resolve any of the ambiguities it contains in either the strategic and tactical senses.

f) The latter: The house of Thomas published some of the pertinent facts in 1963, 1964 and 1966, and that of Little-Brown and Co., in 1964.

g) Ignorance of the supracellular organization, physiology and biology of living, growing bone.

9) The accompanying figure illustrates one common cause: during gait and after heel strike, overcontraction of

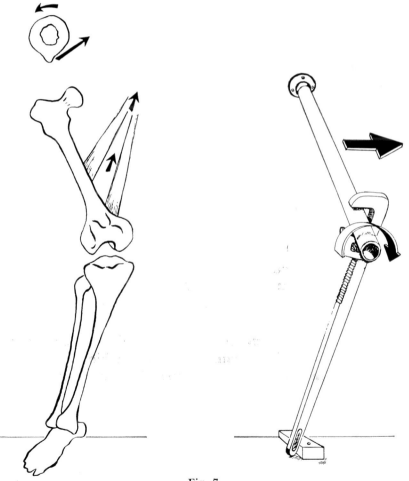

Fig. 7

the adductors on this side pull the knee medially. But the floor restraint holds the foot as shown; while the inertia of the trunk restrains the hip. This adductor pull then develops a torque on the femur, as shown on the right. The growing cartilage regions at the knee will then adapt to it predictably to create the deformity shown.

And any other combination of muscle and/or orthotic forces, which produce a similar torque between the lower and upper ends of the femur, will have similar effects. Such could include overactivity of the anatomical internal rotators and the medial hamstrings.

10) In the figure, top, this child (now an attractive young lady) presented with a waddling gait and onset of hip pain. She had so-called congenital coxa vara, and the x-ray strongly suggests that an overload in vertical shear (here lying parallel to the malaligned epiphyseal plates) could cause the condition (source of that overload???). If true, correction should require only reorienting those planes more perpendicularly to that shearing load. I did this by bilateral pertrochanteric osteotomies, maintained throughout the healing phase in skeletal traction and abduction.

As the lower x-ray shows, this certainly solved the problem. Under normal (i.e., perpendicular) loads the shearing defect on the left healed in and the chondral modeling behavior converted from the positive to the negative (i.e., self perpetuating) and normal feedback mode to maintain epiphyseal alignment thereafter. And the flexure-drift laws account for the restoration of essentially normal external body contours.

Lesson: At least in the direct sense, this disease must arise primarily from biomechanical causes, not biological or biochemical ones. And one must treat it early in the growth period to obtain the best result.

CHAPTER 20:

1) To all: the self repair faculty.

2) Living cells which provide a detection system, a signaling mechanism and a microrepair response mechanism,

plus some means of locating the response in the mechanically damaged tissue.

3) a) No solid evidence exists that such embolism does underlie the condition.

b) We do know of diseases in which repeated micro-embolism occurs, for example bacterial endocarditis. In such diseases varied objective evidence develops of that embolism, including hematuria from small kidney infarcts, petechiae of the skin, splinter hemorrhages of the nails and petechiae of conjunctiva and mucous membranes. *But these phenomena do not associate with aseptic necrosis of the femoral head of any recognized type.*

c) In the known embolic diseases such as bacterial endocarditis, aseptic necrosis of the femoral head does not occur.

d) Since numerous arteries bring blood to the femoral head and free anastomoses exist within the head, how can one in logic expect showers of embolizing fat globules to involve only those vessels and not those in the remainder of the body?

e) In studying another clinical entity known as *fat embolism,* which occurs after trauma, various investigators have injected artificially made suspensions of fat globules into the vascular system of various animals. While clear evidence of small vessel embolism followed (see *b,* above), the clinical syndrome of aseptic necrosis of the femoral head did not.

CHAPTER 21:

This is an erudite "corker". Thus:

1) a) The model system seems good—even very good—for if properly studied it seems it should provide relevant answers.

b) They chose a really bad technique. While *au courant* in that it employs radioisotopes, which seems to impart an aura above the common cut to the whole study, in actual fact fracture healing means regaining mechanical strength following fracture or osteotomy, and its only direct and reliable measure constitutes a study of that strength. A hopeless "vegetable soup" of biological variables could alter deposition of mineral and organic elements in the osteotomy line at four weeks post-osteotomy which would have no reliable relevance at all to the mechanical strength of that line. Thus in terms of fracture healing achieved, the isotope uptakes remain totally uninterpretable. This strategy left something to be desired, even though the tactics greatly impress any bone-biological innocents who might read such a study.

c) The insertion of the implants, like the osteotomy it-self, should (and did) set off the regional acceleratory phe-nomenon in the whole calvarium. But not recognizing that totally independently running phenomenon, they failed to-tally to quantitate it. Now what would you think of a group who compared radioisotope uptake in an operative area to, for example, the surface temperature of the equally indepen-dently determined Mare Christum at high Lunar noon, and concluded that their experimental variable came off well?

d) You can see that their conclusions could prove valid only by the remotest act of providence. Another experiment in which elementary biological ignorance wasted esoteric and quite varied instrumentation, the time of various highly trained Ph.D's and technicians, and more than 130 kilobucks of our tax monies.

2) One uses the dominant hand more, and for tasks re-quiring greater power, than the other, so the strength of its muscles exceed those on the other side. This requires that the muscles stabilizing the spine on the opposite side overdevelop equally. They would include erector spinae, trapezius and intercostals. And when they contract they tend to cause ex-actly the deformity described. Given the underlying chondral pathology, this then forms a plausible explanation for the basic observations.

CHAPTER 23:

1) The smooth one in all three instances. The threads serve as stress risers, and in addition reduce the effective pro-jected cross section area.

2) The large smooth one, to obtain as large a bone-metal

interface as possible, thereby minimizing unit loads on the bone-metal interface in the thin bone cortices. If the traction had to remain on for only a few days the large threaded one would probably serve equally well, but over a period of weeks its threads (which act as stress risers) could cause it to break.

3) While P. Laing and others have shown by radioactive tracer methods that such transfer does occur, it constitutes a purely trivial one for clinical needs, for no single case of implant corrosion due to this phenomenon has become known. Hence an unnecessary precaution.

4) a) The stiff hip means that markedly increased mechanical leverage and force must act upon the fixation device after the operation, for normal hip mobility makes the proximal fragment rather freely mobile to stress relieve an I-T fracture, while a stiff hip transfers all of those unrelieved strains and forces to the fracture. Thus this hip should have received additional protection postoperatively, such as with a 2/3 hip spica, or an equivalent brace or cast-brace. The fault here lay with the surgeon, not the manufacturer.

b) Witness the orthopaedist's prayer, each time he enters the operating room: "Please, God, should I make mistakes today, may they at least be new ones."

5) Not in this country!

6) This author says: The plate would serve only as a temporary internal osseous "suture" anyway, and always requires external mechanical protection during the bone healing time. So go ahead, contour it and protect it postoperatively with a cast or by any other suitable and reliable means.

7) Anatomists often have spoken of tension trabeculae and compression trabeculae in metaphyseal bone. But except for a few special regions possibly such as the tuberosites of the upper femur and humerus, most *trabeculae carry only compression loads*. In the accompanying figure 8, a vertical compression load on a trabecular lattice strains it in compression, and that causes it to bulge laterally. But in real bones the cortical inwaisting phenomenon acts as a rigid restraint to that tendency to bulge, so that the horizontal trabeculae

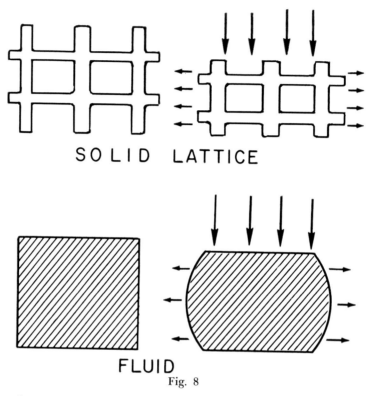

SOLID LATTICE

FLUID

Fig. 8

forced against that cortex came to carry compression loads too. This relationship holds true in regions such as the tuber os calcis, femoral head and neck, condyles about the knee, the hand and wrist bones, and the pelvis. Tension-loaded trabeculae in fact prove uncommon; nature clearly preferred to use better tension-transfer mechanisms than spongy bone. We describe them elsewhere in Part II.

CHAPTER 24:

1) When one pushes a wedge in between two structures, if one ignores friction and any other factors, the upwards force it exerts F, constitutes this relationship between the load P forcing the wedge in, and the angle θ of the wedge:

$$F = \frac{P}{\tan \theta}$$

Now in the problem given, the lateral thrust acting to make the epiphysis slide up the 14° slope or wedge angle must develop a vertical force F, equal to the uniaxial load of 100 kg. Thus we know the value of F, and that of tan θ in the trigonometry tables equals 0.24. So solve for P:

$$P = F \tan \theta; \quad P = 100 \times .24; \quad P = 24 \text{ lb}$$

In other words a vertical load of 100 kg exerts a *shear-locking force* of the epiphysis on the metaphysis of 24 kg or 53 lb. Given that the frictional drag of the knee approximates 1 per cent, then 24 kg of shear resistance exist to withstand the effects of 1 kg of friction induced drag. When you add to this the considerable mechanical shearing strength of the cartilage in the plate (on the order of 1 kg/mm^2) you find a fairly strong junction exists between bone and plate.

2) The relatively high static as well as dynamic compliance of the thick hyaline cartilage structures affords significant protection from impact.

3) a) Wolff, or "Wolff's Law". b) Heuter and Volkmann.

4) Your author.

5) a) A Japanese man named Fukada. b) the Curies, of France.

6) Milch, Rall and Tobie, in 1957.

7) Same as no. 2.

8) a) Rindfleish at Graz, Austria, *ca* 1848. b) Howship (English). c) Clopton Havers (English).

9) Venable and Stuck (U.S.).

10) a) Smith-Petersen of Boston; b) John Charnley of England; c) the Judets of Paris; d) Kuntschner of Germany.

11) Same as for no. 2.

12) a) Dempster, F. G. Evans, Liddicote and Lessner. b) Burstein and Frankel. c) The deceased mathematician, Norbert Wiener. d) L. Euler, a European mathematician.

13) a) Newton and Liebnitz, independently. b) Pythagoras. c) Archimedes. d) Briggs (English). e) Mannheim, an Austrian artillery officer. f) Galileo. g) Newton.

14) All of these developments go so far back in our civilization's antiquity that their inventors remain unknown to us.

15) a) Brandt *ca* 1735. b) Vauquelin *ca* 1797. c) Black in 1755. d) Davy *ca* 1808. e) Wohler and/or Oersted, *ca* 1806. f) Cronstedt, 1751. g) Brand, 1669. h) Ekeberg, 1802. i) Gregor, 1791. j) Scheele, 1783.

16) As to the rectangular moment of inertia, we deal with a hollow cylinder and so need to find the fourth powers of both the outside diameter of the bone D, and its marrow cavity diameter *d*. While not given that, we do know that $D - d = 1.0$ cm (the cortical thickness of 5 mm = 0.5 cm which appears twice across any diameter), and that the cortical cross section area A_c of 3.0 cm² means that when you subtract marrow cavity area A_m, from total cross section area A_t, the result equals 3.0 cm². Thus:

$$A_t = \tfrac{1}{4}\ \pi\ D^2$$
$$A_m = \tfrac{1}{4}\ \pi\ d^2$$
$$A_c = A_t - A_m = 3.0 \text{ cm}^2$$
$$3.0 = \tfrac{1}{4}\ \pi\ D^2 - \tfrac{1}{4}\ \pi\ d^2\ \tfrac{1}{4}\ \pi\ (D^2 - d^2)$$

So: $\dfrac{3.0}{\tfrac{1}{4}\ \pi} = D^2 - d^2$, or $\dfrac{12}{\pi} = D^2 - d^2$, or $3.82 = D^2 - d^2$

and $1.0 = D - d$, or $D = 1.0 + d$

But also, $D^2 = 3.82 + d^2$, so $D = \sqrt{3.82 + d^2}$

$1.0 + d = \sqrt{3.82 + d^2}$, so $(1.0 + d)^2 = 3.82 + d^2$

Square the left hand term thus:
$$
\begin{array}{r}
1.0 + d \\
1.0 + d \\
\hline
d + d^2 \\
1 + d \\
\hline
1 + 2d + d^2
\end{array}
$$

So: $1 + 2d + d^2 = 3.82 + d^2$

Now subtract d^2 from both sides to obtain:

$1 + 2d = 3.82$; thus $2d = 3.82 - 1$; $2d = 2.82$; $d = \dfrac{2.82}{2}$

and we finally have d:

$$d = 1.41 \text{ cm}$$

Then if $D - d = 1.0$, then $D = 1.0 + d$, which comes out to 2.41 cm (whew!). Now we can find the rectangular and polar moments of inertia I_o and J_o from the formulas in Table 17.

The value of I_o will equal 1.46 cm⁴
The value of J_o will equal 2.92 cm⁴
The surface stress will equal

$$\sigma = \frac{My}{I_o}$$

Now we need M, the moments, at midshaft which is 19.5 cm from either end, and to exist in static equilibrium this means that 10 kg $\times$ 10 cm $= x \times$ 19.5 cm; so x equals 5.13 kg. Since y equals distance from the neutral plane or $\frac{1}{2}D$, we have

$$\sigma = \frac{(19.5 \times 5.13) \ 1.20}{1.46} = 95 \text{ kg/cm}^2 = .95 \text{ kg/mm}^2$$

If it will break at 11.0 kg/mm² surface stress (which equals 1100 kg/cm²) the flexural load x required to break the femur becomes:

$$\sigma = \frac{My}{I_o} = \frac{(19.5x) \ 1.20}{1.46}, \text{ or:}$$

$$x = \frac{\sigma I_o}{(19.5) \ 1.2} = \frac{(1100) \ (1.46)}{(19.5) \ 1.2} = 68.6 \text{ kg}$$

Note: This assumes homogeneous E across the whole diameter, and as we noted in Part II the surface fibers of living bone have a lower than average Young's modulus, making the bone some 40 per cent stronger in flexure than calculations such as those just done would suggest. Thus a 240 lb man would have to stand on the middle of this femur to break it.

Biomechanical Problems

QUESTIONS

I append here a few problems for those who wish to try their hand at some fairly tough questions which relate mechanics and skeletal physiology to matters of orthopaedic clinical practice. All were gleaned from material encountered in my own practice during a single week. Answering them correctly requires a fair amount of clinical experience as well as basic "book" knowledge.

1) Some 5 months post fracture this tibia has not healed, although the patient enjoys normal health, the fracture received approved closed treatment and the patient co-operated fully with his orthopaedist.

(*a*) Why has it not healed?

(*b*) The "grainy" tunneling within the compacta on either side of the fracture reflects what?

(*c*) Was it caused by mechanical disuse?

(*d*) Was this nonunion caused by poor blood supply?

(*e*) Does decreased bone formation exist here?

(*f*) By virtue of this tunneling and the associated dynamic process it derives from, what has happened to this tibia's total strength, unit strength, stiffness, compliance and toughness?

(*g*) What would a thermogram of this leg reveal, compared to the good one?

(*h*) You internally fix this with a plate and put the patient in a long leg walking cast. What will probably happen then?

2) This patient has Morquio's disease, a form of chondrodystrophy associated with dwarfism.

(*a*) Why does he waddle when he walks?

(*b*) What does the increased breadth of the femoral

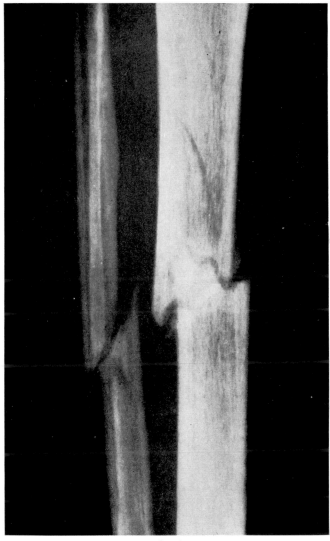

Fig. 9

heads imply about the mechanical properties of the articular cartilage?

(*c*) What does the abnormal vertical spatial relationship of the capital epiphyseal plate region to the plate region of the two trochanters imply about the chondral growth/force-response characteristic in this disease?

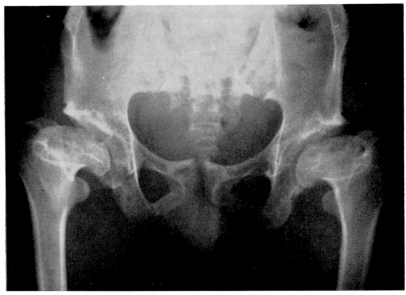

Fig. 10

(*d*) What does the osseous (as opposed to articular) architecture suggest about bone modeling competence?

(*e*) If the answer to (*c*) is right, what does it mean about ultimate growth in height of the vertebral bodies?

3) While this internally fixed intertrochanteric fracture healed properly, the bone screws did not complete the "course" unaffected.

(*a*) What caused extrusion of the top screw?

(*b*) What caused the lower three screws to break?

(*c*) And where did they break?

(*d*) In this particular situation does this breakage cause any harm?

(*e*) If the nail had broken, where would that failure probably have arisen?

(*f*) If this hip had also lacked mobility due to some form of arthritis or because of capsular fibrosis and contracture, how might the outcome have differed?

(*g*) What might the surgeon have done during the operation which enhanced the likelihood that the screws would fail?

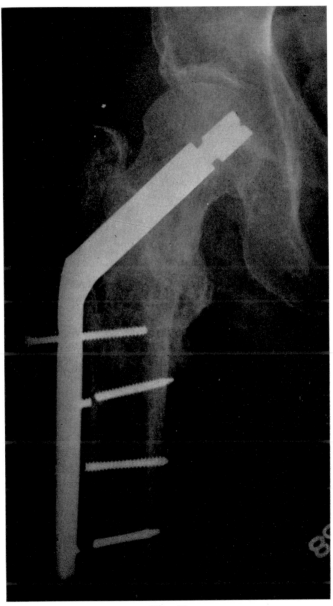

Fig. 11

4) In this lateral x-ray of a weight-bearing foot, assume the length of the plantar fascia (from tuber os calcis to metatarsal heads) equals 11 cm, and that the total load across the ankle joint during the take-off or thrust phase of gait equals 200 kg.

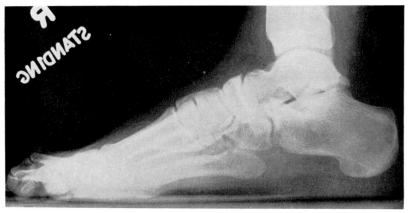

Fig. 12

(a) Compute the total tension load on the plantar fascia, assuming it functions as a bow-string to maintain the vertical arch.

(b) Now assume this foot goes into the pes planus position. In doing so the accompanying forefoot pronation plus heel valgus plus lateral shift of the plantar fascia relative to the line of action of the load coming down the tibia all combine to decrease the vertical distance between plantar fascia and the center of the subtalar joint, in a severe pes planus to less than 50% of normal. What does that do to the total load on the plantar fascia? To the chondral growth centers causing longitudinal bone growth in the foot?

(c) Given the above loads find the approximate total compression load transmitted across the midtarsal joint complex from hindfoot to forefoot. Use a protractor to obtain the necessary angles.

(d) Now find the approximate total compression load acting along the body of the tuber os calcis.

(e) And the unit compression stress at mid tuber, in kg/

mm², given a cross section area of 6.2 cm², of which 20% represents bone and 80% marrow tissue.

5) Using this hand x-ray as a topic of discussion, answer the following questions or requests.

(*a*) Classify in the biomechanical sense the small bones of the wrist joint, and then the metacarpals.

(*b*) The metaphyseal slope of the base of the second metacarpal has an angle of convergence of 36°. As a conse-

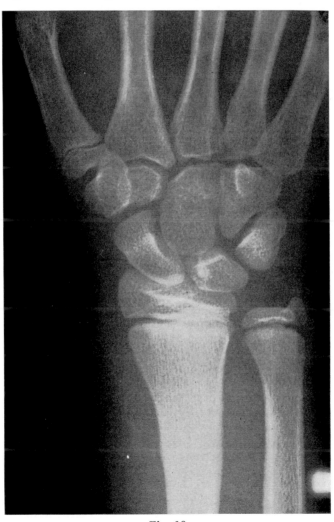

Fig. 13

quence of this inwaisting, what fraction of the longitudinal compression load carried by the cortex represents an inwaisting or imploding or "necking in" force acting on it? And what happens to the size of that fraction as the total longitudinal load changes?

(*c*) When stress fractures (i.e., so called "march fractures") arise in medically healthy persons they usually affect the diaphyseal regions of long bones, not metaphyseal or epiphyseal. And they very rarely affect bone modeling-independent bones. Provide biomechanical explanations for these clinical facts.

(*d*) In the line from the first metacarpal (on your left) to the radial shaft, how many planes of longitudinal skeletal growth appear in this x-ray?

(*e*) On the same line of thought, how many chondral growth planes lie between the hip joint space and the bottom of the os calcis? Do you see why growth prediction charts often overestimate the amount of limb length correction to be gained by epiphyseodesis? And why might they underestimate the correction?

(*f*) If you had to determine how much of the total postnatal growth in limb length derived from articular cartilage growth, how would you do it—quickly, cheaply, easily,—on humans, without laying a hand on them or doing any experiments?

(*g*) With regard to transmission of compression loads from forearm to hand, describe the almost certainly major function or purpose of the complex of carpal bones. Which of the carpal bones does not contribute materially to this function?

(*h*) Explain why more cortical inwaisting appears in the side of the distal ulna facing the radius, than in the apposing radial cortical contour.

6) Recall from Volume II that the sequences in longitudinal bone growth by endochondral ossification include chondroblast proliferation, matrix synthesis, mineralization, partial replacement of the mineralized cartilage to form primary spongiosa, and replacement of that to form the second-

dary spongiosa or "mature" trabecular bone, all processes that were ongoing in the hand x-ray of the previous question.

(a) Which of these steps responds to biomechanical factors in an important way, and how so?

(b) Which responds to known hormonal factors in an important way, and how so? Do we have all the answers to this one yet?

(c) Which depend in an important way upon known dietary factors?

(d) Given those things, then where would you look to find an explanation for increased bone length? dwarfism? and for limb malalignment? articular incongruity? unequal limb lengths?

(e) List some first-order reasons or explanations for finding an abnormal curvature in a bone.

7) In this lateral x-ray view of a weight-bearing but still-flexible flat foot (compare with the normal foot shown in question 4) some of the essential elements of the deformity appear.

(a) List them, and describe their probable effects upon longitudinal growth of these bones.

(b) Now list some further attributes of pes planus not shown in this view, and describe their probable effects on foot growth.

(c) From the above, deduce that time in life when one

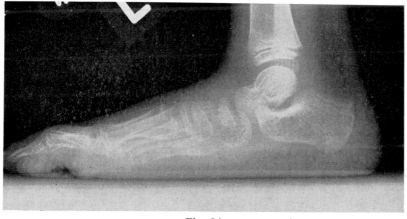

Fig. 14

might most consistently correct pes planus by nonoperative means, and name the basic principles involved in doing so.

(*d*) As to their *effectiveness* in achieving such correction, rate the following: Thomas heels; Thomas heels with medial heel lift; prolonged medial shoe counter; tarsal-supinator last; medial arch "cookie"; medial arch support inserts; combinations of above; Whitman plates.

(*e*) Suppose you elect to treat one of these feet in a non-spastic child by the Frost muscle-balancing procedure (*Clin Orthop 65* :175, 1969), transferring the peroneous longus into the anterior tibial tendon, and lengthening the heel cord. Why might the procedure fail (as it usually does if performed on nonspastics)?

(*f*) All of the previous answers imply that what probably serves as the basic direct cause of pes planus in "normal" children?

8) This x-ray shows the first and second M-P joints of the foot in a young adult. See if you can handle the following challenges to your biomechanical expertise.

(*a*) In what biomechanical situations do most sesamoid bones appear, what kind of loads do they principally carry, and why does mechanical function remain little impaired if you surgically remove one by "shelling" it out of its enveloping soft tissues?

(*b*) What does the differing cross sectional sizes of the first and second metatarsal shafts imply about the loads they normally carry?

(*c*) Why denser subchondral bone on the phalangeal side of the MP joint, relative to the metatarsal side?

(*d*) Upon direct blow the patella often fractures but these sesamoids in the flexor hallucis brevis heads rarely do. Why?

9) In the x-rays of the spine shown in Figure 2.02:

(*a*) The lumbar vertebral bodies clearly demonstrate wedging, the vertical height of the centra on the convex side exceeding that on the concave. Why?

(*b*) Suppose the parents insisted that the child had a perfectly straight back a year before this x-ray. Can you show

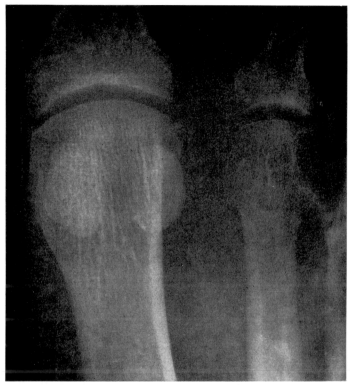

Fig. 15

that this represents lack of perception on their part rather than a "galloping" progression of a scoliosis?

(*c*) The middle x-ray shows the upper Harrington rod fairly clearly. After inspecting it, predict the most likely location of a fatigue fracture, should one occur in it (and they do sometimes). Why would it occur there? And under what type of load, understanding that the rod had a circular cross section and a smooth, polished surface?

(*d*) Assume the spine fusion heals solidly without breakage of the Harrington rod. Could the rod then subsequently break in fatigue?

(*e*) As a joint and biomechanically speaking, how does the intervertebral disc differ from the interphalangeal and other sliding, diarthrodeal joints? And what structure makes this function possible mechanically?

(*f*) The *nucleus pulposus* lacks any innervation. What

then would comprise the "fail safe" mechanism preventing one from overloading the intervertebral disc by voluntary muscle action? What comprises the engineering logic behind such an arrangement?

10) Figure 18.10 middle, shows an arthritic knee seen in x-ray view from the front.

(a) The loss of cartilage space could have occurred by what basic means? Then optimally efficient use of research expertise into this form of arthritis should begin by doing what?

(b) The x-ray configuration of the cartilage space indicates loss of what tissues and structures?

(c) What signifies the bony sclerosis beneath the articular surfaces of the central portions of each condyle, tibial as well as femoral? And why does the tibial sclerosis exceed the femoral?

(d) Why might the act of bearing weight on this knee cause bone pain? And why might weight bearing plus motion cause even more pain?

11) (a) When lower limb paralysis occurs early in life, the affected limb almost always becomes shorter than the unaffected one during subsequent growth. Explain this as a biomechanical phenomenon.

(b) Now name some diseases and affections in which this principle appears to operate, and explain the consistent association of limb length deficiencies with them.

(c) While such shortening in limbs may follow muscular weakness arising from any etiological origin early in childhood, it rarely appears to a magnitude of any clinical concern if the weakness develops after age 10 to 12 years. Why?

(d) Given equal paralysis of the upper and lower extremity on one side, the *relative* shortening of the upper usually exceeds, and respectably so, that of the affected lower. Why?

(e) At various times attempts to stimulate growth in a length-deficient limb have received some experimental and clinical attention, thought and use. Biologically speaking, how do they work? How does a bone screw or an ivory peg or a cortical bone graft inserted in the metaphyseal region stimulate growth of the epiphyseal plate closest to it?

(*f*) You just saw a patient with a shortening of the left lower limb of 3.5 cm as determined on scanograms (special x-rays which measure bone length), and as measured between the hip joint space and the ankle joint space. First, state the ultimate objective of limb length equalization procedures, and the ultimate test of whether your surgical interference has proved successful.

Second, does the scanogram provide all the information necessary to determine your degree of success? Explain.

(*g*) A lower limb paralyzed in early childhood usually reveals a femoral head of smaller diameter than on the normal side. Explain now, should you see a child with such paralysis who has a larger than normal diameter head but no evidence of Perthe's disease: what should you look for?

Biomechanical Problems

1) (a) You see a "biological failure" in which mesenchymal cell reaction and/or cellular differentiation failed to react properly to the injury, so only trivial amounts of fracture callus have materialized.

(b) Extensive, regionally accelerated BMU-based Haversian remodeling, part of the regional acceleratory phenomenon. In Volume III this behavioral entity was named "posttraumatic osteodystrophy"; it is widely but improperly termed disuse osteoporosis.

(c) No, some noxious effect of the original fracture-injury itself caused it.

(d) No; the extensive and accelerated remodeling activity *proves* that supernormal bone perfusion exists here.

(e) Depends on what you mean. The increased cortical tunneling implies increases *lamellar* bone formation (borne out by hot radiostrontium scans done by several investigators in such situations) while the lack of fracture callus reveals depressed *fibrous* bone production.

(f) Total and unit strengths down, stiffness down and compliance up, and toughness down.

(g) Increased temperature due to regionally increased perfusion.

(h) In time the screws will break and/or work loose destroying the internal fixation, and one cannot blame the manufacturer or the design of the devices for this.

2) (a) For two reasons: the growth-related deformity of the femoral heal and neck place the abductor tendon insertion above the hip joint, thereby shortening those muscles and making them "insufficient" mechanically (the muscle length-force relation in action); and the ratio of the lever arms of center of gravity of body/center of hip, and center of

hip/greater trochanter, has altered in such a way that the muscles have lost mechanical advantage on the hip. Consequently the patient's nervous system compensates by swaying the shoulders (and thus the center of mass of the whole trunk) over the center of the stance-phase hip, and alternating this in right-left fashion and so on during walking. This increased swaying constitutes the "waddling" gait.

(*b*) It probably had increased susceptibility to creep, and "flowed" transversely by that means during growth under the influence of the combined forces of muscle contractions and body weight. This could have reflected the increased thickness of articular cartilage during growth (i.e., if one mm. thickness allows 100 microns of creep per year, three mm thickness would allow 300 microns), or an abnormal tendency to creep, or both.

(*c*) The peak of the curve has displaced to the left, and/or has reduced in height relative to the tension-loaded limb.

(*d*) Normal; the distorted bone shapes reflect appropriate adaptations to missteps by the skeletal modeling "conductor", the *chondral* growth and modeling activities.

(*e*) It should reduce relative to transverse growth, causing the configuration known as *platyspondyly* (which in fact does characterize this disease). See Figure (16).

3) (*a*) The bone lying in its thread roots and anchoring it in place failed in fatigue due to cyclic axial extraction loads, allowing additional small tangential motions of the plate rubbing against the femoral shaft then to "walk" the screw out, just as alternately pulling and pushing sideways on the top of a fence post will walk it up out of its hole in the ground.

(*b*) Tangential plate motions on the femur loaded them cyclically in flexure until they failed in mechanical fatigue.

(*c*) At the thread roots close to the lateral periosteal surface of the bone.

(*d*) No. The *purpose* of the device system was to hold things together until bone healing reached the stage that living tissue could take over all mechanical functions. And it did so, after which it became immaterial how many sep-

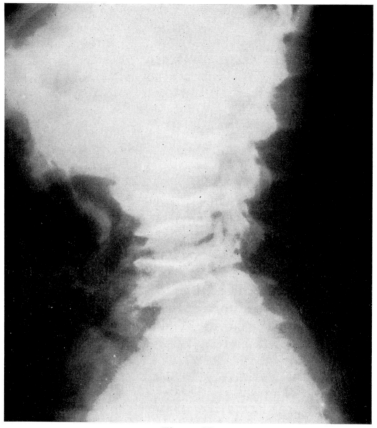

Figure 16

arate parts—and pieces of parts—came to lie in the tissues as inert foreign bodies.

(*e*) Either at the change in contour between nail and plate, or through the upper screw hole; both constitute stress risers.

(*f*) Such stiffness of the hip could increase more than five-fold the flexural and torque loads absorbed by the device, leading to much earlier failure of metal, or of bone in contact with metal, and thus a possible malunion.

(*g*) Turned the screws in or seated them too tightly. First, this preloads them in axial tension, and second, due to the almost inevitable eccentricities between holes in the plate and those in the bone, it would have preloaded their shank regions in flexure. Smaller cyclic loadings thereafter would suffice to cause breakage in fatigue. In addition, over-tightening the screws could strain them excessively, and could do so to the point that strain hardening of the metal developed, which would embrittle the affected parts and thereby locally enhance their susceptibility to fatigue.

4) (*a*) Use of a ruler will show that the horizontal distance—center of ankle joint to the heel contact with the floor—equals 0.25 the length of the plantar fascia; and 11 cm × 0.25 equals 2.74 cm. Thus the torque generated by the 200 kg load on the os calcis and which the plantar fascia must carry to hold the arch up, equals 200 × 2.74, or 550 kg cm. The plantar fascia must exert an equal counter torque for the arch to maintain its shape and relationships. Its fulcrum, or the point about which it tends to rotate the foot, consists of the middle of the talonavicular joint which lies 0.37 the length of the plantar fascia above it, or 4.1 cm. So summing up these moments:

$$500 - 4.1 \text{ x} = 0$$

and x = 134 kg f which is 0.67 times the total ankle load. And in general then the total load on the plantar fascia will approximate 0.67 times that crossing the ankle joint.

(*b*) More than doubles it. And that increases the compression load acting on the chondral longitudinal growth planes of the bones in the arch, often over onto the descending limb of the chondral growth response curve so that in a child a structural pes planus can develop unless one corrects the situation early enough in life ("early enough": around age 3 years).

(*c*) In this x-ray the load on the plantar fascia acts at an angle of approximately 20° to the mean longitudinal axis of the metatarsals. So this relation holds:

Longitudinal component in metatarsals = Plantar fascia load ÷ cos 20° and so:

$$\text{x} = 134/.94 = 143 \text{ kg f}$$

And since that 143 kg load must cross the midtarsal joint complex, it represents the answer we seek.

(*d*) The protractor shows that the vertical 200 kg load has a compression component parallel to the tuber which lies at 125° to the long axis of the tibia. It is offset by three other components: those arising from tendo Achilles pull and the upwards force of the floor on the tuber, plus the 134 kg load on the plantar fascia, which has a tuberal compression component lying at 25° inclination from it. Note that the angle of 125° — 90° = 35°. So the total uniaxial compression load on the tuber equals:

$$200 \cos 35° = \text{tuberal compression load}$$
$$200 \times .82 = 164 \text{ kg f}$$

(*e*) 164 ÷ (6.2 ÷ .20) = 203 kg/cm². And since there are 100 mm² per cm²:

$$\frac{203}{100} = 2.03 \text{ kg/mm}^2, \text{ or about } 1/6 \text{ the breaking load (or}$$

stress).

5) (*a*) The small bones represent bone modeling-independent bones for they lie essentially completely surrounded by articular cartilage and/or ligament insertions (all of which have a layer of cartilage lying between the bone and the fibrous tissues of the ligament). The metacarpals on the other hand form bone modeling-dependent structures, except of course for their articular structures.

(*b*) The angle of each metaphyseal cortex relative to the long axis of the bone equals half of the total angle, or 18°. A longitudinal compression load on this cortex and acting parallel to it then can resolve into two orthogonal components, and the medially directed one (x) will be to the load itself (P), as the sine of the angle of 18°. Or:

$$x = P \sin 18° = P \times .31$$

In other words the necking in load (or stress) will equal 31% of the total longitudinal compression load. And it will remain 31% of that load regardless of any variations in the total load, as long as the bone remains intact. The mathematician calls such a property "an invariant".

(*c*) Recall that reducing a cylinder's diameter causes large increases in surface fiber stresses under both flexural and torque loadings, so the narrow mid shafts of bones should prove more susceptible to fatigue failures than the relatively much wider metaphyses. Such loads probably account for the vast majority of so-called stress fractures (we do not consider pathological fractures here).

As for the bone modeling independent bones, they carry either pure compression loads without significant flexure or torque as in this carpus, or pure tension loads as in the various sesamoids. Thus while they may undergo spontaneous fractures (ex: patella) they rarely develop the clinical entity termed the stress or march fracture.

(*d*) If you said two you need to review the physiology of bone growth, for eight (8) appear. Recall that articular cartilage also grows? These articular growth planes thus constitute the epiphyseal plates of the metacarpal and radius, plus the two apposing articular surfaces each of the metacarpotrapezoidal, trapezoidalnavicular, and naviculoradial joints.

(*e*) A total of eleven (11). They include the epiphyseal plates (4 in number) of upper and lower femur and upper and lower tibia, plus the articular cartilages (7 in number) of the femoral head, and the knee, ankle and subtalar joints. Growth prediction charts often assumed all of the longitudinal growth arose in the epiphyseal plates, thereby leading one to expect more from a particular one than in fact it could deliver, and so leading to undercorrection. As to underestimates, the epiphyseodesis operation initiates a regional acceleratory phenomenon which can affect all of the growth planes in the joint next to the epiphyseodesis. As yet we have no way to predict the magnitude of this effect in a particular child and in some it can prove so large as to nearly undo any reduction in growth provided directly by the epiphyseodesis.

(*f*) Simple: On teleroentgenograms (which reduce the errors of parallax to trivial levels) measure the vertical distance between epiphyseal plate and joint line in adults, and subtract from it that in infants. This growth-derived increase in this distance (which incidentally proves that articular cartilage growth contributes to limb length) reflects the contribution of articular cartilage growth to overall limb length with more than the requisite accuracy.

(*g*) They provide a means of distributing equally among the five metacarpals the compression load transmitted to them (or taken from them) by one bone, the radius. The flexural compliance of this articulated, multibone arrangement also allows that distribution to shift or change instantly according to special situations and/or need. Clearly the mid tarsal bone complex in the foot has a similar function. But the pisiform bone forms in essence a sesamoid in the flexor carpi ulnaris tendon and so does not participate in such a function to any important extent.

(*h*) The pronator quadratus applies an equal flexural load to both of course, and of the static arrangement, but it forms a much lesser fraction of the total longitudinal compression loads carried by the radius than by the ulna. Thus less inwaisting would prove needed in the radial cortex to neutralize it. And also the larger diameter of the radius markedly reduces any flexural strain induced in it by that muscle, relative to that developing in the much narrower ulna.

6) (*a*) Only chondroblast cellular proliferation apparently, as described by the growth/force-response curve.

(*b*) Normal chondroblast division requires STH and thyroxine, while adrenalcorticosteroids definitely and estrogens probably depress it. The cretin demonstrates depressed mineralization (which, by blocking subsequent stages, delays maturation of ossification centers). And we certainly do *not* have all the information yet which we need on this matter for clinical usage.

(*c*) We need vitamin D (actually probably one of its active metabolites 1,25DOHCC) to mineralize cartilage, vitamin C to form the collagen of the matrix (it proves essential to hydroxylate proline in forming tropocollagen molecules), and adequate dietary calcium to retain normal amounts of primary and especially of secondary spongiosa.

(*d*) If *generally* distributed, then for both increased length and dwarfism look in the endocrine area, either in terms of altered amounts of hormones, altered stereochemistry of same, or altered target-cell responsiveness to their normal effects.

For the malalignment and succeeding problems look into abnormal biomechanical milieu, or altered responsiveness of chondral growth or of hyaline cartilage itself to biomechanical factors.

(*e*) Disposing of acquired, postinjury deformities, we would have to include these:

Normal bone modeling responding to abnormal dynamic flexural forces.
Inherently abnormal bone modeling competence.
Normal chondral modeling and growth potential responding to abnormal mechanical forces.
Abnormal chondral modeling and growth competence.

Or some combination of the above. Keep in mind that chondral modeling competence can become abnormal due to increased susceptibility to mechanical shear, as this arises in rickets, or to compression as in Morquio's disease.

7) (*a*) The talus and os calcis (the "hindfoot") lie in relative plantar flexion at the ankle joint while the forefoot has gone into extension relative to the hind foot and at the midtarsal joint complex. As one result the plantar fascia now lies less than half its normal vertical distance below the center of the talonavicular joint. Consequently, and given normal loads across the ankle, the longitudinal tension loads on the plantar fascia must increase, to generate enough inchpounds of torque to offset the counter clockwise torque applied to the hindfoot by the downward-thrusting tibial load. Note that when the hindfoot goes into some equinus as here, the lever arm of the tibial load on it increases, for in essence it represents the *horizontal* distance from center of ankle joint to center of heel support by the floor.

The increased plantar fascia load increases the compression loads on the bony elements of the longitudinal arch,

while the dorsiflexion of the midtarsal joint complex concentrates that load on the upper (i.e., cephalad) portions of the
articular chondral growth planes of the talonavicular and
related joints. And in clinical practice one observes retarded
growth develops there, leading in time and with further
growth to a fixed pes planus deformity.

(b) This drawing illustrates some of the effects as seen
from the rear of the foot. The plantar fascia (cross-hatched
oval) comes to lie laterally to the vertical line of action of the
load crossing the ankle joint. The strap muscles (posterior
and anterior tibial and peroneals) normally exist simply to
tilt the subtalar joint complex in valgus-varus so as to balance
the ankle directly over the plantar fascia, like balancing a
man on top of a barrel, and when the fascia lies in the proper
position it requires little contractile force of posterior and
anterior tibial muscles (P.T.A.T.) or peroneals (P) to maintain it there. But in the pes planus position the posterior
tibial must work much harder and, in point of clinical fact,
it cannot sustain enough contractural force to do so. Rather,
it fatigues quickly. The valgus-tending torque generated by
the illustrated eccentricity between line of action of tibial
load and plantar fascia generates a counterclockwise torque

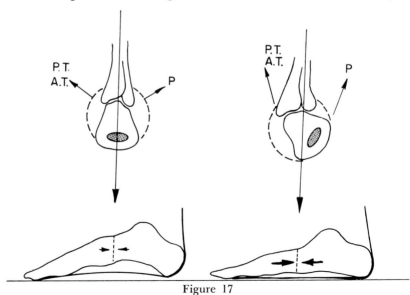

Figure 17

tending to further exaggerate the deformity. And that applies compression to the affected growing chondral articular planes which tends to "freeze in" the deformity as a structurally rigid one in the adult.

Under the subject of "spastic rockerbottom foot", Volume I discussed some further aspects of basic foot mechanics.

(c) Start while most bone growth still lies ahead of you, for the total remaining growth *relative to that already past* determines—and limits—how much growth-related correction you can achieve, an upper limit which you can rarely attain. And you would do it by overloading chondral growth planes in compression in exactly that pattern which tends to lead at the end of growth to a structurally rigid but now normal arch.

(d) While all appear *logical,* only the Whitman plates also prove *effective,* and then only if begun early enough (age 2–3½ years) and used continually and faithfully for the next 3 to 5 years.

(e) In a spastic foot the muscles will retain their original contractural timing during the gait cycle (axiom: "you cannot retrain a spastic muscle"). But the normal youngster has no such limitation in the adaptability and trainability of his nervous system's automaton, and usually unconsciously self-retrains the transferred peroneal to function similarly to his improperly functioning anterior tibial muscle. Thus it comes to *relax* during stance after the transfer, when to correct the subtalar valgus *during stance* it should *contract.*

(f) It becomes a consequence of abnormal muscle activity patterns, which in turn points to some disorder in the neural control over the coordination of the actions of the various muscles controlling posture of the dynamic foot.

8) (a) Where a tension-loaded tendon having a relatively restricted range of excursion changes direction. It carries primarily a tension load of course. And because a respectable tension transfer fan-out envelops all sesamoids, transmission of the tension load remains intact after removing the bone, provided one removes the sesamoid by sharp dissection so as to leave its enveloping, tension-carrying

fascial sheath intact. By this procedure one usually loses only a small fraction of the lever arm of the tendon on the joint it actuates, a fraction insufficient to produce any real disability in most well motivated patients.

(*b*) The larger bone carries the greater loads.

(*c*) The *time averaged* unit loads they respectively carry do not remain equal on each side, although their instantaneous ones do. This happens because of the geometry of their motion, as described in Part II of this text.

(*d*) Upon direct blow the patella has little overlying soft tissue to protect it, and it lies upon a relatively massive "anvil", the femur, so that an impact can lead to momentum transfer over relatively brief time intervals, thereby easily generating internal stresses in excess of its material's properties strength. (If still somewhat foggy on this, review *momentum* and *impact* in Part I.) But the sesamoids lie protected by a much thicker layer of soft tissue, and also on a much less massive and far more compliant anvil, the first metatarsal. Thus the transfer of momentum during an impact becomes sufficiently prolonged in temporal duration that the sesamoid's breaking stress remains above any generated in it by the impact.

9) (*a*) As rotation occurs early in the development of the curve it causes concentration of the vertical compression forces on the sides of the centrae lying nearest the curve's concavity. This loads the horizontal chondral growth planes at top and bottom of each centra into the descending limb of the chondral growth/force-response curve, thereby decreasing growth in height relative to that on the convex side.

(*b*) Yes. The wedging referred to required several years to develop, given the relatively slow vertical growth existing at this child's age of some 15 years at the time of the left hand x-ray.

(*c*) Through the root of one of the notches in the upper third of the rod, because these notches represent sharp changes in contour which create local stress concentrations. Furthermore the rod's diameter reduces in the notch, which further augments the stress concentration. Because of its circular cross section the rod cannot take loading in torque—no equivalent of a pipe wrench to grasp it. So a combination of uniaxial compression and flexure should prove responsible, cyclic in nature because of the biomechanics of gait and normal trunk function.

(*d*) Yes. The fused spine still has appreciable flexural compliance so that normal body function, by causing cyclic flexure of the fused spine, cyclically loads the rod, and it can fail in fatigue as a consequence.

(*e*) The disc contains no joint space or cavity and no gliding surface. It represents a highly compliant, semifluid pressure pad which distributes vertical loads with nearly equal unit loading over the endplates of each vertebral centrum. And somewhat like a meniscus, its high compliance acts to maintain equal unit loading in the face of various mechanical movements of one centrum relative to its neighbor.

To function in this manner some enveloping circumferential container is required to prevent lateral extrusion of the disc or nucleus pulposus under vertical loads, and that container constitutes the *annulus fibrosus.*

(*f*) Nerves in the periphery of the annulus fibrosus signal overload if stretched or bulged too far by an overload, while nerves in the subchondral bone of the vertebral endplates signal overload of those endplates. It seems obvious that, since failure of this flexible pressure-pad function depends upon the mechanical integrity of the walls of its container (rather than upon any risk of collapse of the nucleus pulposus to a degenerate, compressed state of matter as astronomers use that term), the fail-safe mechanism should lie in those walls themselves to indicate *directly*—and thus with maximum reliability—any risk of imminent failure.

10) (*a*) The articular cartilage might have worn off or undergone destruction by some biochemical process; or reactivation of the endochondral ossification sequences might simply have replaced its deeper layers with bone from beneath. Clearly for study of this type of arthritis to proceed with a minimum of false "moves" one should first determine

which of these mechanisms operates there, or which combination, if in fact such combination proves responsible.

(*b*) Obviously articular cartilage has disappeared. Perhaps less obviously but equally unequivocally the menisci have disappeared too, at least in the functional sense, for if present they would float the femur on the tibia and maintain a wider joint space. Surgeons who operate on such knees will recognize the truth of this statement.

(*c*) Lacking the flotation effect of the meniscus, loads across this joint have become unduly concentrated on the central regions of each condyle, and that has existed long enough, and the patient has continued to function physically at a high enough level, to lead to a local adaptational response of the now overloaded subchondral bony regions. That response represents structural reenforcement by the accumulation of additional bone. Because of the geometry of their motion and load transfer behavior and because of the time averaging property, the tibial condyle takes more *cumulative* abuse than an equivalent area of the femoral, so the former develops more bony sclerosis.

(*d*) Lacking a compliant, interposed meniscus and Babbitt to distribute loads evenly over large areas of the articular surfaces, the incongruities of the mating articular surfaces cause high unit loads to concentrate upon small total areas. This generates excessive strain in the bony regions where unloaded and directly loaded bone adjoin, and such strain always generates pain, given a conscious patient and a normal nervous system.

When this weight bearing joint now also moves, the abnormally high coefficient of friction between its damaged articular surfaces (probably 0.3) adds shearing strains to the compression ones; by increasing total strain, this increases total pain.

11) (*a*) Because of the paralysis, the affected limb's chondral growth planes carry reduced time-averaged compression loads; recall that of the total loads on a weight bearing joint, much more than half represents muscle pull, and less than half the superimposed body weight. Given that,

then in the affected limb the growth/response characteristic moves towards the left on the growth/force-response curve, which lies in the direction of reduced growth. Hence in time the affected limb becomes short relative to the normal one.

(*b*) Anterior poliomyelitis; muscular dystrophy; myelodysplasia; myelomeningocele; paralysis and paresis acquired in childhood whether of traumatic, postsurgical, infectious or embolic origin; hemiatrophy of the brain (the opposite side of the body under-develops); spasticity. In all, a reduction occurs of muscle force.

(*c*) First because most of the growth in limb length lies behind rather than ahead of you at that age, and second because even with total paralysis, longitudinal growth does not cease; it merely reduces to some basal level, one which lies around two-thirds of the maximal possible. As a result of these two effects the total difference in limb length acquired by the age of skeletal maturity, given a late onset of the muscle-weakening condition, will rarely exceed the limits presently considered acceptable by our specialty (which lies on the order of 3 cm or so in a male and 2 or more in a female).

(*d*) In both the upper and the lower those compression loads of purely muscular origin carried by and acting on the chondral growth planes reduce equally, so from that aspect alone, equal relative shortening develops. But unlike the upper extremity, the affected lower one also carries the body weight, a load not reduced by the paralysis. This adds an extra element of compression load on its chondral growth planes, which moves their response characteristics somewhat over to the right of where they would lie on the response curve in a nonweight bearing situation. Hence other things remaining equal, in terms of *percentage* growth discrepancy, that in the upper will exceed that in the lower.

(*e*) It almost certainly does so by evoking a regional acceleratory phenomenon. The screw, graft or peg simply serves as an irritant or noxious stimulus which continues to act as such for some months, and the operation adds a further noxious stimulus of shorter duration.

(*f*) First, the purpose and the measure of your success constitutes obtaining a perfectly straight lumbar spine when the patient stands barefooted. Second, *no*, because in one-third or more of the children in whom you make the comparison you will discover that it requires a different amount of lift under the heel of the short limb to straighten the standing lumbar spine than the scanogram reveals. This can come about because the scanogram does not measure that portion of the limb length lying below the ankle joint, nor that between the hip joint and the lumbosacral articulation. And unexpected variations in those two factors can act to enhance, or in other children to subtract, from the length discrepancy revealed by the scanogram alone.

(*g*) Reduced muscle loads on the paralyzed hip moves its growth response characteristic towards the left on the curve which is downwards.

So if the head is larger than normal that forms pretty reliable evidence that something has evoked the regional acceleratory phenomenon and caused it to persist for many months. Look for it; it may constitute a subluxing hip exposed to mechanical abuse on the acetabular rim, or Still's disease, or an osteoid osteoma, or a stress fracture, infection or the like. And some 90% of the time, when you seek you will find.

Glossary

Repeatedly over the years residents have voiced a common complaint about our basic science literature: So many of the scientific terms appearing in it prove foreign to them that they find it difficult to grasp the import of the data, or even of an author's own stated conclusions. These same residents have volunteered appreciation for the glossaries appearing in previous monographs from this desk. And in truth they have the best of it, for an orthopaedist five or more years out of training finds technical jargon constantly changing, enlarging, and departing from meanings he knew as a young resident.

Hence this rather extensive glossary, perhaps more important than its predecessors simply because orthopaedic practice makes more extensive and consistent demands upon engineering concepts and expertise than upon any other nonmedical field ancillary to clinical orthopaedics.

Abscissa: The vertical axis of the graph of Cartesian coordinates.

Acceleration: Changing the speed of motion and/or the direction of motion of a material object. In the broad sense the term includes both positive and negative accelerations, while in the limited sense the acceleration would represent an increasing speed or an increasing change in direction of motion, while the term deceleration would represent the converse.

Acetabulum: The bony socket to the hip joint, which forms a part of the pelvic bone.

Age hardening: This describes a property of some metals whereby they possess a fair amount of ductility or plasticity shortly after cooling from the melt but after a period of time, and because of internal allotropic changes within the metal, increasing resistance to dislocation movements arises so the material demonstrates greater hardness, rigidity, and strength.

Allotropic: A change in crystalline form while in the solid state. Such changes may occur spontaneously with changes in temperature or they may occur following mechanical cold working of the material, or they may occur spontaneously over time.

Alloy: A metal in which two or more metallic elements combine in various ways to produce a bulk material with its own mechanical and physical properties.

Ampere: A measure of the amount of flow of electrical current, very closely analogous to the flow of water in a pipe, i.e., 5 cu ft per min., or 5 amp. In the latter term a particular quantity of electric charge is assumed, and that quantity represents a coulomb.

Anelasticity: Literally, the opposite of elasticity and therefore the property of matter in which it does not return to its original dimension and shape after a strain. The term forms an inclusive one for several different types of anelasticity are recognized by metallurgists.

Anisotropic: In the *mechanical sense* this signifies a material whose mechanical properties differ according to the direction in which one tests it. In the *optical sense* this signifies the fact that light traversing the material in different directions experiences different indices of refraction, usually the hallmark of any material possessing birefringence.

Anodic: The anode designates the more positively charged of two electrodes, the one which collects electrons from some other medium. Anodic therefore means that the material tends to collect electrons from its surroundings, and during metallic corrosion the actual loss of metallic substance due to corrosion usually occurs on anodic surfaces.

Apatite: The crystalline, needle-like form of a major fraction of the bone mineral consisting of calcium, phosphate, and hydroxyll groups arranged in a definite crystalline lattice, although in nature a lattice which contains many, many imperfections.

Arthrodesis: An operation in which one causes bone to bridge a joint completely and solidly, and so to stiffen it permanently.

Austenite: This signifies that crystalline structure of iron and carbon atoms which exist above the critical ferrite-austenite transition temperature of 1183° k.

Bearing: A mechanical arrangement which allows one part to move upon another, usually in a way that minimizes wear, but on occasion, the primary objective may consist of reducing friction.

Bernouilli effect: The fact that the transverse pressure along a moving column of fluid decreases as the velocity of the fluid column increases, and conversely.

Birefringence: This signifies the optical property of polarizing light or, more accurately, the fact that light rays entering such materials experience two separate indices of refraction, break up into two rays within it, and then recombine at the emerging surface somewhat out of phase to produce interference effects. Both a polarizer and an analyzer constitute birefringent materials, and identically so. Their names signify not any differences in their optical properties, but merely differences in their location in the path of a light beam.

BMU: The basic multicellular units of bone remodeling and bone modeling, dealt with extensively in Volumes III and IV of this series.

Bone: The hard and rigid natural building material composed of an organic phase called a bone matrix, and an inorganic phase representing the bone mineral salts, which in part consist of apatite crystals.

Boundary layer lubrication: In essence this represents lubrication of two moving surfaces by a stiff grease which, by virtue of its mechanical stiffness and its chemical adhesiveness to the two materials, prevents their contact, reducing thereby to acceptable levels the amount of wear between them. Usually found primarily in bearings that move at low speeds and infrequently.

Brittle: The property of a material in which it breaks following a small strain. This usually arises because moving any dislocations within the material (if it has a crystalline nature) requires exerting a greater shearing force than will fracture the material in tension.

Callus: The tissues, of somewhat complicated composition, that heal bone and tendon following fractures or ruptures.

Cantilever bending: In ordinary mechanics this represents the situation illustrated for example in figure 19.05. Also, in the bone modeling context it represents a specific and analogous mechanical arrangement for inducing flexure, described adequately in Chapter XIX.

Cartesian coordinates: Two axes drawn perpendicularly to each other, one horizontal, called the ordinate, and one vertical called the abscissa, used for purposes of plotting two variables against each other, the usual form of graphing data found in medical literature.

Cartilage: A rather compliant organic structural material, with a large amount of water, and composed of collagen embedded in an organic gel called mucopolysaccharide or cementing substance.

Cathodic: The more electrically negative or noble metal of two electrodes or two metals lying at different points in the electromotive series. The cathode emits electrons, and since it attracts electrically positive ions in solution, such ions have come to be called cations. Equally those ions attracted to the anode and which therefore carry negative charges, have come to be called anions. The more cathodic of two metals forming such a battery does not actually corrode.

Cement substance: See mucopolysaccharide.

Chondral growth force response characteristic: This signifies the relative changes in speed of growth of growing cartilage under the action of normal forces. Volume II describes it in some detail. It and its corollaries represent an original contribution of the author's.

Chondroitin sulfate: These form three of the specific muco-polysaccharides found in skeletal tissues, and include chondroitin sulphates A, B, and C.

Clavicle: The collar bone.

Collagen: A crystalline organic fiber composed of amino acids and having a fairly well defined amino acid sequence. By end-to-end as well as side-to-side bonding, the basic, helical and triply wound tropocollagen molecule can serve as a mer to build up collagen polymers into fibers of varying size, at all levels of resolution from the naked eye to the electron microscopic. This constitutes one of nature's basic building blocks or structural materials which, on the evolutionary scale, apparently already had come into existence by the time fossilization of recognizable multicellular organisms began some 600 million years ago.

Compacta: This constitutes the outer wall or cortex of most of the bones in the body, and constitutes a complex tissue synthesized out of the simple tissue termed lamellar bone.

Compression: That which tends to squeeze together or, when one discusses stresses, that which tends to resist such a squeeze.

Complex tissue: Any tissue not sufficiently highly organized to justify the designation of an organ, but which does contain more order within it than one finds in a simple tissue. A complex tissue may consist of one or more simple tissues.

Compliance: In one static definition this consists of the inverse of rigidity, or the amount of strain developing under uniform constant load. In another somewhat more complicated dynamic context it represents the readiness with which a structure or material accelerates under an external load. Either method of usage serves quite well but obviously one must specify which he uses in order to avoid misunderstandings.

Corrosion: The capacity of materials to undergo chemical attack as a consequence of which loss of the bulk material occurs. It may occur within gasses and liquids but does not occur in a vacuum or in the interior of solid matter.

Cortex: See compacta.

Coulomb: A quantity of electric charge, which in fact constitutes a particular number of electrons. Appendix 6 defines it more precisely.

Couple: A rotatory force acting upon an object and created by two forces acting in parallel, equal in magnitude but acting in opposite directions, and separated from each other by some perpendicular distance between their lines of action.

Covalent bond: A chemical bond between atoms in which some of the electrons in the outer shell of one atom become shared by adjacent atoms so that the electrons in question exert attractions on the positively charged atomic nucleii of each. One of the strong, so-called primary bonding forces of matter.

Creep: The capacity of matter under a constant load to undergo a very slow and progressive plastic deformation. It constitutes an anelastic phenomenon.

Crystalline: That state of matter in which various atoms and molecules array regularly with respect to each other in space, so that long range order exists within the crystal. The antithesis of the crystalline state constitutes the amorphous state.

Damping: The capacity of a material to absorb energy upon impact and to dissipate it by means other than the rebound or resilience phenomenon.

Deceleration: That form of acceleration in which a body in motion decreases its rate of motion with respect to the observer, or decreases its previous rate of change in direction. When one applies the brakes of a car on the expressway, he (hopefully) decelerates the car.

Diaphysis: The mid-shaft portion of a long bone, usually constituting the middle two thirds approximately.

Dielectric: A material constituting an electrical insulator which has the capacity to localize positive or negative charges upon its surface.

Dielectric constant: That figure of merit which signifies how much better than a vacuum a given material increases the capacity of a capacitor for storing electric charge, when it serves as a medium intervening between the two conducting plates of the capacitor.

Dislocation: In orthopaedic surgery of course, this refers to the joint between two bones coming completely apart, and we also call such a phenomenon a luxation or, if incomplete, a subluxation. In metallurgy however, a dislocation represents a lattice defect within a crystal, usually running for some distance through the crystal along one of its inherent planes, which prestresses or strains the surrounding lattice networks in such a way that a relatively small externally applied load will cause one plane of the crystal to move in shear on the next one. These dislocations account for the bulk mechanical properties of metals, which possess only one-thousandth or so of the strength of perfectly pure small crystals of the metals.

Ductile: The capacity of a metal or other material to flow under tension. This property serves to produce finer and finer wires by the drawing process, and it sometimes serves to strain-harden wire rope.

Dyne: That unit of force which, when acting for one second upon a mass of one gram, will give to it a speed of 1 cm per second. It consttutes approximately 1/980 of the pull of the earth on a one gram weight.

Elasticity: The capacity of a material to return to its original shape and dimension following a deformation, regardless of how rapidly or slowly the restitution of shape and dimension occur.

Elastic limit: The limiting amount of internal stress above which some permanent deformation of the material occurs.

Elastomer: Those polymeric materials which exhibit elastic behavior. They usually constitute plastics which at room temperature lie within their glass transition state or temperature range.

Energy: A quantity of work, which may represent potential or kinetic energy and which may exist as heat, as mechanical work, as a chemical state, as an amount of electricity brought to a particular potential, etc.

Epiphysis: The usually somewhat spherical or quasi-spherical bone center at the end of the long bone, and separated from the body of that bone by a plate of cartilage called the epiphyseal plate. The bulk of growth in length occurs in the epiphyseal plate, while the bulk of the chondral modeling which determines the architecture of the joint surface occurs in the articular cartilage that usually covers the epiphysis. By definition an epiphysis usually has a joint on one side of it, while an analogous structure called an apophysis does not.

Equilibrium: In the mechanical sense this constitutes a body carrying a number of loads but which nevertheless does not exhibit acceleration. Consequently all of the loads acting upon it must cancel each other out, permitting it to remain in mechanical, static equilibrium. In dynamic chemical and analogous contexts, equilibrium constitutes that stage in which the input into a system equals its output, and it represents a special case of the steady state in which the relationship between input and output of the system remains constant over some arbitrary unit of time.

Erg: A unit of work representing that done upon a mass of one gram by accelerating it to a speed of one centimeter per second.

Farad: A measure of electrical capacitance, and analogous to the volume of a tank which stores air under pressure.

Fascia: A natural, living fabric woven of collagen fibers which possesses tensile rigidity in two directions lying in a common plane but remains compliant in shear and flexure in all orientations, and consequently does not possess significant rigidity in compression.

Fatigue: In the mechanical sense, the property of structural materials in which they develop fractures after cyclic loading and deloading which remain well within the static stress design limits. It has become fairly generally accepted by now that the basic phenomenon causing this represents a group of phenomena which tend to concentrate mechanical stress in local regions within the material so that locally the strength of the material becomes exceeded, even though averaged throughout the bulk of the structure it lies well below its fracturing strength.

Feedback: This signifies the transmission of information about the behavior of a system back to the facilities that control its behavior. Positive feedback acts in the sense that a change in the system's behavior signals enhancement of that change, so the system tends to act in a "vicious cycle" or runaway or explosive manner. Negative feedback systems, the rule in animal physiology, act in that sense or mode which tends to reduce any change in the controlled parameter. Negative feedback systems therefore serve very well to maintain things within desired limits, such as the temperature of the body, the shape of a bone relative to the mechanical loads it carries, or the level of the calcium and magnesium ion concentrations in the blood.

Femur: The thigh bone.

Ferrite: A particular eutectic form of iron and carbon which exists at room temperature and has greater hardness, strength and resistance to shearing deformation than pure iron.

Fibrocartilage: A type of cartilage, containing the same chemical building blocks as hyaline cartilage but with greater proportions of collagen and somewhat less water than hyaline cartilage. It usually possesses great tensile rigidity and strength along its well defined grain, while remaining quite compliant in both shear and flexure in all orientations.

Fibrous bone: A primitive type of bone produced during repair or as a defensive reaction. It appears to have the property of automatically self-initiating its subsequent replacement by lamellar bone. Except for studies of the fracture and allied healing processes, the structural and material properties of fibrous bone have relatively little concern to biomechanicians.

Fibula: The small non-weight bearing bone on the outer part of the lag.

First order: Referring to a relationship or a function, it represents the direct and immediate thing. Thus the first order function of the human joint consists of allowing motion between two rigid parts of the body. A second order function consists of maintaining that capacity over the life span of a man which leads to a third order function, that of minimizing wear of the two sliding surfaces.

Flexure: Bending.

Flexure drift law: That bone modeling activity in which bones affected by a stereotyped series of flexural strains then begin to shift all of their affected surfaces towards the concavity that arises during the act of dynamic flexure. Discussed at length in Volume IV, credit for formulating it and its corollaries belongs to your author.[92]

Force: In physics and mechanics, that which can accelerate matter.

Fracture: A break of a material, whether of a bone or beam, a glass rod, or any other solid body. But when a tendon or ligament breaks in tension, rather than saying that it fractures we usually say that it ruptures.

Fragile: The property of a material in which it breaks following minimum absorption of work or strain energy. Fragile materials usually therefore also exhibit considerable brittleness, but it does not follow that brittle materials of necessity are also fragile.

Free body: This constitutes an artiface in which one draws a diagram of a small portion of a system, or of its mechanical essence so that all of the forces acting upon that abstracted system, and all of the reactions to those forces, appear in their proper direction and magnitude so that one may analyze some or several aspects of the system's behavior and response to those forces. Described in Appendix 9.

Fretting: Microscopic rubbing motions or working of one hard object upon another which tend to produce microscopic regions of wear at the contacting surfaces. Fretting motions between a screw head and a bone plate can mechanically disrupt their surface oxide film to expose potentially corrosive material underneath.

Friction: The resistance of one body of matter to sliding on or rubbing against another. When discussing two solid objects, the starting friction constitutes that force required to initiate relative motion, and the moving friction (usually but not always less than the starting) represents that force required to maintain uniform motion thereafter. The friction of a fluid constitutes viscosity. Other types of friction also exist, such as rolling, pneumatic, magnetic.

Function: In these volumes, that action supplied by one part of a system to another. While this constitutes a highly restricted meaning of the term, it defines accurately its meaning wherever one finds it in these five volumes.

Gas: That phase of matter which lacks rigidity in tension, compression, and shear. If unconfined, a gas therefore will expand indefinitely and does not possess a rigid volume.

Glass transition temperature: That range of temperatures within which a polymeric material exhibits rubber-like behavior, as opposed to solid crystalline behavior below the transition temperature, and fluid behavior above.

Grain: In metallurgy this represents a small region made up of a single crystal having the same long range atomic order and orientation of its lattice planes existing throughout.

Grain boundary: This simply represents the perimeter which envelops a particular grain and which separates it from adjoining grains within a metal.

Gram: The unit of mass in the cgs system of units, and essentially equal to the mass of one cubic centimeter of pure water.

Gram force: That force exerted by the pull of the earth on a mass of one gram and equal to 980 dynes approximately.

Growth: The process of enlarging the size of the body from that of an embryo to that of the adult, independently of those additional processes which control the architecture of the final product.

Growth process: All of those cellularly driven processes recognizable as distinct entities which contribute to the overall growth in size of the body. Most anatomists lump the modeling processes in with the growth processes.

Hamstring muscles: The muscles in back of the thigh which, because of their anatomy, simultaneously act to extend the hip and flex the knee.

Hardness: The resistance of solid matter to penetration by a pointed object. Various hardness scales have been conceived, such as Brinell, Rockwell, Vickers, Moh, etc. In Special Table 15, Part III, find a table which converts the various hardness scales.

Haversian system: A small moiety of bone usually produced within the substance of the compacta, composed of lamellar bone, and possessing tubular geometry with its long axis paralleling the resultant of the compression and/or tension strains on the part.

Heat treatment: The process of treating metals or other materials with carefully controlled temperatures and rates of heating and cooling in order to modify their physical properties. A very important body of expertise in metallurgy, and in the processes of fabricating machines and other objects out of metals of all kinds.

Hook's law: The state in which varying stress remains proportional to the strain.

Hookean: A material which at least over some portions of its stress/strain curve demonstrates a constant proportionality between stress and strain.

Hyaline cartilage: The basic tissue comprising articular cartilage and the epiphyseal plates, and consisting of collagen embedded in mucopolysaccharides and containing a large amount of water. It constitutes one of the basic skeletal building materials, or one of the basic "letters" of the skeletal "alphabet".

Hyaluronic acid: A mucopolysaccharide found in the soft tissues of the body as a gel. It embeds cells and collagen. It also appears in synovial fluid attached to a protein backbone molecule to form the mucin polymer molecule.

Hydrodynamic lubrication: A bearing arrangement in which one somehow pumps fluid in between the two sliding solid surfaces in such a way that they float upon the fluid without actually touching each other.

Impact: Signifying a blow, as a hammer blow. It represents a physical process by means of which kinetic energy acquired in a somewhat leisurely manner by some object then becomes transferred very rapidly to another object, thereby generating very large although briefly acting stresses within the second object.

Impulse: In mechanics this relates to impact but it signifies transfer of momentum from one object to another during a collision, and it remains independent of how rapidly that transfer occurs.

Inertia: The property of mass which represents its resistance to acceleration or deceleration by externally applied forces.

Infarct: To kill a mass of tissue by cutting off its blood supply.

Ionic bond: A strong chemical bonding mechanism between different atoms in which one atom "steals" one of the outer electrons of another to fill a vacancy in its own electron shell. As a consequence the deprived and now positively charged second ion becomes strongly attracted to the thief. This type of bond exists in ordinary table salt, in the hydroxyapatite of the skeleton and in most gem stones.

Isotropic: In the mechanical sense this identifies a material in which mechanical properties remain the same regardless of the orientation along which one tests them. In the optical sense it identifies a material which treats light rays passing through it in an identical manner regardless of the direction in which they traverse it. Thus optically isotropic materials lack birefringence and will not polarize light.

Joint: A biological bearing allowing one rigid bone and its attendant soft tissues to move upon another.

Joule: A unit of work equal to ten million or 10^7 ergs and also to .737 foot-pounds.

Keratan: Another of the mucopolysaccharides found in skeletal tissues, usually in amounts below 1% of the dry mass.

We do not yet know its function or role but one finds it in skin, cartilage, and bone. It differs from the skin protein, keratin.

Kilogram: A mass of one thousand grams.

Kilogram force: That pulling force which the earth exerts upon a mass of one kilogram.

Kinetic energy: This signifies energy in motion, whether it represents moving matter, moving electricity, moving mechanical processes or whatever. It can also represent radiant energy.

Lamellar bone: One of the basic simple tissues of the skeleton having long range order in such a way that its mechanical strength in one direction significantly exceeds that in all others.

Laminar flow: That flow of gases and liquids in which turbulence or eddy currents within the portions of the fluid in contact with walls of its container does not occur. Above a certain critical value laminar flow converts to turbulent flow, and maintaining continued flow in that state requires disproportionately larger amounts of pumping work put into the system.

Lever: A mechanical arrangement which multiplies the force put into the system, at the expense of an inversely proportional decrease in tne distance over which that force acts or moves, as well as in the speed of its motion.

Lever arm: This represents the actual mechanical advantage (or disadvantage) of the lever.

Ligament: An anatomical structure composed of fibrous tissue which serves to limit motion of some joint, usually only within particular planes which muscles do not exist to control.

Liquid: That state of matter exhibiting rigidity in tension and compression but a total lack of rigidity in shear. As a consequence the liquid will flow to adopt the shape of its container but even in a vacuum it has a rigid, characteristic volume, provided, of course, one ignores evaporation.

Load: A force applied to some structure or structural material from without. One of the subcategories of forces. Note that when Howard Duncan, Boy Frame or Mike Parfitt load a patient with ammonium chloride or D-xylose they do an analogous thing to him.

Lubricant: A solid, liquid, or gas which serves the function of minimizing both wear and friction between two moving surfaces.

Magnitude: Meaning how large a particular value has become, and serves in the sense of distinguishing that value from any other additional value appropriate to the parameter, such as its direction or polarity.

Malleable: The property which allows solid matter to flow under hammer blows. It relates closely to ductility, and represents a temporary transition from rigidity in shear to the fluid state. Observe that while in that temporarily fluid state, it still possesses stiffness in shear, described as the shearing stress needed to produce unit shearing strain.

Martensite: That particular phase of iron which occurs when austenite becomes very quickly cooled. It consists of carbon atoms trapped in the interstitial position between iron atoms in the tetragonal lattice, and it possesses great hardness, great strength, and great resistance to the motion of dislocations. It is also very brittle.

Mass: That property of matter which resists acceleration by an externally applied force, and it specifically does not represent the weight of the material. See weight.

Mean skeletal age: The average age of all the separate moieties of bone in one bone or the whole skeleton, weighted according to their individual sizes. Many important mechanical properties of bone depend upon the MSA for their particular values.

Mechanical advantage: Equivalent to the lever arm. Thus if one applies ten pounds of force on a lever to lift a load, the load lying one third of the distance from the fulcrum that the point of application of the force does, the load will experience a three-fold multiplication of the force acting on it, but at the expense of only one-third as much displacement.

Mer: The chemical building block or molecule of a polymer.

Mesenchymal cell: The primitive or pluripotent or parent cell which, usually by the process of cell division, gives rise to the new specialized cells which supply on a moment-to-moment basis all of the biomechanical functions required to maintain the body in a healthy state.

Metallic bond: The still not too clearly understood mechanism which bonds atoms of metal to each other in a crystalline lattice in such a way that some of their peripheral electrons remain perfectly free to move throughout the crystal lattice. Thus the metallic bond associates with the ability to conduct electricity.

Metaphysis: This signifies that part of the bone usually lying at the ends, distinct from the shaft or diaphysis, and which contains significant amounts of spongy or trabecular bone within encased by a thin cortex.

Modeling: This signifies all of those cellularly driven activities which determine the architecture of the growing skeleton.

Modeling processes: Those particular cellular systems and activities affecting cartilage, bone and fibrous tissues which, in combination, determine the architecture of the mature skeleton.

Moments: In mechanics, the stresses generated within the material of a shaft, beam, or column as a consequence of external loads which tend to rotate it, either as a whole or of one of its regions relative to another.

Mucin: A basic molecule of the synovial fluid, and represents chondroitin sulfate molecules attached to a protein backbone and looking very like a test tube bristle brush. Some degree of polymerization of these basic mers can and usually does occur.

Mucopolysaccharide: This signifies one of the biological gels, of which a group exist. Chemically one usually finds the same specific kinds in a particular type of tissue, and they usually embed or surround collagen and sometimes other fibrillar material, probably by some type of chemical bonding force.

Newton: This equals 9.8 joules, i.e., a measure of work equal to that in lifting one kg a distance of one meter against the earth's gravitational pull.

Newtonian fluid: The shearing stress or resistance to fluid motion increases in direct proportion to the speed of the motion of one lamina of the fluid relative to another.

Notch effect: The ability of small notches or cracks in the surfaces of structures or machine parts to cause stress concentrations at their roots which, by exceeding in the minute local region the material's strength, can initiate a crack which will gradually propagate through the material until it finally fails in fatigue.

Ordinate: This signifies the horizontal line of the Cartesian coordinates.

Osteoblast: A cell which manufactures new bone—discussed at some length in Volumes II, III and IV.

Osteoclast: A cell which can solubilize both the organic and inorganic phases of bone. Discussed at some length in Volumes II, III and IV.

Osteon: A synonym for a secondary haversian system. We need not worry about primary haversian systems in this book.

Photoelasticity: A method of measuring strain in birefringent plastics in order to infer the distribution of stresses within plastic models of some structure or some mechanical arrangement.

Plasticity: The ability of solid matter to flow under an applied load, and representing a semi-fluid type of behavior.

Poisson's ratio: The reduction in diameter of a test sample divided by its elongation per unit length at the stress level of fracture in tension.

Polymer: A material composed of chemical molecular units called mers, which assemble end-to-end and/or side-to-side, in order to build up long chains or felt works which can have mechanical and physical properties totally different from those of solutions of the basic mer.

Potential: A difference in voltage, or a difference between two potential energy states.

Potential energy: The amount of energy temporarily stored within a system but which it can release as kinetic energy under proper conditions. Lifting a pound three feet above the floor represents the process of expending three foot-pounds of kinetic energy. Once the pound has reached its three foot level and one holds it there, it then has three foot pounds of potential energy, and if one then releases it this again converts to kinetic energy, this time of the negative sense mathematically.

Pound: The unit of mass in the English system of units.

Pound force: That amount of force exerted by the earth's gravitational pull upon a mass of one pound.

Poundal: That force which when acting upon a mass of one pound will give it an acceleration of one foot per second after a duration of one second.

Power: The rate at which one expends work. It remains independent of the total amount of work spent.

Pressure: In the mechanics of fluids, that compression force acting equally in all directions within a fluid.

Proportional limit: That point upon the stress/strain curve of some material within which its deformation remains proportional to stress; in other words, this term remains synonymous with the term "Hookean limit".

Pseudarthrosis: A failure of bone healing leading to a false joint.

Quenching: The process of rapidly cooling a hot metal in order to freeze into it a crystalline and/or chemical phase which at room temperature will possess desirable mechanical properties, but whch under conditions of slow cooling would automatically convert to another more stable state in the thermodynamic sense at room temperature, but a less desirable one in the mechanical sense.

Reaction: In mechanics a force acting upon a structure which, as a "reaction" to other direct forces acting upon it, establishes the condition of mechanical equilibrium.

Remodeling: In these texts, specifically used in the limited sense of a BMU-based kind of bone turnover, which has the effect of renewing the material in a tissue without producing any great changes in its architecture or total amount. This word has varied meanings beyond these five volumes. Some (including most biochemists) use it to designate all growth, modeling, remodeling and repair phenomena which can cause turnover of any skeletal tissue. Others (including most embryologists and anatomists) use it to signify growth and modeling phenomena primarily.

Resilience: The ability of a material to return as mechanical work all of the mechanical work done in deforming it. Any loss occurring during the process represents damping, or as engineers sometimes call it, "hysteresis".

Resistor: An electronic component which resists the flow of direct current.

Resultant: When two or more forces act upon a single solid body it moves in response to them as though under the pressure of a single force representing some combination of them. That single force has become termed the resultant.

Rigidity: The capacity of a material to maintain its dimensions in compression, tension, or shear under some applied external force, even if only very small. Note that a composite material can possess rigidity in tension and yet in essence lack it in compression and shear, as, for example, one finds in tendon and ligaments. Or it can possess rigidity in both compression and tension but lack it totally in shear, which characterizes the liquid state of matter. Or it can remain rigid in all three, which characterizes the solid state of matter. Thus rigidity in this text means a different thing than stiffness.

Scalar: A number or parameter which contains only one dimension, usually and throughout this book, that of magnitude. In this book as in other textbooks of elementary mechanics, a vectorial quantity is sometimes defined as one which has direction. But rigorously speaking, in good mathematics direction alone also represents a scalar property, and a vectorial property represents any which requires two or more numbers or terms to specify.

Second order: A second order function represents one provided within the system to subserve the needs of a more directly important first order function. Because in biomechanical physiology we have not yet identified all of the functions of the body, or even thought too much about the first, second, third, and higher order structures of such functions, our knowledge of such matters at the moment remains elementary.

Sharpey's fibers: Fibers of collagen running into bone, and thereby attaching to it tension loading structures such as ligament, tendon, fascia, muscle and joint capsule.

Shear: As a motion this represents sliding of one object upon another. As a stress, it represents the resistance of the intermolecular bonds of the materials to such motion.

Sigma: This represents a temporal property of any dynamic system, and its particular value for such systems specifies the amount of time required for its transients to disappear following a challenge, and for its steady state response thereto to appear. Extensively discussed in Volume III of this series.

Simple tissue: One of the elementary tissue building blocks or letters of the skeletal alphabet, outlined at some length in Volume II of this series.

Spongy bone: The trabecular or cancellous bone found within the ends of most long bones, and left behind as a result of longitudinal growth processes.

Static bending: In ordinary mechanics this constitutes the bending arrangement seen in Figure 11.10, and implies that the beam exists in dynamic equilibrium. But in the flexure-drift law this term specifies a mechanical arrangement for inducing bending moments within a bone, an arrangement which can and practically invariably does coexist with dynamic forces of various kinds acting on the bone.

Stiffness: The amount of resistance to mechanical deformation which characterizes a given material. Young's modulus expresses the property. It does not mean the same thing in this book as rigidity.

Strain: The deformation of matter under an applied external load. Strain may occur in the gaseous, liquid, and solid states of matter.

Strain energy: The amount of mechanical work put into a material in deforming it.

Strain hardening: The property of some metals and plastics of becoming harder and usually more rigid in shear, following straining or mechanical working. Sometimes a desirable property deliberately produced at the end of a manufacturing stage, and sometimes an undesirable one which one can often correct by annealing the material, provided the annealing temperature does not harm other more important characteristics of the material.

Stress: The intermolecular resistance of a material to deformation or strain.

Stress riser: The property of any surface notch or crevice, of locally concentrating stresses above the ultimate or yield strength of the material, so that a crack can commence which can ultimately lead to a fatigue failure.

Stresscoat: A brittle lacquer which cracks upon a minimum amount of tensile deformation, and which when sprayed upon the surfaces of some structure, will reveal by its patterns of cracks, the distribution of tensile strain in the material. Useful as a means of evaluating the behavior of structures under load, and in trying to design more durable structures.

Subchondral bone: That bone lying immediately beneath and supporting mechanically the articular cartilage of a joint.

Synovia: The soft tissue lining of a joint which creates of it a closed cavity within which the sliding articular surfaces move and which contains the usually small amount of synovial fluid contents.

Synovial fluid: The water-based lubricant of animal joints.

System: Any construct or machine containing two or more interrelated parts.

Tempering: Heat treating previously heated and then quenched steel, in order to reduce the great hardness and brittleness of the martensite phase, and to add to the material's toughness.

Tendon: An anatomical structure made largely of collagen with some hyaluronic acid embedding it, which serves to transmit tension loads from a muscle to some other anatomical structure, usually a bone.

Tendon transfer: An operation in which one moves the insertion of a tendon to some new location.

Tension: A pulling apart.

Thixotropy: The optical property of a material in which in the unstrained condition it does not exhibit birefringence but during strain or flow it does become birefringent.

Tibia: The shin bone which bears almost all of one's weight during standing, walking and running.

Torque: A twist.

Toughness: The ability of a material to withstand impact or, equally, the ability of a material to absorb a great deal of energy before fracturing.

Trabecular bone: Synonymous with spongy bone.

Triple arthrodesis: Arthrodesis of the articulations of the talus with the major foot bones.

Uniaxial: When speaking of mechanical loads this signifies a compression or tension load very accurately centered over the neutral axis or neutral plane of a material and very accurately aligned parallel to it. A laboratory ideal seldom if ever actually realized.

Unit strain: That manner of specifying the strain of a material in terms of the fundamental units of measurement, rather than in terms of the total deviation of an intact structure.

Unit stress: Specifying the stress within a material as the amount per unit of cross section area, rather than as the total stress within the intact structure.

van der Waal's forces: Those weak forces between molecules which arise when geographic asymmetry of the centers of their positive and negative charges causes one end of the molecule to remain slightly positive with respect to the other. Thus the more positive end of one molecule can become attracted to the more negative end of an adjacent one. A much weaker bonding force than the ionic, covalent and metallic bonds.

Vector: In mechanics this represents a parameter specified by three terms: the magnitude of the force or load, the orientation of this line of action in three dimensional space, and the directional sense on that line of action along which the load or the stress acts. Most books simply combine the orientation and directionality terms into a single one called the line of action.

Vectorial quantity: In this book, a parameter which contains a statement both of magnitude and of direction, as just noted.

Viscoelasticity: The ability seen in many plastics or other materials to deform rather slowly and in a non-linear manner following the application of a load but yet, following deloading, to return to the original shape and dimension, although again slowly and in a non-linear manner.

Viscosity: This signifies the resistance of fluids to flow or to shearing motion. Often called fluid friction, it implies force acting over a distance converting mechanical work into equivalent amounts of heat. In the bearings of rapidly moving machine parts that heat can attain values high enough to destroy the chemical and physical properties of the lubricant as well as of the machine, were provisions not made to dissipate the heat by some cooling device or radiator.

Volt: A unit of electrical potential or pressure, and representing that pressure required to drive one ampere of current through a resistance of one ohm.

Weight: This represents the force of the earth's attraction or pull upon an object.

Work: A force acting over a distance, or the equivalent. Thus one ampere flowing for a finite period of time against a finite resistance constitutes electrical work.

Chlorophyl uses photons from the sun to perform the chemical work that synthesizes cellulose out of atmospheric carbon dioxide and oxygen, while the amount of heat required to raise a given mass of water from the freezing to the boiling point represents also a definite calorimetric equivalent of mechanical work.

Work hardening: See strain hardening.

Woven bone: See fibrous bone.

Yield strength: That point upon the stress/strain curve at which the material begins to flow plastically.

References

1) Aegerter, E., and Kirkpatrick, J. A.: *Orthopaedic Diseases,* 2nd ed., Philadelphia, W. B. Saunders Co., 1962.
2) Adams, R. D., Denny-Brown, D., and Pearson, C. M.: *Diseases of Muscle,* 2nd ed. New York, Harper Brothers, 1962.
3) Agna, J. W., Knowles, H. C., and Alverson, G.: The mineral content of normal human bone. *J Clin Invest, 37:* 1357, 1958.
4) *American Institute of Physics Handbook* (Ed.) : Gray, D. E., New York, McGraw-Hill Book Co., Inc. 1957.
5) Amprino, R.: Microhardness testing as a means of analysis of bone tissue biophysical properties; in: *Biomechanical and Biophysical Studies of the Musculoskeletal System.* Springfield, Ill., Charles C Thomas, 1961, p. 20.
6) Amprino, R., and Marotti, G.: A topographic quantitative study of bone formation and reconstruction. In *Bone and Tooth Symposium.* (ed.) : Blackwood, H. J., New York, Macmillan Co., 1964, p. 21.
7) Anderson, W. A. D.: *Pathology*; 4th ed. St. Louis, C. V. Mosby Co., 1961.
8) Anderson, D. R.: The ultrastructure of elastic and hyaline cartilage in the rat. *Am J Anat, 114:* 403, 1964.
9) Armelagos, G. J.: Disease in ancient Nubia. *Science, 163:* 255, 1969.
10) Armstrong, W. D., and Singer, L.: Composition and constitution of the mineral phase of bone. *Clin Orthop, 38:* 179, 1965.
11) Arnold, J. S., Bartley, M. H., Tont, S. A., and Jenkins, D. P.: Skeletal changes in aging and disease. *Clin Orthop, 49:* 17, 1966.
12) Arnold, J. S.: The quantitation of bone mineralization as an organ and tissue in osteoporosis. In *Dynamic Studies of Metabolic Bone Disease,* Philadelphia, F. A. Davis, 1964, p. 59.
13) Arnold, J. S., Frost, H. M., and Buss, R. O.: The Osteocyte as a bone pump. *Clin Orthop, 78:* 47, 1971.
14) Arnold, J. S.: Quantitation of mineralization of bone as an organ and tissue in osteoporosis. *Clin Orthop, 17:* 167, 1960.
15) Arnold, J. S., and Jee, W. S. S.: Bone growth and osteoclastic activity as indicated by radioautographic distribution of plutonium. *Am J Anat, 101:* 367, 1957.
16) Ascenzi, A., and Bonucci, E.: A quantitative investigation of the birefringence of the osteon. *Acta Anat, 44:* 236, 1961.
17) Ascenzi, A., and Bonucci, E. A.: The ultimate tensile strength of single osteons. *Acta Anat, 58:* 160, 1964.

621

18) Ascenzi, A.: Etude du tissu osseux par la microscopie électronique. *L'Osteoporose*. Paris, Masson and Co., 1964, p. 42.

19) Ashby, W. R.: *An Introduction to Cybernetics*. New York, John Wiley and Sons, 1963.

20) Avis, V.: The significance of the angle of the mandible: An experimental and comparative study. *Am J Phys Anthrop, 1:* 55, 1961.

21) Baer, M. J.: Patterns of growth of the skull as revealed by vital staining. *Human Biol, 26:* 80, 1964.

22) Bailey, J. A.: Forms of dwarfism recognizeable at birth. *Clin Orthop, 76:* 150, 1971.

23) Barnett, C. H., Davis, D. V., and MacConaill, M. A.: *Synovial Joints: Their Structure and Mechanics*. Springfield, Ill., Charles C Thomas, 1961.

24) Bartel, D. L., and Johnston, R. C.: Mechanical analysis and optimization of a cup arthroplasty. *J Biomech, 2:* 97, 1969.

25) Bartley, M., Arnold, J. S., Haslam, R. K., and Jee, W. S. S.: Relationship between bone strength and bone quantity in health, disease and aging. *J Gerontol, 21:* 517, 1966.

26) Bassett, C. A. L., and Becker, R. O.: Generation of electric potentials by bone responding to mechanical stress. *Science, 137:* 1063, 1962.

27) Bassett, C. A. L.: Biological significance of piezoelectricity. *Calcif Tiss Res, 1:* 252, 1968.

28) Bechtol, C. O., Ferguson, A. B., and Laing, P. G.: *Metals and Engineering in Bone and Joint Surgery*. Baltimore, Williams and Wilkins Co., 1959.

29) Becker, R. O., Bassett, C. A., and Bachman, C. H.: Bioelectrical factors controlling bone structure. In *Bone Biodynamics*. Boston, Little-Brown and Co., 1964, p. 209.

30) Benninghoff, A.: Spaltinien am knochen, eine methods zur Ermittlung der Architektur platter Knochen. *Verh Anat Ges Suppl, 60:* 189, 1925.

31) Best, C. H., and Taylor, N. B.: *The Physiological Basis of Medical Practice*, 7th ed. Baltimore, Williams and Wilkins Co., 1961.

32) Blaimont, P.: Contribution a l'etude biomécanique du femur humain. *Acta Orthop Belg, 34:* 675, 1968.

33) Block, B., and Dintenfass, L.: Rheological study of human synovial fluid. *Aust N Z J Surg, 33:* 108, 1963.

34) *Bone and Tooth Symposium*, Blackwood, H. J. J. (Ed.). New York, Macmillan Co., 1964.

35) *Bone As a Tissue*, K. Rodahl, Nicholson J. T., and Brown, E. M. Jr., (Eds.). New York, Blakiston Div., McGraw-Hill Book Co., Inc. 1960.

36) *Bone Biodynamics*, Frost, H. M., (Ed.) Boston, Little-Brown and Co., 1964.

37) Bowden, F. P., and Tabor, D.: *Friction and Lubrication*. New York, John Wiley and Sons, Inc., 1956.
38) Boyes, J. H.: *Bunnell's Surgery of The Hand*, 4th ed. Philadelphia, J. B. Lippincott Co., 1964.
39) Brady, G. S.: *Materials Handbook*, 9th ed. New York, McGraw-Hill Book Co., 1963.
40) Bromley, R. G., Dockum, N. L., Arnold, J. S., and Jee, W. S. S.: Quantitative histological study of human lumbar vertebrae. *J Gerontol, 21:* 537, 1966.
41) Browman, G. E., Trotter, M., and Peterson, R. R.: The density of selected bones of the human skeleton. *Am J Phys Anthrop, 16:* 197, 1958.
42) Burdi, A. R., and Faist, K.: Morphogenesis of the palate in normal human embryos, with special emphasis on the mechanisms involved. *Am J Anat, 120:* 149, 1967.
43) Bures, M. F., and Wuehrmann, A. H.: Bone remodeling dynamics following local x-irradiation. *J Dent Res, 48:* 376, 1969.
44) Burstein, A. H., Currey, J. D., Frankel, V. H., and Reilly, D. T.: The ultimate properties of bone tissue. *J Biomech, 5:* 35, 1972.
45) *Calcification in Biological Systems,* Sognnaes, R. F., (Ed.) Washington, AAA Science, 1960.
46) Caniggia, A., Stuart, C., and Guideri, R.: Fragilitas Ossium hereditaria tarda. *Acta Med Scand, 162:* 1, 1958.
47) Cantarow, A., and Schepartz, B.: *Biochemistry,* 2nd ed. Philadelphia, W. B. Saunders Co., 1957.
48) Carlstrom, D.: Microhardness measurements on single haversian systems in bone. *Experientia, 10:* 171, 1954.
49) Casagrande, P. A., and Frost, H. M.: *Clinical Fundamentals of Orthopaedics.* New York, Grune and Stratton, 1953.
50) Colletti, J. M., Akeson, W. H., and Woo, S. L.: A comparison of the physical behavior of normal articular cartilage and the arthroplasty surface. *J Bone Joint Surg, 54A:* 147, 1972.
51) Conrad, J. A., and Frost, H. M.: Evaluation of subcutaneous heel cord lengthening. *Clin Orthop, 64:* 121, 1969.
52) Cottrell, A. H.: *Theoretical Structural Metallurgy,* 2nd ed. London, Edward Arnold, 1955.
53) Crenshaw, A. H.: *Campbell's Operative Orthopaedics,* 4th ed. St. Louis, C. V. Mosby Co., 1963.
54) Currey, J. D.: The adaptations of bones to stress. *J Theor Biol, 20:* 91, 1968.
55) Dempster, W. T.: Free-Body diagrams as an approach to the mechanics of human posture and locomotion. In *Biomechanical and Biophysical Studies of the Musculoskeletal System.* Springfield, Ill., Charles C Thomas, 1961, p. 81.

56) Dempster, W. T., and Liddicoat, R. T.: Compact bone as a non-isotropic material. *Am J Anat, 91:* 331, 1952.

57) Dintenfass, L.: Lubrication in synovial joints: a theoretical analysis. *J Bone Joint Surg, 45A:* 1241, 1963.

58) Donisch, E. W., and Trapp, W.: The cartilage endplates of the human vertebral column. *Anat Rec, 169:* 705, 1971.

59) Duncan, H.: Paget's disease of bone (osteitis deformans). *Tice's Practice of Medicine.* Maryland, Harper Row, 1969, Vol. 5, Chap. 54.

60) Duncan, H., and Jaworski, Z. F.: Osteoporosis. *Tice's Practice of Medicine.* Maryland, Harper Row, 1970, Vol. 5, Chap. 52.

61) Eastoe, J. E., and Eastoe, B.: The organic constituents of mammalian compact bone. *Biochem J, 57:* 453, 1954.

62) Eisberg, R. M.: *Fundamentals of Modern Physics.* New York, John Wiley and Sons, Inc., 1961.

63) Enlow, D. H., and Brown, S. O.: A comparative histological study of fossil and recent bone tissues. *Tex J Sci, 10:* 187, 1958.

64) Enlow, D. H.: A study of the postnatal growth and remodeling of bone. *Am J Anat, 110:* 475, 1962.

65) Enlow, D. H.: Functions of the Haversian system. *Am J Anat, 110:* 269, 1962.

66) Enlow, D. H.: *Principles of Bone Remodeling.* Springfield, Ill., Charles C Thomas, 1963.

67) Enlow, D. H.: Wolff's law and the factor of architectonic circumstance. *Am J Orthod, 54:* 803, 1968.

68) Epker, B. N., and Frost, H. M.: Correlation of patterns of bone resorption and formation with physical behavior of loaded bone. *J Dent Res, 44:* 33, 1965.

69) Epker, B. N., and Frost, H. M.: The direction of transverse drift of actively forming osteons in human rib cortex. *J Bone Joint Surg, 47A:* 1211, 1965.

70) Eshback, O. W.: *Handbook of Engineering Fundamentals,* 2nd ed. New York, John Wiley and Sons, Inc., 1952.

71) Evans, F. G.: *Stress and Strain in Bones.* Springfield, Ill., Charles C Thomas, 1957.

72) Evans, F. G.: *Biomechanical Studies of the Musculoskeletal System.* Springfield, Ill., Charles C Thomas, 1961.

73) Evans, F. G., and King, A. I.: Regional differences in some physical properties of human spongy bone. In *Biomechanical and Biophysical Studies of the Musculoskeletal System.* Springfield, Ill., Charles C Thomas, 1961, p. 49.

74) Ferguson, A. B.: *Orthopaedic Surgery in Infancy and Childhood,* 3rd ed. Baltimore, Williams and Wilkins Co., 1968.

75) Firschein, H. E.: Collagen and mineral dynamics in bone. *Clin Orthop, 66:* 212, 1969.

76) Fleming, J. L.: *Polio Lectures*. Henry Ford Hospital, 1960–1964.

77) Frame, B., and Smith, R. W.: Phosphate diabetes: a case study of osteomalacia. *Am J Med, 25:* 771, 1958.

78) Frame, B., Arnstein, A. R., Frost, H. M., and Smith, R. W.: Resistant osteomalacia. *Am J Med, 38:* 145, 1964.

79) Frankel, J. P.: *Principles of the Properties of Materials*. New York, McGraw-Hill Book Co., Inc., 1957.

80) Frankel, V. H., and Burstein, A. H.: *Orthopaedic Biomechanics*. Philadelphia, Lea & Febiger, 1970.

81) Frankel, V. H.: Biomechanics of the knee. *Orth Clin N Am, 2:* 175, 1971.

82) Friedenberg, Z. B., and Brighton, C. T.: Bioelectric potentials in bone. *J Bone Joint Surg, 48A:* 915, 1966.

83) Frost, H. M.: Introduction to joint biomechanics. *Henry Ford Hosp Med Bull, 8:* 415, 1960.

84) ———: Micropetrosis. *J Bone Joint Surg, 42A:* 144, 1960.

85) ———: Observations on fibrous and lamellar bone. *Henry Ford Hosp Med Bull, 8:* 199, 1960.

86) ———: Presence of microscopic cracks *in vivo* in bone. *Henry Ford Hosp Med Bull, 8:* 25, 1960.

87) ———: Observations on the fundamental nature of otosclerosis. In *Otosclerosis*. Boston, Little-Brown and Co., 1962, p. 43.

88) ———: Measurement of bone formation by means of tetracycline labeling. *Can J Biochem Physiol, 41:* 31, 1963.

89) ———: *Bone Remodelling Dynamics*. Springfield, Ill., Charles C Thomas, 1963.

90) ———: *Mathematical Elements of Lamellar Bone Remodeling*. Springfield, Ill., Charles C Thomas, 1964.

91) ———: The etiodynamics of aseptic necrosis of the femoral head. In *Proceedings Conference on Aseptic Necrosis of the Femoral Head*, Surgery Study Section, N.I.H., 1964, p. 383.

92) ———: *The Laws of Bone Structure*. Springfield, Ill., Charles C Thomas, 1964.

93) ———: The dynamics of bone remodeling. In *Bone Biodynamics*. Boston, Little-Brown and Co., 1964, p. 315.

94) ———: *Introduction to Biomechanics*. Springfield, Ill., Charles C Thomas, 1966.

95) ———: *Bone Dynamics in Osteoporosis and Osteomalacia*. Springfield, Ill., Charles C Thomas, 1966.

96) ———: *Orthopaedic Lecture Series. Orthopaedic Surgery in Spasticity*. Springfield, Ill., Charles C Thomas, 1972, vol. I.

97) ———: *Orthopaedic Lecture Series*. Springfield, Ill., Charles C Thomas, 1972, vol. II.

98) ———: *Orthopaedic Lecture Series*. Springfield, Ill., Charles C Thomas, 1973, vol. III.

99) ———: *Orthopaedic Lectures.* Springfield, Ill., Charles C Thomas, 1973, vol. IV.

100) ———: Tetracycline-based histological analysis of bone remodeling. *Calcif Tiss Res, 3:* 211, 1969.

101) ———: Form and function. In *Craniofacial Growth in Man.* R. E. Moyers and W. M. Krogman, (Eds.), New York, Pergamon Press, 1971. p. 252.

102) Frost, H. M., and Guise, E. R.: A replacement prosthesis for the hip. *Henry Ford Hosp Med J, 19:* 3, 1971.

103) Frost, H. M.: Unpublished observations.

104) Frost, H. M., Roth, H., and Villanueva, A. R.: Physical characteristics of bone IV: Microscopic prefailure and failure patterns. *Henry Ford Hosp Med Bull, 9:* 163, 1961.

105) Fukada, E., and Yasuda, I.: On the piezoelectric effect of bone. *J Phys Soc Jap, 12:* 1158, 1957.

106) Galante, J. O.: Tensile properties of the human lumbar annulus fibrosus. *Acta Orthop Scand Suppl, 100:* 1, 1967.

107) Garn, S. M.: *The Earlier Gain and The Later Loss of Cortical Bone.* Springfield, Ill., Charles C Thomas, 1970.

108) Gendreau, C. L.: Osteogenesis of the capital femoral epiphysis of the dog. (thesis). Univ. Guelph, Ontario, 1, 1970.

109) Gillis, L., (Ed.): *Modern Trends in Surgical Materials.* London, Butterworth and Co., Ltd., 1958.

110) Glimcher, M. J.: Specificity of the molecular structure of organic matrices in mineralization. In *Calcification in Biological Systems.* Washington, AAA Science, 1960.

111) Goldman, J. E.: *The Science of Engineering Materials.* New York, John Wiley and Sons, Inc., 1957.

112) Gong, J. K., Arnold, J. S., and Cohn, S. H.: The density of organic and volatile and nonvolatile inorganic components of bone. *Anat Rec, 149:* 319, 1964.

113) ———: Composition of trabecular and cortical bone. *Anat Rec, 149:* 325, 1964.

114) Goss, C. M.: *Gray's Anatomy of the Human Body,* 27th ed. Philadelphia, Lea and Febiger, 1959.

115) Goss, R. J.: Hypertrophy vs. hyperplasia. *Science, 153:* 1615, 1966.

116) Greenwald, A. S., and O'Connor, J. J.: The transmission of load through the human hip joints. *J Biomech, 4:* 507, 1971.

117) Haack, D. C., and Weinstein, S.: Geometry and mechanics and relative tooth movement studied by a two dimensional model. *J Am Dent Assoc, 66:* 158, 1963.

118) Haas, H. G., Muller, J., and Schenk, R. K.: Osteomalacia: Metabolic and quantitative histologic studies. *Clin Orthop, 53:* 213, 1967.

119) Haines, R. W., and Mohiuddin, A.: *Handbook of Human Embryology.* Baltimore, Williams and Wilkins Co., 1965.

120) Hall, B. K.: Histogenesis and morphogenesis of bone. *Clin Orthop, 74:* 249, 1971.

121) Hall, M. C.: *The Locomotor System: Functional Anatomy.* Springfield, Ill., Charles C Thomas, 1965.

122) Ham, A. W., and Leeson, T. S.: *Histology,* 4th ed. Philadelphia, J. B. Lippincott Co., 1961.

123) *Handbook of Chemistry and Physics.* Cleveland, Chemical Rubber Publ. Co., 1965.

124) Hanson, C. A., Sagrin, J. W., and Duncan, H.: The osteoporosis of ankylosing spondylitis. *Clin Orthop, 74:* 59, 1971.

125) Harris, W. H., and Heaney, R. P.: *Skeletal Renewal and Metabolic Bone Disease.* Boston, Little, Brown and Co., 1969.

126) Hicks, J. H.: The function of the plantar aponeurosis. *J Anat, 85:* 414, 1957.

127) Hattner, R., Epker, B. N., and Frost, H. M.: Suggested sequential mode of control of changes in cell behavior in adult bone remodeling. *Nature, 206:* 489, 1965.

128) Hert, J.: Regulace Rusto dlouhych kosti do delky. *Plezsky Lekarsky Sbornik, Suppl, 12:* 12, 1964.

129) Hirsch, C., and Schajowicz, F.: Studies on structural changes in the lumbar annulus fibrosus. *Acta Orthop Scand, 22:* 184, 1952.

130) Hirsch, C.: Personal communication. 1964.

131) Hitt, O., Jaworski, Z. F., Shimizu, A. G., and Frost, H. M.: Tissue-level bone formation rates in chronic renal failure, measured by means of tetracycline bone labeling. *Can J Physiol Pharmacol, 48:* 824, 1970.

132) Hunter, C. J.: The correlation of facial growth with body height and skeletal maturation at adolescence. *Angle Orthodont, 36:* 44, 1966.

133) Huddleston, J. V.: *Introduction to Engineering Mechanics.* Reading, Addison-Wesley Publ. Co., Inc., 1961.

134) Hurxthal, L. M., Dotter, W., Baylink, D. J., and Clerkin, E. P.: Two new methods for the study of osteoporosis and other metabolic bone disease. *Lahey Clin Bull, 13:* 155, 1964.

135) Huxley, H. E., and Hanson, J.: The molecular basis of contraction in cross striated muscles. In *Structure and Function of Muscle.* New York, Academic Press, 1960.

136) Ingelmark, B. E.: Functionally induced changes in articular cartilage. In *Biomechanical Studies of the Musculoskeletal System.* 1961, p. 3.

137) Inman, V. T.: Functional aspects of the abductor muscles of the hip. *J Bone Joint Surg, 29:* 607, 1947.

138) Jacqueline, F., and Rutishauser, E.: Idiopathic necrosis of the femoral head. In Zinn, W. M. (Ed.): *Idiopathic Ischemic Necrosis of the Femoral Head in Adults.* 1971, p. 34.

139) Jaffe, H. L.: *Tumors and Tumorous Conditions of Bones and Joints.* Philadelphia, Lea and Febiger, 1958.

140) Jarcho, S.: *Human Paleopathology.* New Haven, Yale Univ Press, 1966.

141) Jee, W. S. S.: The influence of reduced vasecularity on the rate of internal reconstruction in adult long bone cortex. In *Bone Biodynamics.* Boston, Little-Brown and Co., 1964, p. 259.

142) Jee, W. S. S., and Arnold, J. S.: Haversian system growth and formation in rabbits. *Anat Rec, 115:* 276, 1953.

143) ———: Rate of individual haversian system formation. *Anat Rec, 118:* 315, 1954.

144) ———: The toxicity of plutonium deposited in skeletal tissue of beagles. *Lab Invest, 10:* 797, 1961.

145) Jessop, H. T., and Harris, F. C.: *Photoelasticity.* New York, Dover Publications, 1949.

146) Johnson, L. C.: Joint remodeling as the basis for osteoarthritis. *J Am Vet Med Assoc, 141:* 1237, 1962.

147) ———: Morphologic analysis in pathology: The kinetics of disease and general biology of bone. In *Bone Biodynamics.* Boston, Little-Brown and Co., 1964, p. 543.

148) ———: Bone density and the relation of structure to function. In *Proc. Conf. on Aseptic Necrosis of The Femoral Head.* Surgery Study Section, N.I.H., 1964, p. 25.

149) ———: Genetics and growth. In Moyers, R. E. and Krogman, W. M. (Eds.): *Craniofacial Growth in Man.* New York, Pergamon Press, 1971, pp. 258–283.

150) Johnston, F. E., and Malina, R. M.: Age changes in the composition of the upper arm. *Pa Children Human Bull,* 38, 1966.

151) ———: Correlations of midshaft breadths and compact bone thickness among bones of the upper and lower extremities in children aged 6 to 16 years. *Am J Phys Anthrop, 32:* 323, 1970.

152) Karpovich, P. V.: *The Physiology of Muscular Activity,* 5th ed. Philadelphia, W. B. Saunders Co., 1959.

153) Katake, K.: The strength for tension and bursting of human fasciae. *J Kyoto Pref Med Univ, 69:* 484, 1961.

154) Kendrick, G. S., and Risinger, H. L.: Changes in the antero posterior dimension of the human male skull during the 3rd and 4th decade of life. *Anat Rec, 159:* 77, 1967.

155) Kempson, G. E., Spivey, C. J., Swanson, S. A. V., and Freeman, M. A. R.: Patterns of cartilage stiffness on human femoral heads. *J Biomech, 4:* 597, 1971.

156) Kimura, H.: On the mechanical properties of the compact bone of a horse. *J Kyoto Pref Med Univ, 51:* 447, 1952.

157) Klein, L., Vessely, J. C., and Heiple, K. G.: Quantification of 3H collagen loss of rat allografted and isografted tendon. *J Bone Joint Surg, 51A:* 891, 1963.

158) Koch, J. L.: The laws of bone architecture. *Amer J Anat, 21:* 177, 1917.

159) Kolav, J., Babicky, A., and Vrabec, R.: *The Physical Agents and Bone.* Prague, The Publ. House of the Czechoslovak Acad. of Sciences, 1965.

160) Knese, K. H., Hahne, O. H., and Bierman, H.: Festig keitsuntersuchungen an menschlichen Extremit a tenknochen. *Morph Jahrbuch, 96:* 141, 1954.

161) Krogman, W. M.: *The Human Skeleton in Forensic Medicine.* Springfield, Ill., Charles C Thomas, 1962.

162) Kubo, K.: Study on the abraision test of human hard tissues. *J Jap Stomatol Soc, 8:* 497, 1959.

163) Kummer, B.: Principles of the biomechanics of the human supportive and locomotor system. In Proceedings of the Ninth Congress, International Society of Surgery, Orthopaedics and Trauma, *2:* 60, 1963.

164) Kuntscher, G.: Die Bedeutung der Darstellung des draftflusses in knochen fur die Chirurgie. *Arch Klin Chir, 182:* 489, 1935.

165) Kuruma, R.: Studies on the impulsive bending test upon the compact bone. *J Kyoto Pref Med Univ, 59:* 21, 1956.

166) Lacroix, P.: *The Organization of Bones.* London, Churchill, 1951.

167) Lagier, R.: Idiopathic aseptic necrosis of the femoral head. In *Idiopathic Ischemic Necrosis of the Femoral Head in Adults.* W. M. Zinn, (Ed.), Stuttgart, George Thieme, 1971, p. 49.

168) Laing, P. G.: The significance of metallic transfer in the corrosion of orthopaedic screws. *J Bone Joint Surg, 40A:* 853, 1958.

169) Landeros, O., and Frost, H. M.: A cell system in which rate and amount of protein synthesis are separately controlled. *Science, 145:* 1323, 1964.

170) Ledley, R. S.: A computer model for bone growth. In *Craniofacial Growth in Man,* R. E. Moyers and W. M. Krogman, (Eds.), New York, Pergamon Press, 1971, p. 219.

171) Lee, W. R., Marshall, J. A., and Sissons, H. A.: Calcium accretion and bone formation in dogs. *J Bone Joint Surg, 47B:* 157, 1965.

172) Lee, B. W.: Relationship between tooth movement rate and estimated pressure applied. *J Dent Res, 44:* 1053, 1965.

173) Long, C.: *Biochemist's Handbook.* New York, D. Van Nostrand Co., 1961.

174) Long, R. R.: *Mechanics of Solids and Fluids.* Englewood Cliffs, Prentice-Hall, Inc., 1961.

175) Luck, J. V.: *Bone and Joint Diseases.* Springfield, Ill., Charles C Thomas, 1950.

176) Mankin, H. J., and Lippiello, L.: The turnover of adult rabbit articular cartilage. *J Bone Joint Surg, 51:* 862, 1969.

177) McLean, F. C., and Urist, M. R.: *Bone*. Chicago, University of Chicago Press, 1961.

178) McLean, W. G., and Nelson, E. W.: *Engineering Mechanics*. New York, Schaum Publishing Co., 1960.

179) Marotti, G.: Quantitative studies on bone reconstruction. *Acta Anat, 52:*291, 1963.

180) Matthews, L. S., and Hirsch, C.: Temperatures measured in human cortical bone when drilling. *J Bone Joint Surg, 54A:*297, 1972.

181) Martz, C. D.: Stress tolerance of bone and metal. *J Bone Joint Surg, 38A:*827, 1956.

182) Maximow, A. A., and Bloom, Wm.: *A Textbook of Histology*, 6th ed. Philadelphia, W. B. Saunders Co., 1955.

183) McElhaney, J. H.: The charge distribution on human femur due to load. *J Bone Joint Surg, 49A:*1561, 1967.

184) McMaster, J. H., and Weinert, C. R. Jr.: Effects of mechanical forces on growing cartilage. *Clin Orthop, 72:*308, 1970.

185) *Mechanisms of Hard Tissue Destruction;* R. F. Sognnaes, (Ed.) Washington, AAA Science, 1963.

186) Meema, H. E., and Schatz, D. L.: Simple radiologic demonstration of cortical bone loss in thyrotoxicosis. *Radiology, 97:*9, 1970.

187) Mendenhall, C. E., Eve, A. S., Keyes, D. A., and Sutton, R. M.: *College Physics;* 4th ed. Boston, D. C. Heath and Co., 1956.

188) Meunier, P., Vignon, G., and Vauzelle, J. L.: Methodes histologiques quantitatives en pathologie osseuse. *La Rev Lyonnaise de Med, 28:*133, 1969.

189) Meunier, P., Aaron, J., Edouard, C., and Vignon, G.: Osteoporosis and the replacement of cell populations of the marrow by adipose tissue. *Clin Orthop, 80:*147, 1971.

190) Meunier, P., Bernard, J., and Vignon, G.: The measurement of periosteocytic enlargement in primary and secondary hyperparathyroidism. *Isr J Med Sci, 7:*482, 1971.

191) Meunier, P.: Personal communication.

192) Milch, R. A., Rall, D. P., and Tobie, J. E.: Fluorescence of tetracycline antibiotics in bone. *J Bone Joint Surg, 40A:*897, 1958.

193) Millington, P. R., Gibson, T., Evans, J. H., and Barbenel, J. C.: Structural and mechanical aspects of connective tissue. In *Advances in Biomedical Engineering*. R. M. Kenedi, (Ed.) Academic Press, 1971, p. 189.

194) Miller, M. R., and Kashara, M.: Observations on the innervation of human long bones. *Anat Rec, 145:*13, 1963.

195) Moffett, B.: The morphogenesis of the temporomandibular joint. *Am J Orthod, 52:*401, 1966.

196) Moffett, B. C., Johnson, L. C., McCabe, J. B., and Askew, H. C.: Articular remodeling of the adult human temperomandibular joint. *Am J Anat, 115:*119, 1964.

197) Morris, J. M., Lucas, D. B., and Bresler, B.: Role of the trunk and stability of the spine. *J Bone Joint Surg, 43A:* 327, 1961.

198) Morris, J. M.: Biomechanical aspects of the hip joint. *Orthop Clin N Am, 2:* 33, 1971.

199) Moss, J. B.: *Properties of Engineering Materials.* Cleveland, C R C Press, 1971.

200) Moss, M. L.: Functional analysis of human mandibular growth. *J Prosthet Dent, 10,* 1960.

201) Moss, M. L., and Salentijn, L.: The primary role of functional matrices in facial growth. *Am J Orthod, 55:* 566, 1969.

202) Moyers, R. E., and Krogman, W. M.: *Craniofacial Growth in Man.* New York, Pergamon Press, 1971, p. 15.

203) Nachemson, A.: Some mechanical properties of the lumbar intervertebral disc. *Bull Hosp Joint Dis, 23:* 130, 1962.

204) Nachemson, A., and Morris, J. M.: *In vivo* measurements of intradiscal pressure. *J Bone Joint Surg, 46A:* 1077, 1964.

205) Nachemson, A.: The load on the lumbar disks in different positions of the body. *Clin Orthop, 45:* 107, 1966.

206) Nachemson, A., and Elfstrom, Gosta: Intravital dynamic pressure measurements in lumbar discs. *Scand J Rehab Med (Suppl. 1),* 5, 1970.

207) Nanda, S. K., Merow, H. W., and Sassouni, V.: Repositioning of the masseter muscle and its effect on skeletal form and function. *Angle Orthod, 37:* 304, 1967.

208) Nordin, B. E. C., Young, M. M., Bulosu, L., and Horsman, A.: Osteoporosis reexamined. In *Osteoporoses,* U. S. Barzel, (Ed.) New York, Grune and Stratton, 1970, p. 47.

209) Odegaard, J.: Growth of the mandible studied with the aid of metallic implants. *Am J Orthod, 57:* 145, 1970.

210) Olsen, G. A.: *Strength of Materials.* Englewood Cliffs, Prentice Hall, Inc., 1956.

211) Owen, M.: Cell population kinetics of an osteogenetic tissue. *J Cell Biol, 9:* 19, 1963.

212) Paul, J. P.: The effect of walking speed on the force actions transmitted at the hip and knee joints. *Proc R Soc Med, 63:* 200, 1970.

213) Pauwels, Fr.: The importance of biomechanics in orthopaedics. In Proceedings of the 9th Congress of the International Society of Surgery Orthopaedics and Trauma, Vienna 1, 1963.

214) Perry, H. T.: Relation of occlusion to temporomandibular joint dysfunction: the orthodontic viewpoint. *J. Am Dent. Assoc, 79:* 137, 1969.

215) Polanyi, M.: Life's irreducible structure. *Science, 160:* 1308, 1968.

216) Popov, E. P.: *Mechanics of Materials.* Englewood Cliffs, Prentice Hall, Inc., 1952.

217) Rasch, P. J., and Burke, R. K.: *Kinesiology and Applied Anatomy.* Philadelphia, Lea and Febiger, 1963.

218) Robinson, R. A.: An electron microscopic study of the crystalline inorganic component of bone and its relationship to the organic matrix. *J Bone Joint Surg, 34A:* 389, 1952.

219) Robinson, R. A., and Elliott, S. R.: The water content of bone. *J Bone Joint Surg, 38A:* 324, 1956.

220) Robinson, R. A.: Chemical analysis and electron microscopy of bone. In *Bone as a Tissue.* New York, McGraw-Hill Book Co., Blakiston Div., 1960, p. 196.

221) Rojkind, M., and Perez-Tamayo, R.: Studies on reabsorption of connective tissues. *Arch Pathol, 74:* 455, 1962.

222) Ropes, M. W., and Bauer, W.: *Synovial Fluid Changes in Joint Disease.* Cambridge, Harvard Univ Press, 1953.

223) Romer, A. S.: *Vertebrate Paleontology,* 3rd ed. Chicago, Univ. Chicago Press, 1966.

224) Roth, H., Frost, H. M., and Villanueva, A. R.: Physical characteristics of bone: In The Existence of Plastic Flow *in vitro. Henry Ford Hosp Med Bull, 9:* 149, 1961.

225) Rubin, P.: *Dynamic Classification of Bone Dysplasias.* Chicago, Year Book Publishers, Inc., 1964.

226) Rutishauser, E., and Majno, G.: Lesion osseuses par surcharge dans la squellette normal et pathologique. *Bull Schweiz Akad der Medic Wissenschaften, 5:* 333, 1950.

227) Rydell, N.: Forces acting on the femoral head-prosthesis. *Acta Orthop Scand Suppl,* 88, 1966.

228) Salter, R. B.: *Textbook of Disorders and Injuries of the Musculoskeletal System.* Baltimore, Williams and Wilkins Co., 1970.

229) Schaeffer, J. P.: *Morris' Human Anatomy,* 10th ed. Philadelphia, The Blakiston Co., 1942.

230) Schmid, F. R., and Ogata, R. I.: Synovial fluid evaluation in joint disease. In *Symposia for Orthopaedic Surgeons.* (Eds.) : M. A. Entin, E. F. Rosenberg, and H. G. Sofield, W. B. Saunders Co., 1965, p. 196.

231) Scott, J. H.: Muscle growth and function in relation to skeletal morphology. *Am J Phys Anthrop, 15:* 197, 1957.

232) Sedlin, E. D.: Uses of bone as a model system in the study of aging. In *Bone Biodynamics.* Boston, Little-Brown and Co., 1964, p. 655.

233) Segmuller, G., Cech, O., and Bekier, A.: Diagnostic use of strontium in the preoperative evaluation of nonunion. *Acta Orthop Scand, 41:* 150, 1970.

234) Sedlin, E. D., and Hirsch, C.: Factors affecting the determination of the physical properties of femoral cortical bone. *Acta Orthop Scand,* 1966.

235) Seliger, W. G.: Tissue fluid movement in compact bone. *Anat Rec, 166:* 247, 1970.

References 633

236) Selye, H.: *Stress*, Chicago, Univ. Chicago Press, 1963.
237) Semb, H.: Experimental limb disuse and bone blood flow. *Acta Orthop Scand, 40:* 552, 1969.
238) Shamos, M. H., and Lavine, L. S.: Physical basis for bioelectric effects in mineralized tissues. *Clin Orthop, 36:* 177, 1964.
239) Shannon, C. E., and Weaver, W.: *The Mathematical Theory of Communication.* Chicago, Univ. Illinois Press, 1963.
240) Shifrin, L. Z.: Correlation of serum alkaline phosphatase with bone formation rates. *Clin Orthop, 70:* 212, 1970.
241) ———: The lateral position for spine fusion and Harrington Instrumentation for scoliosis: a brief report. *Clin Orthop, 81:* 48, 1971.
242) ———: Recognizing scoliosis early. *Family Phys, 4:* 76, 1971.
243) ———: Giant cell tumor of bone. *Clin Orthop, 82:* 59, 1971.
244) ———: Personal communication.
245) Simmons, D. J., Simmons, N. B., and Marshall, J. H.: The uptake of calcium-45 in the acellular-boned toadfish. *Calc Tiss Res, 5:* 206, 1970.
246) Singer, F. L., Milch, H., and Milch, R. A.: Distribution of strain in paired human femurs. *Nature, 202:* 206, 1964.
247) Sissons, H. A.: Osteoporosis of Cushing's syndrome. In *Bone As A Tissue.* (Eds.) : K. Rodahl, J. T. Nicholson, and E. M. Brown Jr., New York, Blakiston Div., McGraw-Hill Book Co., 1960, p. 3.
248) Slaymaker, R. R.: *Bearing Lubrication Analysis.* New York, John Wiley and Sons, Inc., 1955.
249) Smith, R. W., Eyler, W. R., and Mellinger, R. C.: On the incidence of senile osteoporosis. *Ann Int Med, 52:* 773, 1960.
250) Smith, R. W., and Walker, R. R.: Femoral expansion in aging women: implications for osteoporosis and fractures. *Science, 145:* 150, 1964.
251) Smith, J. W.: The relationship of epiphyseal plates to stress in some bones of the lower limb. *J Anat (London), 90:* 58, 1970.
252) Soni, N. N.: Quantitative study of bone activity in alveolar and femoral bone of the guinea pig. *J Dent Res, 47:* 584, 1968.
253) Stanisavljevic, S.: *Diagnosis and Treatment of Congenital Hip Pathology in the Newborn.* Baltimore, Williams and Wilkins Co., 1964.
254) Stanisavljevic, S., and Mitchell, C. L.: An anatomical-pathological study of congenital hip dysplasia, subluxation and dislocation of the hip in stillborn and newborn infants. *J Bone Joint Surg, 54A:* 1147, 1963.
255) Steendjik, R.: Metabolic bone disease in children. *Clin Orthop, 77:* 247, 1971.
256) Stein, I., Stein, R. O., and Beller, M. L.: *Living Bone.* Philadelphia, J. B. Lippincott Co., 1955.
257) Stoker, N., and Epker, B. N.: Age changes in endosteal bone remodeling and balance in the rabbit. *J Dent Res, 50:* 1570, 1971.

258) Sutherland, D. H., Schottstaedt, E. R., Larsen, L. J., Ashley, R. K., Callander, J. N., and James, P. M.: Clinical and electromyographic study of seven spastic children with internal rotation gait. *J Bone Joint Surg, 51:* 1070, 1969.

259) Swanson, S. A. V.: Biomechanical characteristics of bone. In *Advances in Biomedical Engineering.* (Eds.) R. M. Kenedi, New York Academic Press, 1971, p. 137.

260) Takahashi, H., Epker, B. N., and Frost, H. M.: Resorption precedes formative activity. *Surg Forum, 15:* 437, 1964.

261) ———: The relation between age and size of osteons in man. *Henry Ford Hosp Med Bull, 13:* 25, 1965.

262) Takahashi, H., and Frost, H. M.: Age and sex related changes in the amount of cortex in normal human ribs. *Acta Orthop Scand, 37:* 122, 1966.

263) Takahashi, H., Ota, M., and Norimatsu, H.: A tetracycline based study of the linear rate of bone matrix mineralization in canine bone. *Acta Med et Biol, 18:* 269, 1971.

264) Talmage, R. V.: Calcium homeostasis—calcium transport—parathyroid action: the effects of parathyroid hormone on the movement of calcium between bone and fluid. *Clin Orthop, 67:* 211, 1969.

265) Tipei, N.: *Theory of Lubrication.* Stanford, Stanford Univ. Press, 1962.

266) Tonna, E. A.: The cellular complement of the skeletal system studied autoradiographically with tritiated thymidine during growth and aging. *J Biophys Biochem Cytol, 9:* 813, 1961.

267) Trotter, M., and Peterson, R. R.: Ash weight of human skeletons in per cent of their dry, fat free weight. *Anat Rec, 123:* 314, 1955.

268) Trueta, T.: The dynamics of bone circulation. In *Bone Biodynamics.* Boston, Litttle-Brown and Co., 1964, p. 245.

269) Trueta, T.: *Studies of the Development and Decay of the Human Frame.* Philadelphia, W. B. Saunders Co., 1968.

270) Turek, S. L.: *Orthopaedics.* Philadelphia, J. B. Lippincott Co., 1959.

271) Turner, C. D.: *General Endocrinology,* 3rd ed. Philadelphia, W. B. Saunders Co., 1960.

272) Urist, M. R., Silverman, B. F., Buring, K., Dubuc, F. L., and Rosenberg, J. M.: The bone induction principle. *Clin Orthop, 53:* 243, 1967.

273) Van Vlack, L. H.: *Elements of Materials Science,* 2nd ed. Reading, Addison-Wesley Publ. Co., Inc., 1964.

274) Varadacheri, Rangeasami: Personal communication.

275) Venable, C. S., and Stuck, W. G.: *The Internal Fixation of Fractures.* Springfield, Ill., Charles C Thomas, 1947.

276) Vose, G. P., and Kubala, A. L.: Bone strength; its relationship to x-ray determined ash content. *Human Biol, 31:* 261, 1959.

277) Vose, G. P.: Quantitative microradiography of osteoporotic compact bone. *Clin Orthop, 24:* 206, 1962.

278) Vose, G. P., and Lockwood, R. M.: Femoral fracture—its relationship to radiographic bone density. *J Gerontol, 20:* 300, 1965.

279) Washburn, S. L.: Effect of the temporal muscle on the form of the mandible. *J Dent Res, 21:* 174, 1947.

280) Weast, R. C.: *Handbook of Tables for Applied Engineering Science.* Cleveland, Chemical Rubber Co., 1970.

281) Weast, R. C.: *Handbook of Chemistry and Physics,* 52nd ed. Cleveland, Chemical Rubber Co., 1971.

282) Wei, J., and Arnold, J. S.: Staining osteoid seams in thin slabs of undecalcified trabecular bone. *Stain Tech, 45:* 193, 1970.

283) Weinman, J. P., and Sicher, H.: *Bone and Bones,* 2nd ed. St. Louis, C. V. Mosby Co., 1955.

284) White, R. K.: The cause of nonunion of femoral neck fractures. In *Proc Conf. Aseptic Necrosis of the Femoral Head.* Surgery Study Section, N.I.H., 1964, p. 381.

285) White, Campbell: Personal communication.

286) White, R. K.: The rheology of the synovial fluid. Personal communication.

287) Wiener, N.: *Cybernetics,* 2nd ed. Cambridge, M. I. T. Press, 1961.

288) Wilkins, L.: *Endocrine Disorders in Childhood and Adolescence.* Baltimore, Williams and Wilkins, 1969.

289) Williamson, J. B. P.: The metallurgical problems in surgery. In *Modern Trends in Surgical Materials.* (Ed.) : L. Gillis, London, Butterworth and Co., Ltd., 1958.

290) Williams, M., and Lissner, H. R.: *Biomechanics of Human Motion.* Philadelphia, W. B. Saunders Co., 1962.

291) Woodard, H. O.: Composition of human cortical bone. *Clin Orthop, 37:* 187, 1964.

292) Young, R. W.: Specialization of bone cells. In *Bone Biodynamics.* Boston, Little-Brown and Co., 1964, p. 117.

293) Yamada, H.: *Strength of Biological Materials.* Baltimore, Williams and Wilkins Co., 1970.

Postscript

In reading a particularly good novel, one regretfully comes to the last sentence of the last paragraph of a particularly good chapter. The regret, and perhaps nostalgia, this evokes appears little tempered by the knowledge that another and probably even better one begins on the next page, or by the ability to savor the one just ended at will in memory.

So with this author: After fifteen years at Henry Ford Hospital I have resigned the Chairmanship of its Department of Orthopaedic Surgery (an independent department thanks to the foresight of C. Leslie Mitchell, my predecessor in that position) and prepare to move and begin a new life chapter. Whatever and wherever it may lead, certain things will go along which already evoke nostalgia and seem surrounded by an aura of gold and warmth:

The more than 100 residents, orthopaedic and otherwise, fine young men all, with whom I worked a while, lived among, discoursed with. Teaching them made me useful (if they thought sometimes I was overuseful, I sometimes thought the contrary!), and their respect immensely honors and enriches this recipient as that testimonial, that talisman of effort of which I am proudest.

Our department's permanent staff, an exceptional collection of personalities and talents with whose help and cross-talk our daily activities became much more fun and pleasure than duty and penalty. We all tried to take good care of patients and residents, and to practice high quality orthopaedics.

Our research laboratory, a gift of providence, of the institution and of its full and part time personnel, everyone who ever worked in it and contributed to its success. These too were—still are!—wonderful people, dedicated, capable, honest and warm in their dealings with me and others. It may take a generation to measure the real value of our collective efforts, and that measure may not lie as high as my personal one at this writing, but I am content, for I loved it and them, and every minute, every thought, every datum.

The institution of Henry Ford Hospital itself. It began as a nebulous concept of the senior Mr. Henry Ford which, by remaining adaptable and by attracting dedicated men, grew into something excellent and worthwhile; then troubles beset it, and a troubleshooter/builder named Robin Buerki was brought in who built of it something even bigger and much, much better than before. It was my good fortune and privilege to arrive there near the zenith of his efforts, and in some measure to contribute towards them.

With those circumstances and people in mind, I bid adios. Barring an unexpected turn in the road ahead, this book constitutes the last installment of a debt to all the staff and residents who made possible the time to do it, and whose needs directed its conception and execution.

Index